Cancer of the Larynx

Volume II

Editor

Alfio Ferlito, M.D.
Professor of Otolaryngology
Department of Otolaryngology
University of Padua School of Medicine
Padua, Italy

CRC Press, Inc.
Boca Raton, Florida

Library of Congress Cataloging in Publication Data
Main entry under title:

Cancer of the larnyx.

Bibliography: p.
Includes index.
1. Larynx--Cancer. I. Ferlito, Alfio. [DNLM:
1. Laryngeal Neoplasms. WV 520 C215]
RC280.T5C36 1985 616.99'422 84-9509
ISBN 0-8493-6587-2 (v. 1)
ISBN 0-8493-6588-0 (v. 2)
ISBN 0-8493-6589-9 (v. 3)

Direct all inquiries to CRC Press, Inc., 2000 Corporate Blvd., N.W., Boca Raton, Florida, 33431.

International Standard Book Number 0-8493-6587-2
International Standard Book Number 0-8493-6588-0
International Standard Book Number 0-8493-6589-9

Library of Congress Card Number 84-9509
Printed in the United States

PREFACE

It was for me a great honor and pleasure to be entrusted with the editing of *Cancer of the Larynx*, and I express my thanks to all contributors from several countries who have shown great interest in the important oncologic prob ems of cancer in this site.

The purpose of this book is to enforce measures and therapeutic modalities allowing a better prognosis and a better survival of patients with this disease. In order to reach this goal it is necessary to have a deep knowledge of laryngeal cancer in all its aspects, ranging from epidemiology to carcinogenesis, immunology, pathology, clinical presentation, diagnosis, management, and rehabilitation.

Being both a clinician and a pathologist by training, I work daily in these two specialized basic fields and have felt the need of gathering in one single book the different aspects of a single problem, not only in order that any readers interested in the study and treatment of laryngeal cancer may have a comprehensive view of the disease they are to manage, but also, and above all, for proposing the most recent advances in the multidisciplinary therapeutic approach to the condition. And thus, as editor of the book, I have assigned each single chapter to a highly qualified investigator of international renown capable of bringing an actual contribution of knowledge and experience to the subject dealt with.

A. Ferlito

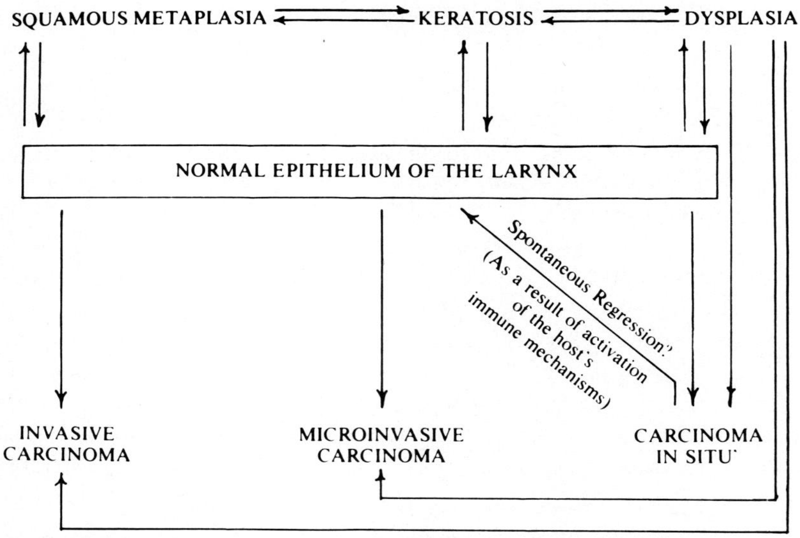

All the above pathological processes may be present simultaneously, though rarely, in a single laryngeal specimen. They do not represent compulsory successive phases in carcinogenetic modalities.

ACKNOWLEDGMENTS

I wish to thank I. Friedmann, Emeritus Professor of Pathology, University of London and V. J. Hyams, M.D., Chairman ENT Pathology Department of the Armed Forces Institute of Pathology, Washington, D.C., for reading the various parts of my chapters, and am grateful for their comments and suggestions.

It is a pleasant duty to thank the Editors of the *Acta Otorhinolaryngologica (Stockholm)*, of the *Acta Otorhinolaryngologica Belgica*, of the *American Journal of Otolaryngology*, of the *Annals of Otology, Rhinology and Laryngology* (*St. Louis*), of the *Archives of Oto-Rhino-Laryngology*, of *Cancer*, of the *Journal of the American Geriatrics Society*, of the *Journal of Clinical Pathology*, of the *Journal of Laryngology and Otology*, of the *Journal for Otorhinolaryngology and its Related Specialties*, and of the *Laryngoscope* (*St. Louis*) for permission to refer to my papers and to reproduce some of the illustrations published in their journals.

I would also like to thank the Editors and publishers of the reviews referred to in the legends of the illustrations for allowing me to reproduce their pictures.

Sincerest thanks are due to those colleagues whose illustrations and specimens have enhanced the quality of the relevant chapters.

My grateful thanks are also expressed to Vania Landucci and to Giuliano Grandi, who assisted me, respectively, in shaping the English of the chapters I had assigned myself and in supplying the best photographic material.

Finally, I am indebted to my publishers, CRC Press, Inc., for their assistance in the planning and execution of the book. Ms. Sandy Pearlman, Managing Editor, has given inestimable assistance in its compilation.

DEDICATION

To my wife, Gianna, whose encouragement
and sacrifice helped to make it all possible.

THE EDITOR

Alfio Ferlito, M.D., is Professor of Otolaryngology at the University of Padua School of Medicine. After graduating at the University of Bologna, he did his post graduate training first in pathology at Trieste University, then in otolaryngology at Padua University, completing these specialties. He worked for 2 years in the Pathology Department of Trieste University where he started his university career as a lecturer. Since 1970 he has been working in the ENT Department of Padua University as a clinician and has continued his research work in the field of ENT pathology. He has trained many postgraduate trainees and has been active in cancer research for many years. His contributions to the literature are in all fields of otolaryngology. In particular, his efforts have focused upon laryngeal cancer investigations. He has authored more than 150 scientific papers and chapters, of which 110 are published in Anglo-Saxon medical literature. In 1984 Prof. A. Ferlito was selected by Prof. C. R. Pfaltz to become a co-editor of the *Journal for Oto-Rhino-Laryngology and Its Related Specialties (Basel).*

One of his chief interests is promoting international cooperation in cancer research and education.

CONTRIBUTORS

Alfio Ferlito
Professor of Otolaryngology
Department of Otolaryngology
University of Padua School of Medicine
Padua, Italy

Jan Olofsson
Associate Professor
Department of Otolaryngology
Linköping University Hospital
Linköping, Sweden

H. J. Shaw
Director, Head and Neck Unit
Royal Marsden Hospital
London, England

H. Sökjer
Associate Professor
Department of Diagnostic Radiology
Linköping University Hospital
Linköping, Sweden

TABLE OF CONTENTS

CANCER OF THE LARYNX

Alfio Ferlito

Volume I

Epidemiology of Cancer of the Larynx
Experimental Laryngeal Carcinogenesis
Immunologic Aspects of Cancer of the Larynx
The Role of Smear Cytology in Cancer of the Larynx
Malignant Epithelial Tumors of the Larynx

Volume II

Soft Tissue Sarcomas of the Larynx
Malignant Lymphomas and Related Conditions of the Larynx
Secondary Tumors of the Larynx
Spread of Cancer of the Larynx
Clinical Manifestations of Cancer of the Larynx
Diagnostic Procedures in Cancer of the Larynx
The Radiologic Diagnosis of Cancer of the Larynx

Volume III

Classification and Staging of Cancer of the Larynx
Evaluation of the Patient with Cancer of the Larynx
Cancer of the Larynx in Unusual Hosts
The Role of Surgery in the Treatment of Cancer of the Larynx
The Use of CO_2 Laser in the Treatment of Cancer of the Larynx
The Role of Irradiation in the Treatment of Cancer of the Larynx
The Role of Chemotherapy in the Treatment of Cancer of the Larynx
The Role of Immunotherapy in the Treatment of Cancer of the Larynx
Vocal Rehabilitation after Total Laryngectomy
Complications in Cancer of the Larynx and their Treatment
Prognosis of Cancer of the Larynx

Chapter 1

SOFT TISSUE SARCOMAS OF THE LARYNX

A. Ferlito

TABLE OF CONTENTS

I. GENERAL CONSIDERATIONS

Soft tissue sarcomas of the larynx include all nonepithelial malignant tumors, with the exception of the neoplasms of lymphoreticular origin.

These tumors are rare[1] and form less than 1% of all malignant neoplasms of the larynx. Of a total number of 6067 malignant laryngeal tumors treated in five Yugoslavian teaching hospitals, Krajina[2] reported only 20 sarcomas (0.32%). During the period from 1949 to 1974, approximately 3100 patients with cancer of the larynx were examined at the Mayo Clinic, of which only 17 had sarcomas (0.55%), excluding lymphomas involving the larynx and sarcomatous invasion of the larynx from other primary sites.[3]

In the material of the Section of Pathology of the ENT Department of Padua University, gathered over an 18-year period from January 1966 through December 1983, 27 cases of sarcomas were found out of a total number of 3012 primary and secondary malignant neoplasms of the larynx and hypopharynx. These included malignant fibrous histiocytoma (7), malignant lymphoma (7), plasmacytoma (3), chrondrosarcoma (3), hemangiopericytoma (2), angiosarcoma (1), leiomyosarcoma (1), liposarcoma (1), rhabdomyosarcoma (1), and synovial sarcoma (1).

Soft tissue sarcomas of the larynx reported in the literature exceed the true incidence, as several lesions (i.e., spindle cell squamous carcinoma, pseudolymphoma, and some reparative or inflammatory lesions) have been included.

Special histochemical stains and immunocytochemical, biochemical, and ultrastructural investigations play an ancillary role in the diagnosis of these tumors and serve to confirm the diagnosis suggested by light microscopy.

Table 1 shows the classification of soft tissue sarcomas of the larynx, which is mainly based on the histological features of the tumors.

II. FIBROSARCOMA

A. Introduction

Fibrosarcoma is the oldest known malignant mesenchymal neoplasm of the larynx. In the past, a large variety of lesions, both neoplastic (benign and malignant) and pseudoneoplastic, have been indiscriminately labeled as fibrosarcoma. Moreover, fibrosarcoma was once a term applied to almost any spindle cell tumor,[4] such as schwannoma, malignant schwannoma, malignant neurofibroma, leiomyosarcoma, rhabdomyosarcoma, monophasic synovial sarcoma, malignant fibrous histiocytoma, and in particular, spindle cell squamous carcinoma. Thus, any old series of laryngeal fibrosarcoma cannot be relied on. As an example, one may agree with Davies[5] that many of the 27 cases of laryngeal fibrosarcoma found in the review by Flanagan et al.[6] were probably epithelial in origin. In addition, some of the reported *congenital* or *infantile* fibrosarcomas should be reclassified as fibromatosis.[6a] Only occasional cases have been reported in recent years.[7-9]

B. Terminology

The most common term adopted is ''fibrosarcoma''. In the past other terms have been used, such as fibromyxosarcoma, fibrosarcoma myxomatoides, angiofibrosarcoma, neurofibrosarcoma, and spindle cell sarcoma. Recently, Ghadially[10] suggested that fibrosarcomas should be divided into two groups, and proposed that when a high proportion of myofibroblasts is present, the lesion should be referred to as ''myofibrosarcoma''.

C. Definition

It is a malignant mesenchymal neoplasm derived from fibroblasts and composed of spindle-shaped cells which produce reticulin and collagen.

Table 1
HISTOLOGICAL CLASSIFICATION OF SOFT TISSUE SARCOMAS OF THE LARYNX

1. Fibrosarcoma
2. Malignant fibrous histiocytoma
3. Liposarcoma
4. Leiomyosarcoma
5. Rhabdomyosarcoma
6. Angiosarcoma
7. Hemangiopericytoma
8. Kaposi's sarcoma
9. Synovial sarcoma
10. Chondrosarcoma
11. Osteosarcoma
12. Malignant schwannoma
13. Malignant granular cell tumor

D. Incidence

Fibrosarcoma was, and still is, thought to be the most common malignant mesenchymal tumor of the larynx,[11-13] and it has altogether been stated that more than half of the sarcomas are fibrosarcomas. On the contrary, fibrosarcoma is a much less common tumor than previously thought.[14] In 17,325 patients with laryngeal cancer collected from data presented by several investigators,[2,3,14-16] only 9 cases (0.05%) were fibrosarcomas.

E. Age and Sex

Fibrosarcoma shows a predilection for the male sex and is more frequent above age 50. However, it may be seen in all ages.

F. Site

These tumors are mostly located in the anterior third of the vocal cords or on the anterior commissure or both. However, they may affect other laryngeal sites, such as the cricoid cartilage or the ventricles.[17]

G. Etiology

The etiology of fibrosarcoma is unknown. It seems, however, that prior radiation therapy may be taken into consideration as the causative agent, at least in some cases. It is worth mentioning a case of laryngeal fibrosarcoma which occurred in a patient previously treated by radiation therapy for a squamous cell carcinoma of the left vocal cord.[8] Another factor often implicated is trauma, but it is not convincing.

H. Histogenesis

The neoplasm derives from fibroblasts. In some tumors myofibroblasts have also been seen[18-20] and defined as modified fibroblasts, which have acquired some morphological and functional features of a smooth muscle cell.[21]

I. Pathology

Gross pathology — The neoplasm forms a hard, greyish tumor lesion, often nodular or polypoid in appearance, and may appear circumscribed but not encapsulated.[17]

Light microscopy (Figures 1 to 4)— These tumors have been divided into two, three, or four groups, ranging from grade I (most differentiated) to grade IV (least differentiated) according to their degree of cellular differentiation.

The neoplasm consists of uniform, spindle-shaped cells which form interlacing bundles, often arranged in a "herringbone" pattern. Rarely, the neoplasm may display a suggestive attempt at reproducing an indistinct focal storiform pattern. The cells have a slightly eosinophilic cytoplasm. Their nuclei are elongated, fusiform, and hyperchromatic. Mitoses are present and may be numerous, but marked pleomorphism of cells is not a feature of this neoplasm.

In the well-differentiated lesion, abundant collagen is present among tumor cells, whereas the poorly differentiated lesions are highly cellular. Tumors often show intervening cleft-like vascular spaces. Necrotic foci are usually numerous in the less differentiated forms. Fibrosarcoma does not show differentiation into other types of tissue. Scattered chronic inflammatory cells, particularly lymphocytes and plasma cells, may be seen. Myxoid changes are also occasionally observed. The trichrome stains (Mallory's stain, Masson's stain) and PAS are useful for recognizing the amounts of intercellular collagen, while reticulin stain shows argyrophilic fibrils surrounding individual tumor cells.

Electron microscopy — Shin and Abramson[7] reported the first electron microscopic studies of laryngeal fibrosarcoma. Another case was investigated by Tobey et al.[9] The tumor shows fusiform malignant mesenchymal cells. Dilated cisternae of rough endoplasmic reticulum contain abundant floccular material of medium electron density.[9] The potentially useful subdivision of fibrosarcomas into those with and without a major component of myofibroblasts can only be achieved ultrastructurally.[22]

J. Diagnosis and Differential Diagnosis

The diagnosis of fibrosarcoma must be made only when other tumors which may demonstrate fibrous tissue and collagen production have been excluded.[17,23] Of the first 119 consecutive sarcomas reviewed by the ECOG Pathology Review Committee on Soft Tissue Tumors, only 4 of the cases were confirmed as fibrosarcomas.[4]

In differential diagnosis, various lesions should be considered: fibromatosis,[9a,14] malignant schwannoma, spindle cell amelanotic melanoma, synovial sarcoma, malignant fibrous histiocytoma, leiomyosarcoma, pleomorphic liposarcoma, pleomorphic rhabdomyosarcoma, and osteosarcoma. In particular, however, the tumor must be distinguished from spindle cell squamous carcinoma. A thorough examination of serial sections from the whole surgical specimen may reveal an area of carcinoma *in situ* or early invasive squamous carcinoma.

Mononuclear or multinuclear giant cells are usually absent or scarce even in the most undifferentiated fibrosarcoma. If they are present, malignant fibrous histiocytoma, pleomorphic liposarcoma, pleomorphic rhabdomyosarcoma, or leiomyosarcoma have to be considered.

The differential diagnosis from leiomyosarcoma may be difficult. In fibrosarcoma, nuclei are vesicular, elongated, fusiform and some have prominent nucleoli, whereas in leiomyosarcoma there are plump, nonpointed nuclei. Furthermore, in leiomyosarcoma, reticulin stain reveals reticular fibers arranged parallel to the long axis of cells, while in fibrosarcoma there is a strict relationship between cells and reticular fibers. Ultrastructural studies are useful in differentiating the spindle cell tumors and consequently in confirming the diagnosis.[7,9,22]

K. Behavior and Prognosis

Dissemination occurs by the blood stream, and secondary deposits develop in the lungs.

Fibrosarcoma seldom metastasizes to the cervical lymph nodes, although the regional lymph nodes may be involved by direct extension. Pritchard et al.[24] reported that of 199 fibrosarcomas of the soft tissues of the extremities and trunk, 92 had metastasized and 62 had not. In 45 patients the presence of metastases could not be accurately ascertained. Metastases were blood-borne, and in only one case was a regional lymph node clinically involved with tumor. The prognosis varies according to cellular differentiation.

In consideration of the uncertainty as to the true nature of the cases published as fibrosarcomas, at present it is difficult to assess the behavior of this neoplasm in the larynx.

III. MALIGNANT FIBROUS HISTIOCYTOMA

A. Introduction

Malignant fibrous histiocytoma is a mesenchymal tumor which was recognized as a distinctive entity in the early 1960s.[25,26] This lesion usually occurs in the soft tissues, tendons, and joints of the upper and lower extremities,[27-30] but it can arise not uncommonly also in the head and neck.[31]

B. Terminology

This neoplasm has been designated by various terms, such as fibrous histiocytoma, histiocytic fibrosarcoma, malignant fibroxanthoma, xanthofibrosarcoma, xanthosarcoma, malignant fibrous xanthoma, pleomorphic malignant fibrous histiocytoma, fibroxanthosarcoma, and malignant xanthoma, but the most common term adopted is "malignant fibrous histiocytoma".

C. Definition

It is a malignant mesenchymal neoplasm characterized by proliferation of fibroblasts and histiocytes with spindle cells showing varying degrees of storiform pattern and production of collagen fibers.

D. Incidence

This tumor is rare, but it is the most common malignant neoplasm of the soft tissue of the larynx encountered in our material. The first case of fibrous histiocytoma of the larynx was reported by Rolander et al.,[32] and was interpreted as benign; Ferlito,[33] in a critical review of the literature, considered this neoplasm as malignant fibrous histiocytoma. Since then, some additional cases have been reported.[34-40] Ferlito et al.[41] have recently described seven cases of primary laryngeal fibrous histiocytoma and reviewed critically all cases previously published. In this review they included also the cases of "giant cell tumor"[42,43] and of "malignant giant cell tumor"[44] of the larynx, at present more correctly classified as a subtype of malignant fibrous histiocytoma.[45-47] Kleinsasser[47a] mentioned a case of laryngeal malignant fibrous histiocytoma. Other cases have been reported.[47b-d]

E. Age and Sex

The neoplasm occurs most frequently in elderly patients and appears to have a predilection for the male sex.

F. Site

The tumor does not present any predilection for a particular laryngeal location.

G. Histogenesis

The question of the origin of the malignant fibrous histiocytoma, though seemingly nearing solution, is not fully understood in detail as yet. Several authors[26-28,48] state that this tumor is most probably of histiocytic origin. The hypothesis is confirmed by ultrastructural studies[49] and by tissue cultures.[25] The fibroblastic component of this neoplasm is explained by the fact that the histiocyte has the potential to become a fibroblast. According to other inves-

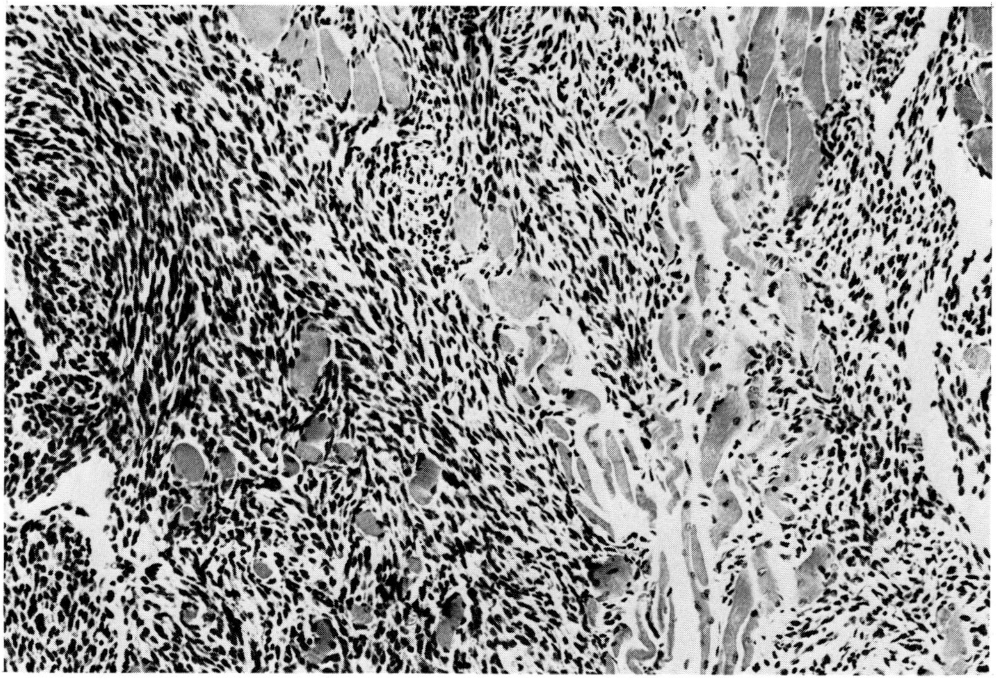

FIGURE 1. Fibrosarcoma. The neoplasm invades muscles tissues. (H.E.; Magnification × 40.) (Specimen given by Prof. I. Friedmann.)

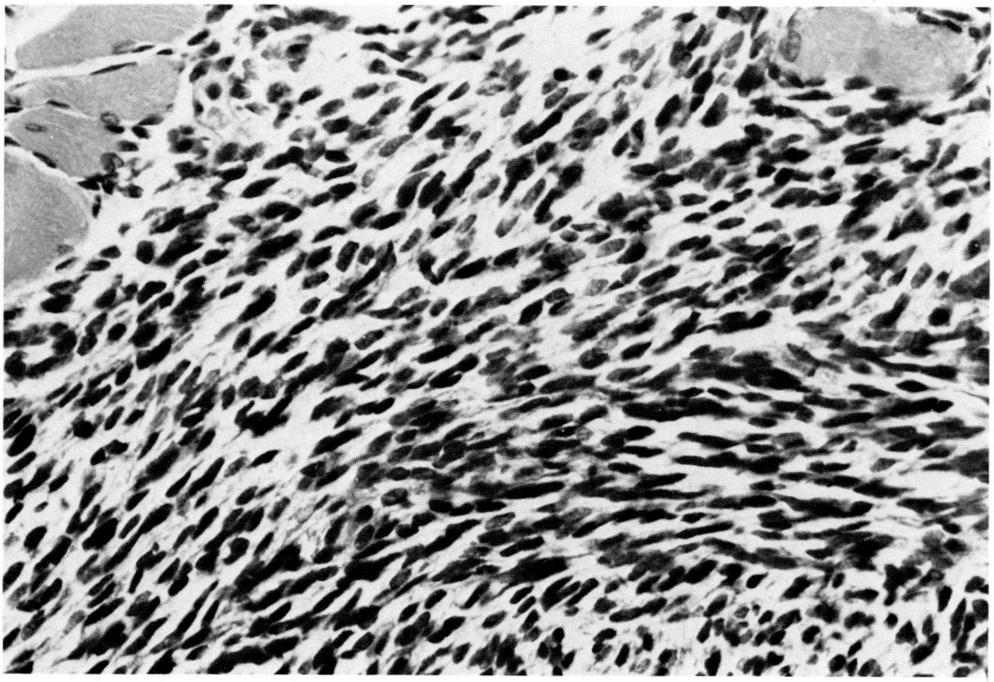

FIGURE 2. Fibrosarcoma. Detail of Figure 1. The neoplasm is composed of uniform spindle cells. (H.E.; Magnification × 100.) (Specimen given by Prof. I. Friedmann.)

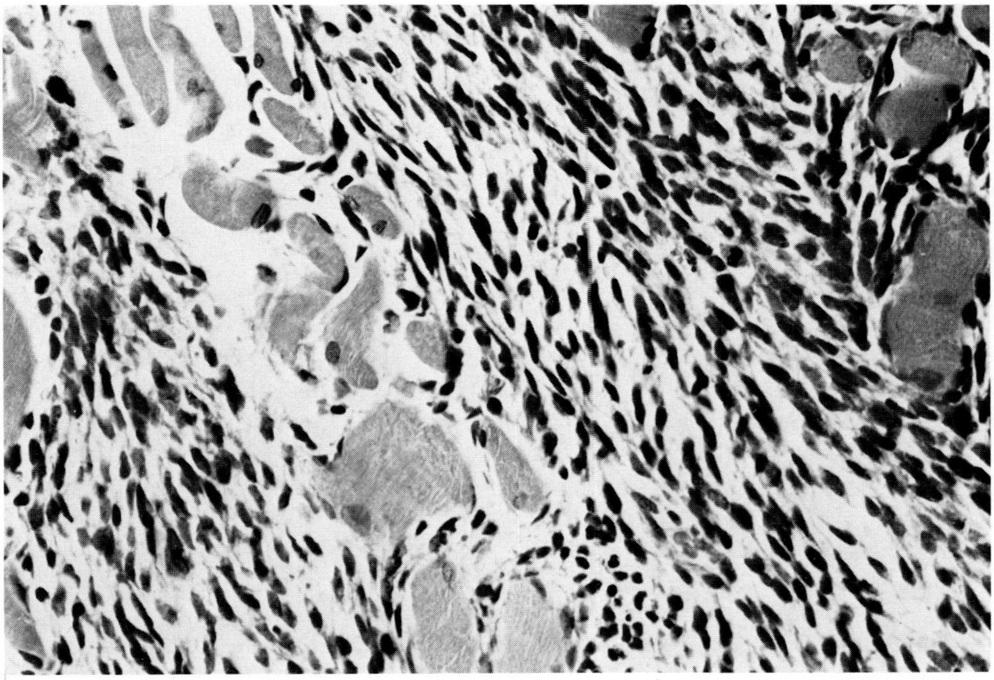

FIGURE 3. Fibrosarcoma. Another area of the neoplasm. (H.E.; Magnification × 100.) (Specimen given by Prof. I. Friedmann.)

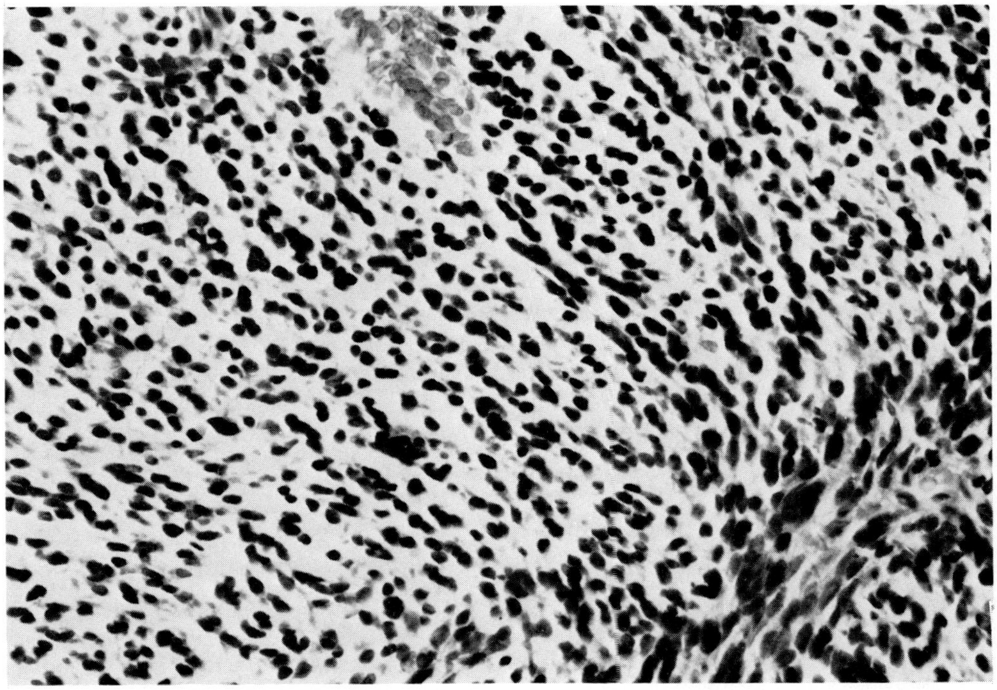

FIGURE 4. Fibrosarcoma. In this area the neoplasm is densely cellular and undifferentiated. (H.E.; Magnification × 100.) (Specimen given by Prof. I. Friedmann.)

tigators,[29,50,51] this tumor originates from a primitive mesenchymal cell. Ultrastructural investigations[52] confirmed the results obtained by Fu et al.[50] Alguacil-Garcia et al.[52] believe that malignant fibrous histiocytoma is a sarcoma of undifferentiated mesenchymal origin, which differentiates along a broad fibroblastic and histiocytic (fibrohistiocytic) spectrum and has a predominant ''fibroblastic'' component.

H. Pathology

Gross pathology — The tumor often presents as a soft tissue mass, usually of fibrous consistency, which could mimic a variety of lesions.

Light microscopy and classification — The neoplasm is composed mainly of numerous spindle cells arranged in short fascicles in a so-called ''storiform'' pattern. This appearance is more evident with reticulin stain. Bizarre, multinucleated giant cells with abundant strongly eosinophilic cytoplasm are often present and show atypical mitoses. Several Touton-type giant cells may also be seen. Areas of necrosis, hemorrhage, and amounts of lipid are uncommon. Because of its variegated histological picture, the neoplasm may be classified into six different subtypes:

1. The **pleomorphic** variant (Figures 5 to 8)[29] is composed of bizarre tumor cells, mononucleated or multinucleated, and of a highly malignant spindle cell stroma. The neoplasm shows a cartwheel or storiform pattern. This variant resembles microscopically pleomorphic liposarcoma and pleomorphic or adult rhabdomyosarcoma or even anaplastic carcinoma. This is the most common type of malignant fibrous histiocytoma of the larynx.
2. The **fibrous** variant is composed of numerous spindle cells and resembles fibrosarcoma.
3. The **giant cell** variant (Figures 9 to 12)[45-47,53] is characterized by the presence of osteoclast-like multinucleated giant cells, fibroblasts, and histiocytes.
4. The **angiomatoid** variant (Figures 13 to 21)[54] displays focal areas of hemorrhage or hemorrhagic cyst-like spaces and aggregates of chronic inflammatory cells, chiefly lymphocytes and plasmacytes.
5. The **myxoid** variant (Figures 22 and 23)[55] shows a mixture of round, stellate, and multinucleated giant cells within a myxoid and well-vascularized stroma.
6. The **inflammatory** variant[56] is characterized by a diffuse and intense neutrophilic infiltrate unassociated with tissue necrosis, in combination with atypical cells of histiocytic appearance with phagocytized neutrophils within their cytoplasm.

At times, however, different morphologic aspects may be simultaneously present in the same tumor if enough sections are examined, and it is correct to designate it on the basis of the predominant feature. All the above subtypes have been described in the larynx, except the inflammatory variant.[41]

Löbe and Katenkamp[47d] described the first electron microscopic findings of laryngeal malignant fibrous histiocytoma.

I. Diagnosis and Differential Diagnosis

The diagnosis of malignant fibrous histiocytoma may be problematic, particularly with limited biopsy material. Electron microscopy may be an ancillary procedure in diagnosis.

Differential diagnosis must be made from several neoplasms, i.e., from fibrosarcoma, pleomorphic rhabdomyosarcoma, pleomorphic and myxoid liposarcoma, spindle cell squamous carcinoma, angiosarcoma, hemangiopericytoma, histiocytic lymphoma, and Hodgkin's disease. None of these neoplasms, however, displays a distinct storiform pattern, which is a typical feature of malignant fibrous histiocytoma but not a reliable criterion per se. Rarely, the fibrosarcoma may present an abortive and indistinct storiform pattern.

Special stains, such as Masson trichrome or PTAH (for myofibrils) and reticulin stain may help in difficult cases. In particular, cross-striations are never seen in malignant fibrous histiocytoma, whereas they may be present in rhabdomyosarcoma. It is also necessary to distinguish clearly the foam cells of the malignant fibrous histiocytoma from the lipoblasts of the pleomorphic liposarcoma. In malignant fibrous histiocytoma the vacuoles are not intracytoplasmatic but rather in the stroma, whereas in liposarcoma the vacuoles are in the cytoplasm. Furthermore, liposarcoma contains a lesser amount of stromal collagen as compared to histiocytic neoplasm. Moreover, in the latter the characteristic lipoblasts are never present. In addition, staining of the apparent "lipoblast-like" cells in histiocytic tumors indicates that the vacuoles contain acid mucopolysaccharides rather than neutral fat, characteristic of lipoblasts.[55] In order to demonstrate acid mucopolysaccharides, special stains may be used, such as Alcian blue or colloidal iron. These stains are completely removed by prior treatment with hyaluronidase. Sometimes it is particularly difficult for the pathologist to distinguish a malignant fibrous histiocytoma from spindle cell squamous carcinoma, in particular when the latter does not show areas of carcinoma *in situ* or microinfiltrative carcinoma, or when lymph node metastases display only pseudosarcomatous appearances, or again when the malignant fibrous histiocytoma does not exhibit a distinct storiform pattern, as sometimes in the pleomorphic subtype. Weiss and Enzinger[55] state that stains for mucin or glycogen may be helpful in differential diagnosis. Glycogen may be present in the spindle cell squamous carcinoma, whereas it is usually absent in malignant fibrous histiocytoma. This tumor must also be differentiated from angiosarcoma: the Weibel-Palade bodies and intracellular lumina, which may be seen in the ultrastructure of angiosarcoma, are never present in malignant fibrous histiocytoma.

J. Behavior and Prognosis

Even though the number of these neoplasms observed in the larynx is limited, it may be said that in this organ the tumor has an aggressive biological behavior,[31,41] because not only does it frequently recur, but it also metastasizes to various sites (lung, brain, arachnoid, kidney, liver, spleen musculoskeletal system, subcutaneous tissues, pelvis). In spite of the presence of visceral metastases, only in one case[32] were cervical lymph node metastases seen.

IV. LIPOSARCOMA

A. Terminology

The most common term for indicating this tumor is "liposarcoma", but others have sometimes been used, such as lipomyxosarcoma, myxoliposarcoma, fibroblastic liposarcoma, epithelioid liposarcoma, undifferentiated liposarcoma, and myxosarcoma.

B. Definition

Liposarcoma is a malignant mesenchymal neoplasm composed of atypical lipoblasts at various stages of differentiation.

C. Incidence

Only solitary cases of laryngeal liposarcoma have been described.[9,57-65a] The first case was observed by von Urfer,[57] who described a case of "myxolipoma" of the aryepiglottic fold with focal sarcomatous changes. This case must actually be considered as a true liposarcoma, not unlike that reported later by Kapur[58] as recurrent lipomata of the larynx and pharynx with late malignant changes.

In the case reported by Miller et al.,[59] the patient had developed another liposarcoma on

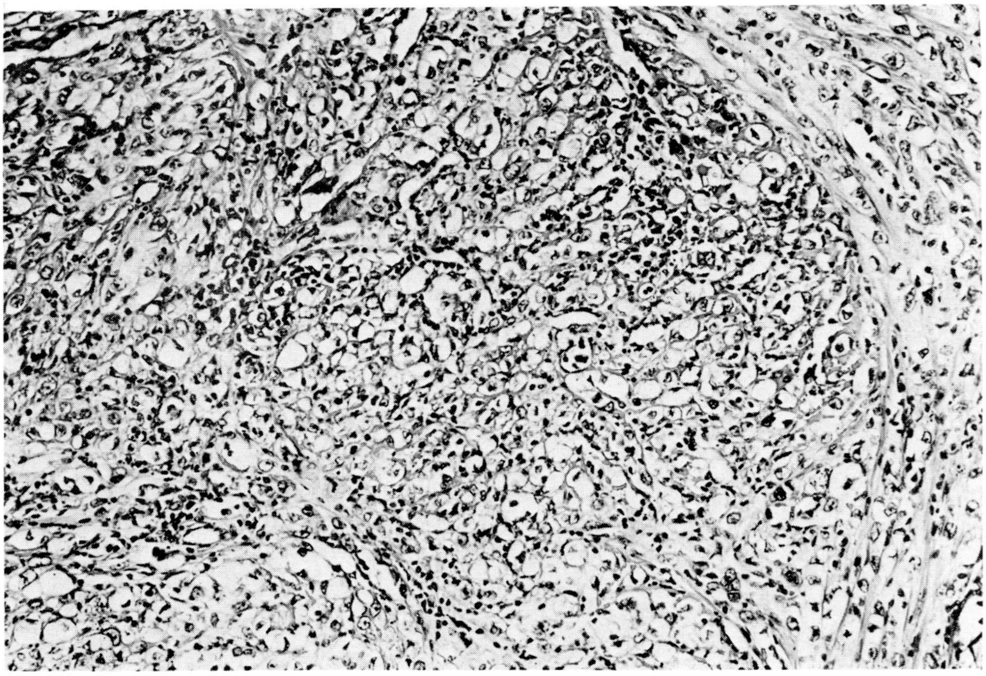

FIGURE 5. Malignant fibrous histiocytoma, pleomorphic variant. In this area the neoplasm is characterized by the presence of abundant closely packed foam cells. (H.E.; Magnification × 40.) (From Ferlito, A., *Cancer*, 42, 611, 1978. With permission.)

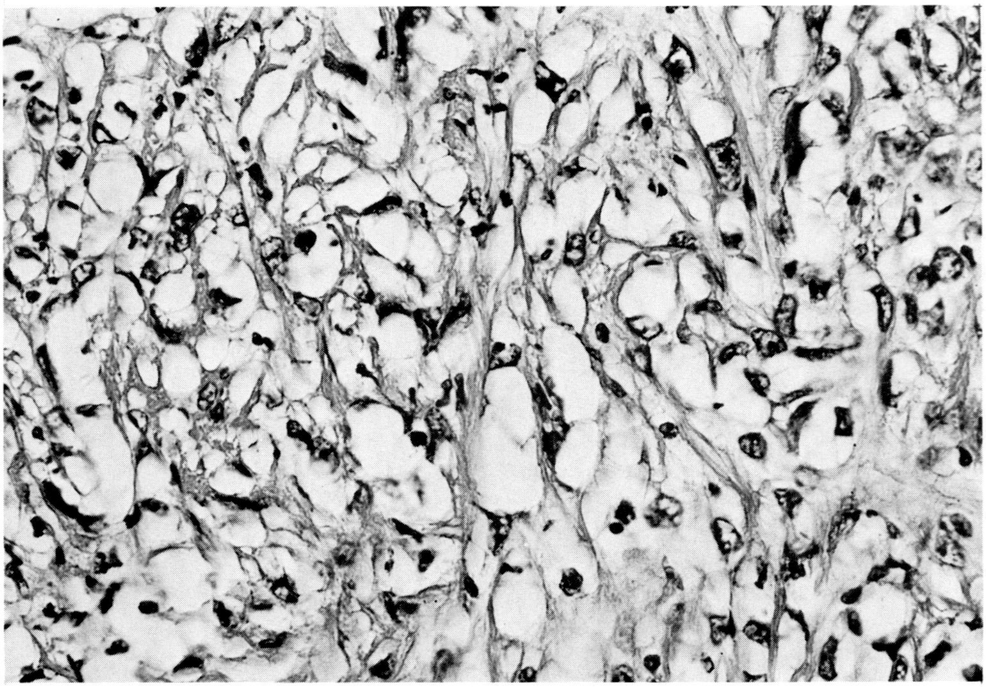

FIGURE 6. Malignant fibrous histiocytoma, pleomorphic variant. Higher magnification shows better the characteristics of foam cells. (H.E.; Magnification × 100.) (From Ferlito, A., *Cancer*, 42, 611, 1978. With permission.)

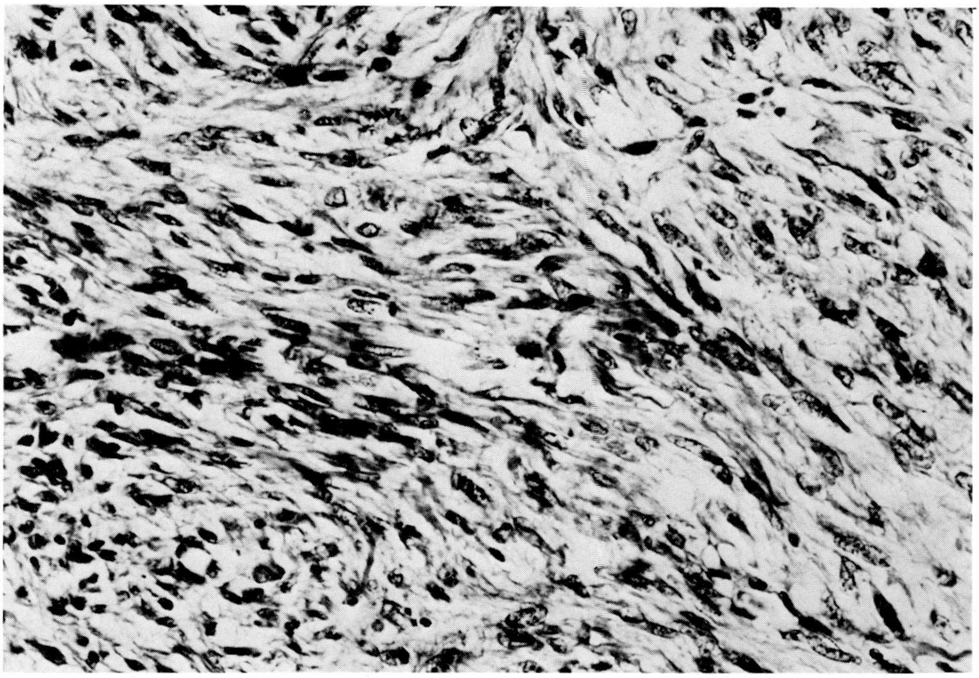

FIGURE 7. Malignant fibrous histiocytoma, pleomorphic variant. Another microscopic field of the same case as in Figure 5 simulating the pattern of fibrosarcoma. (H.E.; Magnification × 100.) (From Ferlito, A., *Cancer*, 42, 611, 1978. With permission.)

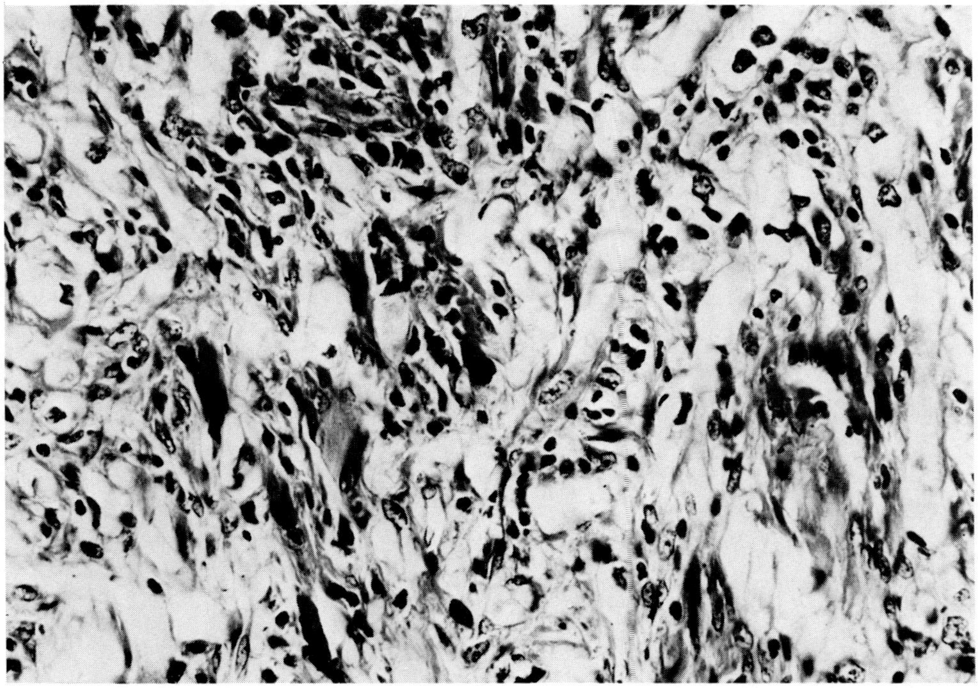

FIGURE 8. Malignant fibrous histiocytoma, pleomorphic variant. Note the pleomorphic malignant multinucleated giant cell. (H.E.; Magnification × 100.) (From Ferlito, A., *Acta Otorhinolaryngol. Belg.*, 30, 390, 1976. With permission.)

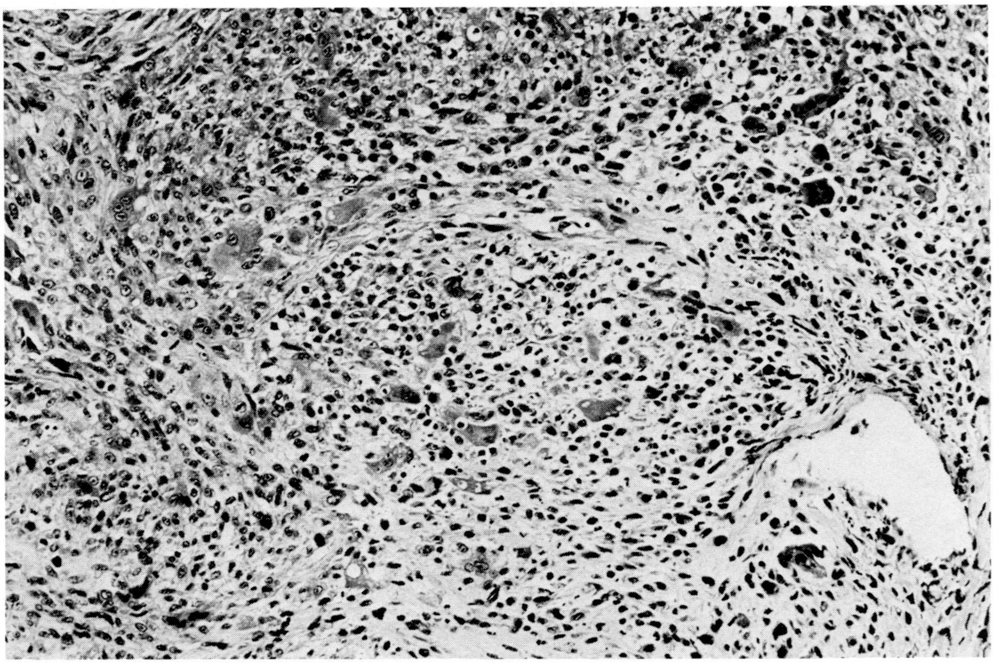

FIGURE 9. Malignant fibrous histiocytoma, giant cell variant. Note the typical pattern of the neoplasm. (H.E.; Magnification × 40.)

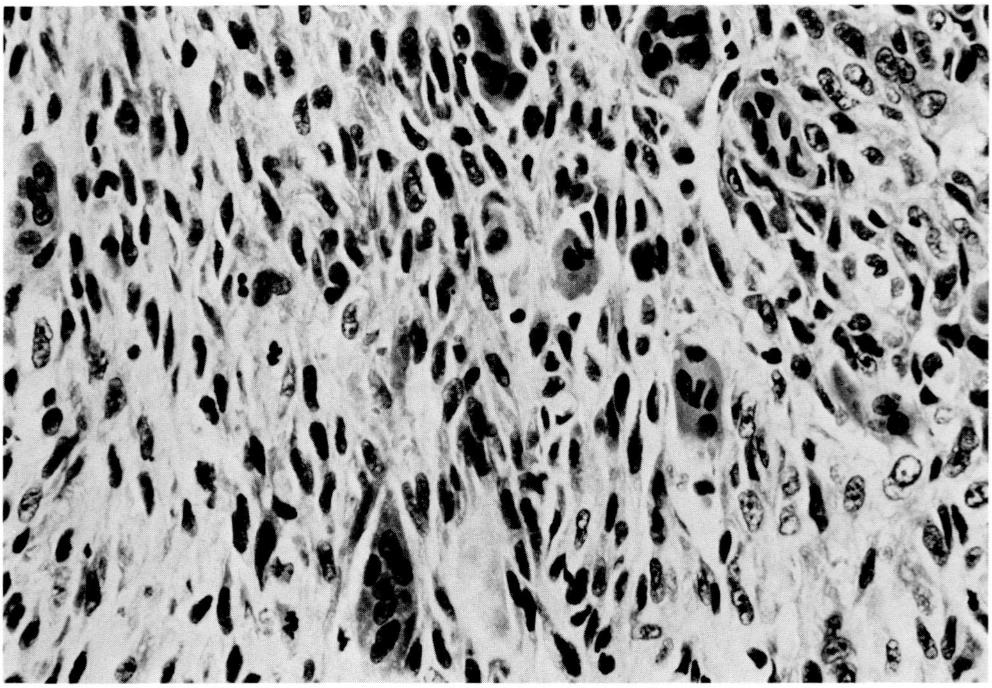

FIGURE 10. Malignant fibrous histiocytoma, giant cell variant. Another area of the tumor. (H.E.; Magnification × 100.)

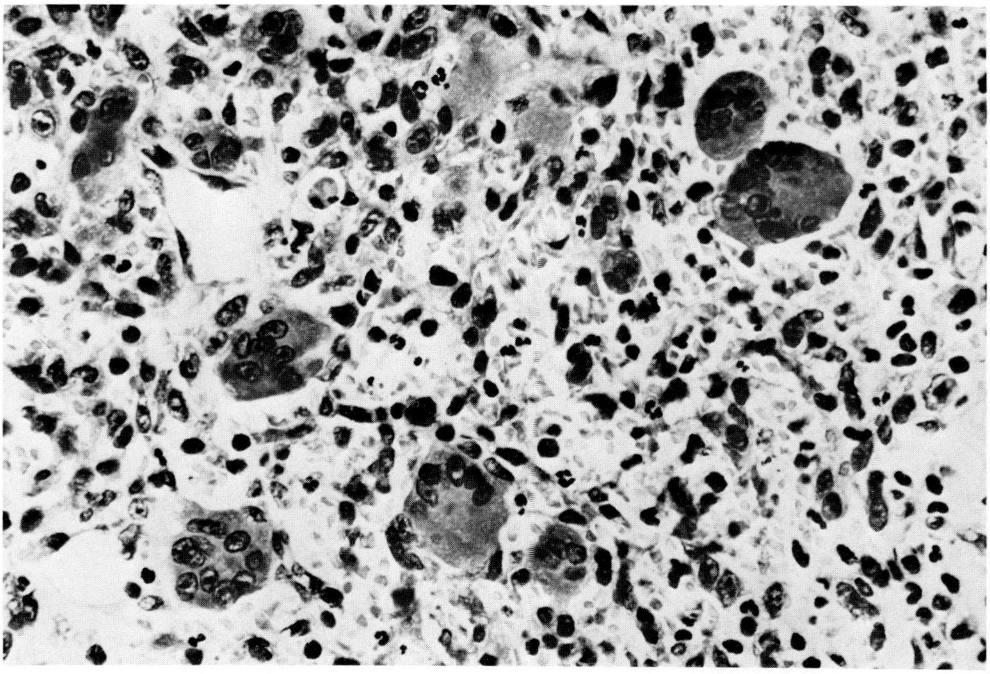

FIGURE 11. Malignant fibrous histiocytoma, giant cell variant. The neoplasm is composed of mononuclear histiocyte-like cells and osteoclast-type giant cells. (H.E.; Magnification × 100.)

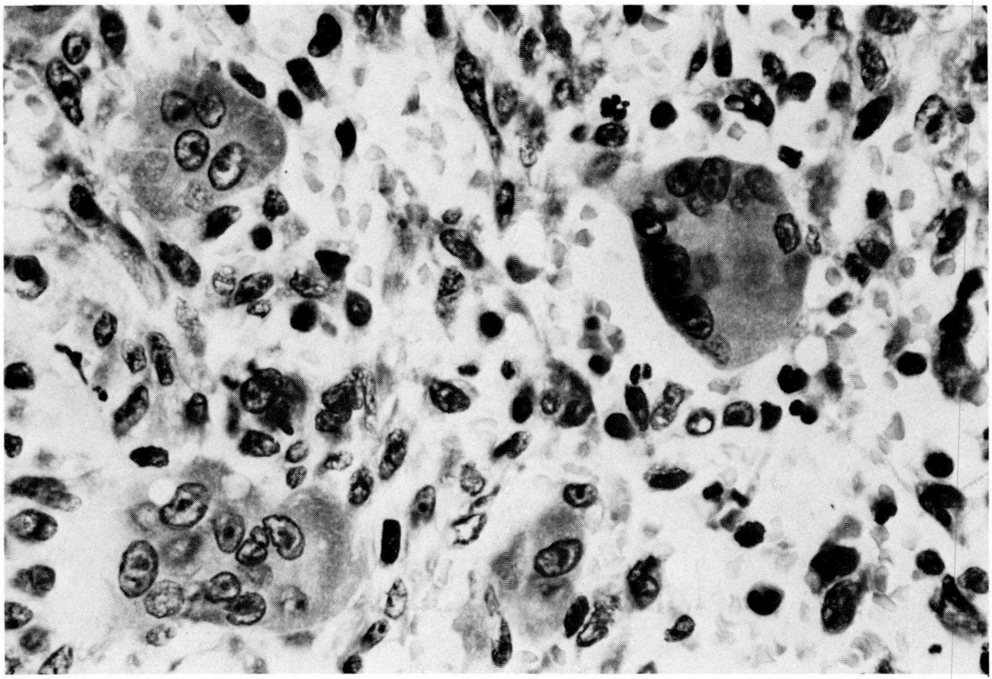

FIGURE 12. Malignant fibrous histiocytoma, giant cell variant. Note the cytologic details of some osteoclast-type giant cells. (H.E.; Magnification × 160.) (From Ferlito, A. et al., *Laryngoscope*, 93, 1351, 1983. With permission.)

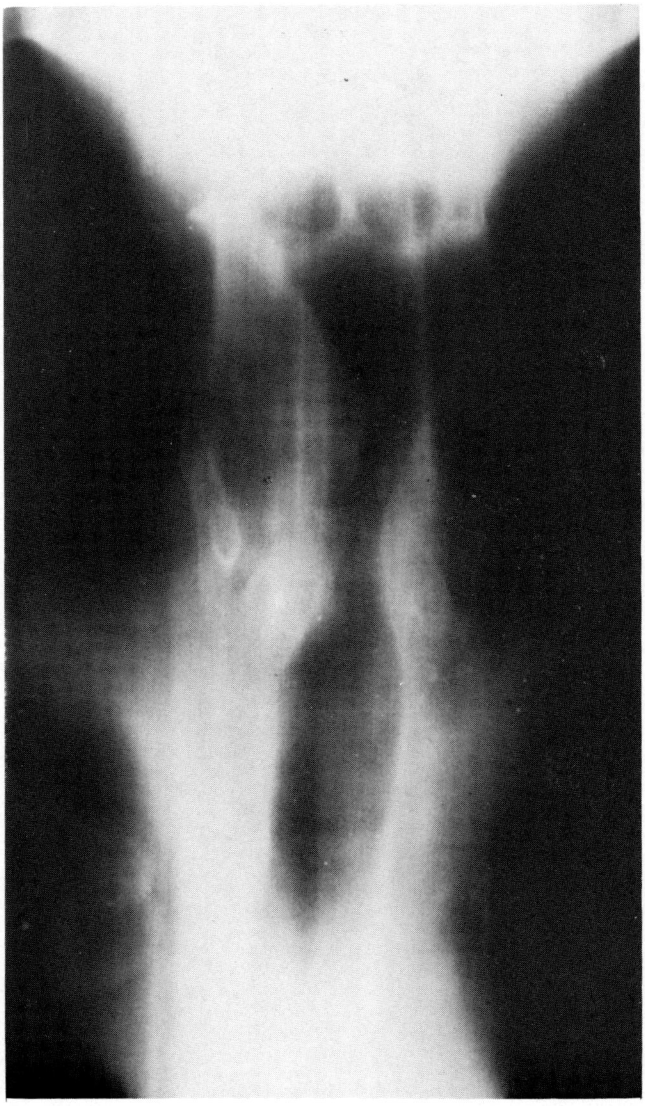

FIGURE 13. Malignant fibrous histiocytoma, angiomatoid variant. Frontal tomogram of the larynx revealing an extensive neoplastic lesion. (From Ferlito, A. et al., *Laryngoscope*, 93, 1351, 1983. With permission.)

his back a few months later,[60] and in the case described by Krausen et al.,[61] the patient had been previously treated for a liposarcoma involving the left thigh.

Dockerty et al.[63a] described a case of pleomorphic liposarcoma orginating from the parapharyngeal area in which the intrinsic larynx, the left aryepiglottic fold, and the left pyriform sinus were secondarily infiltrated. This occurred in a 33-year-old man and surgical ablation and radiation therapy failed to control the primary lesion. The neoplasm recurred and the patient died with pulmonary metastases.

D. Age and Sex

Liposarcoma is essentially a tumor of adult life,[66] and also, in the larynx it appears to have a predilection for elderly male patients.

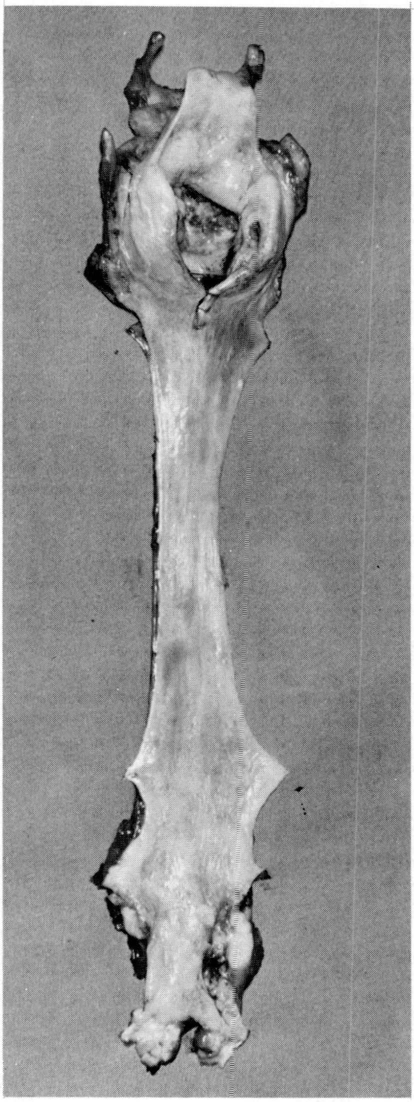

FIGURE 14. Malignant fibrous histiocytoma, angiomatoid variant. Surgical specimen from a 63-year-old man with malignant fibrous histiocytoma of the larynx and a squamous cell carcinoma of the esophagus. (From Ferlito, A. et al., *Laryngoscope*, 93, 1351, 1983. With permission.)

E. Site

The most common location is the aryepiglottic fold.

F. Etiology

The etiology is unknown. Morton et al.[67] noted that in tissue cultures from liposarcoma cells, intracellular particles resembling RNA containing C virus particles were present. Györkey et al.[68] evidenced at electron microscopy that in various malignant mesenchymal neoplasms, and among them also three liposarcomas, cytoplasmatic structures resembling ribonucleoprotein strands of paramyxovirus were present. Furthermore, immunologic studies

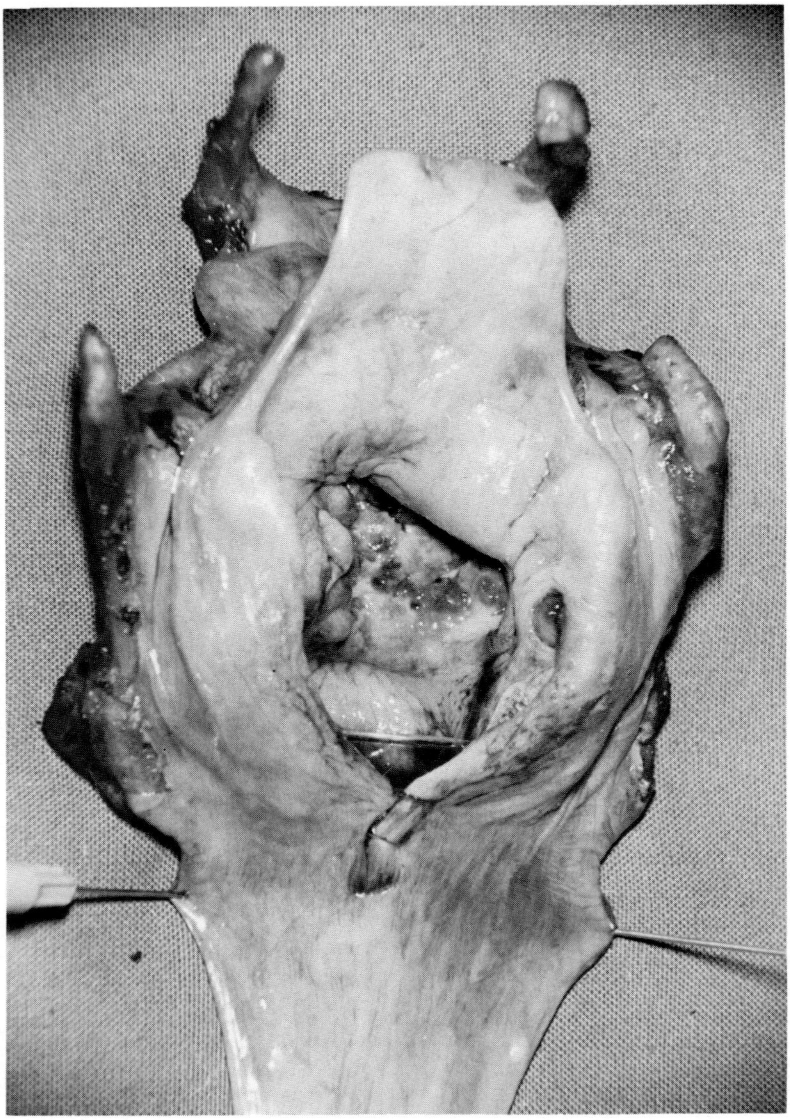

FIGURE 15. Malignant fibrous histiocytoma, angiomatoid variant. Detail of Figure 14 in which the extensive laryngeal neoplasm may be seen. (From Ferlito, A. et al., *Laryngoscope*, 93, 1351, 1983. With permission.)

have revealed a high incidence of antibody to sarcoma-specific antigen in patients with liposarcoma.[69] These studies would suggest a viral origin of liposarcoma, but this fact needs further investigations.

G. Histogenesis

The histogenesis of the tumor is not clear, though one is inclined to believe that it may originate from lipoblasts or totipotential mesenchyme.

H. Pathology

Gross pathology — Macroscopically, the neoplasm is often of polypoid shape.

Light microscopy and classification — The microscopical features of liposarcoma were

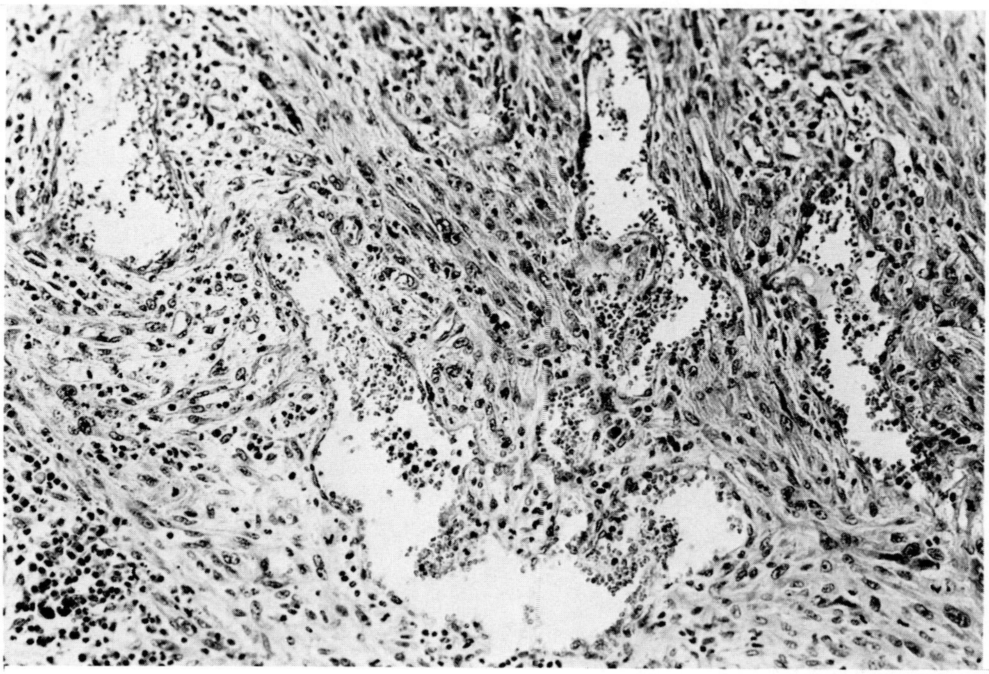

FIGURE 16. Malignant fibrous histiocytoma, angiomatoid variant. Note neoplastic cells simulating a vascular neoplasm. (H.E.; Magnification × 40.) (From Ferlito, A. et al., *Laryngoscope*, 93, 1351, 1983. With permission.)

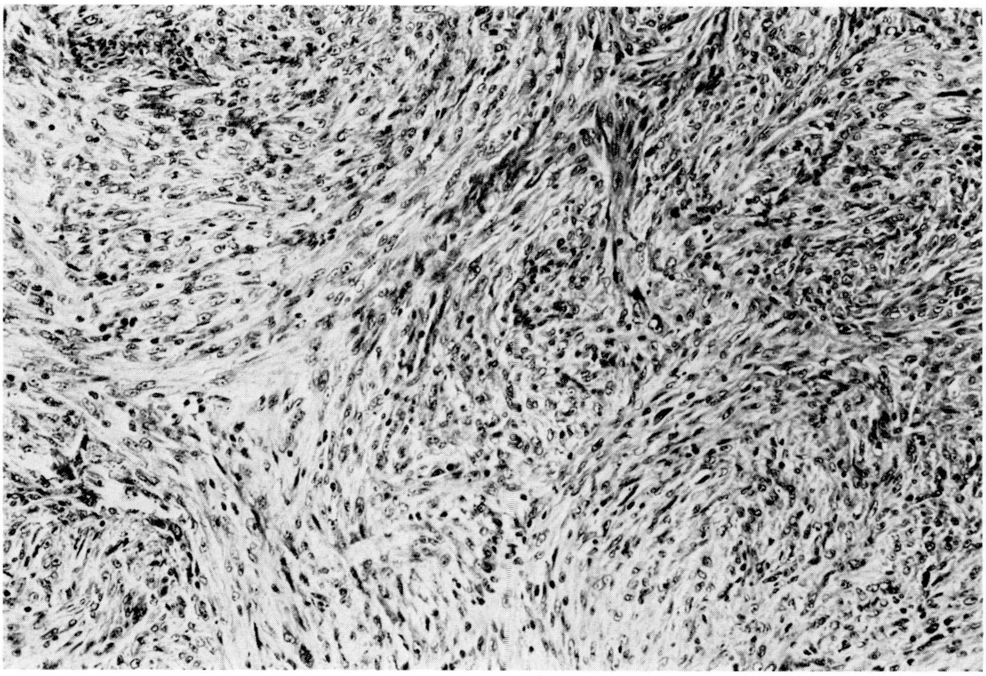

FIGURE 17. Malignant fibrous histiocytoma, angiomatoid variant. Note the storiform pattern. (H.E.; Magnification × 40.) (From Ferlito, A. et al., *Laryngoscope*, 93, 1351, 1983. With permission.)

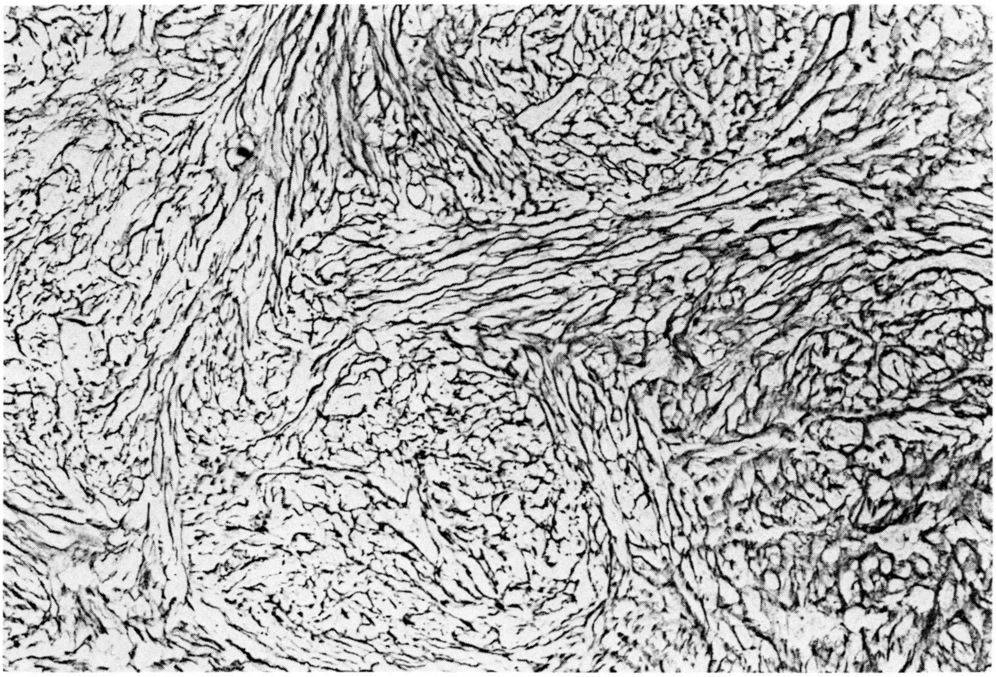

FIGURE 18. Malignant fibrous histiocytoma, angiomatoid variant. Reticulin stain accentuates the storiform pattern. (Gomori's stain; Magnification × 100.)

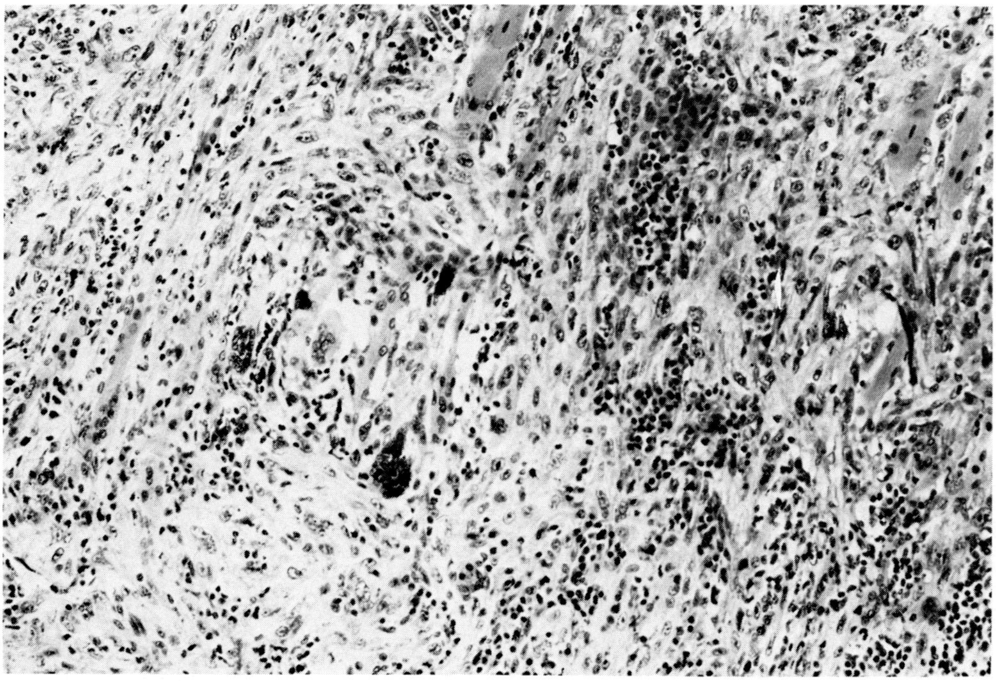

FIGURE 19. Malignant fibrous histiocytoma, angiomatoid variant. Note several and different multinucleated giant cells. (H.E.; Magnification × 40.)

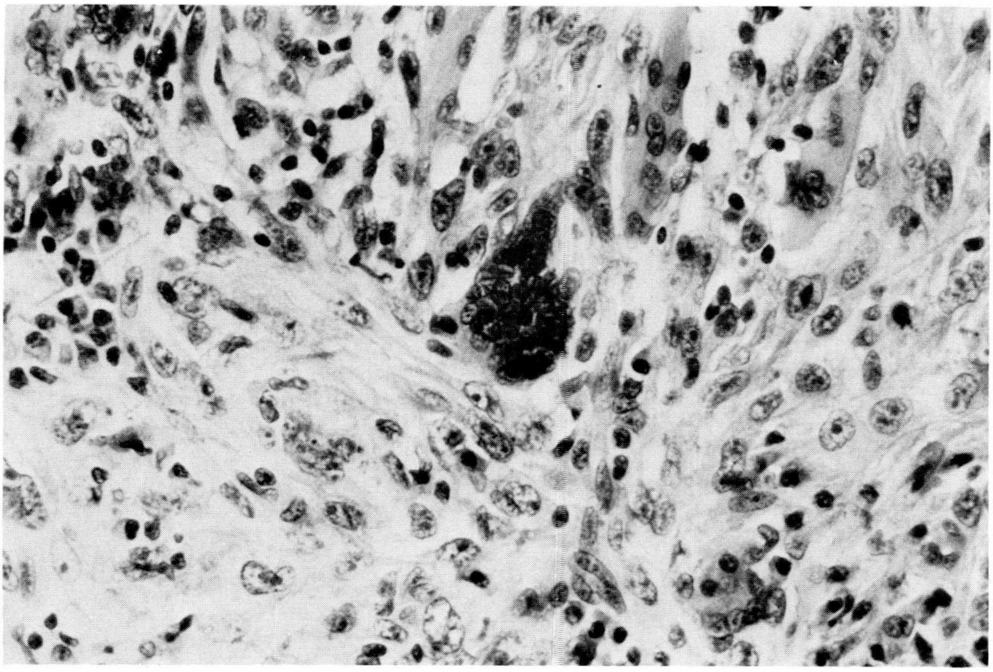

FIGURE 20. Malignant fibrous histiocytoma, angiomatoid variant. Detail of the Figure 19. Note in the center of the photomicrograph a bizarre and multinucleated giant cell. (H.E.; Magnification × 100.) (From Ferlito, A. et al., *Laryngoscope*, 93, 1351, 1983. With permission.)

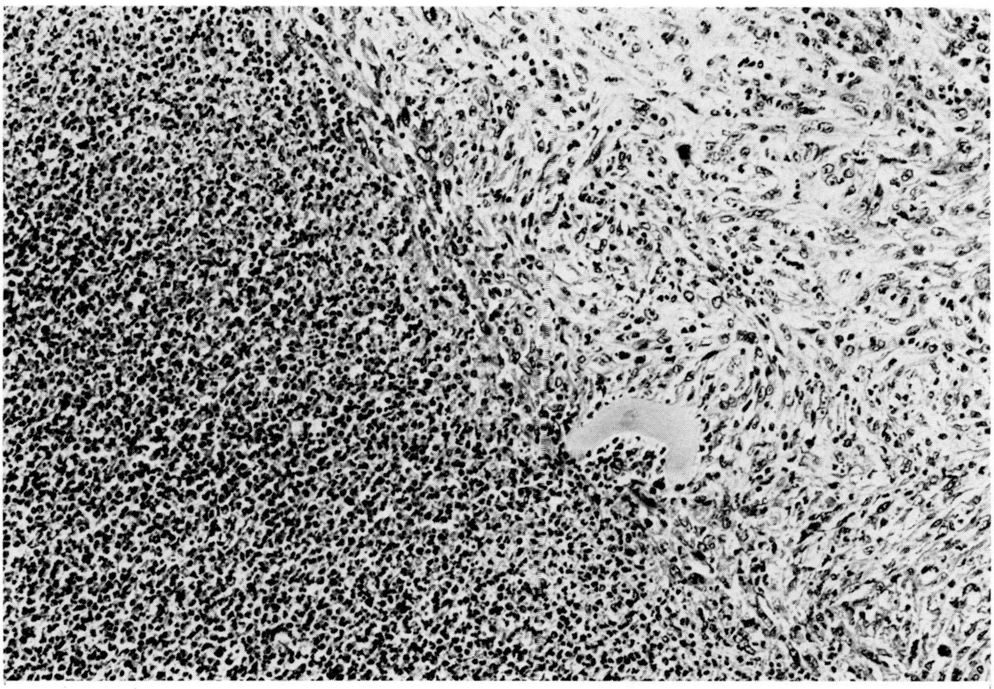

FIGURE 21. Malignant fibrous histiocytoma, angiomatoid variant. In this area there are numerous inflammatory cells surrounding the neoplasm. (H.E.; Magnification × 40.)

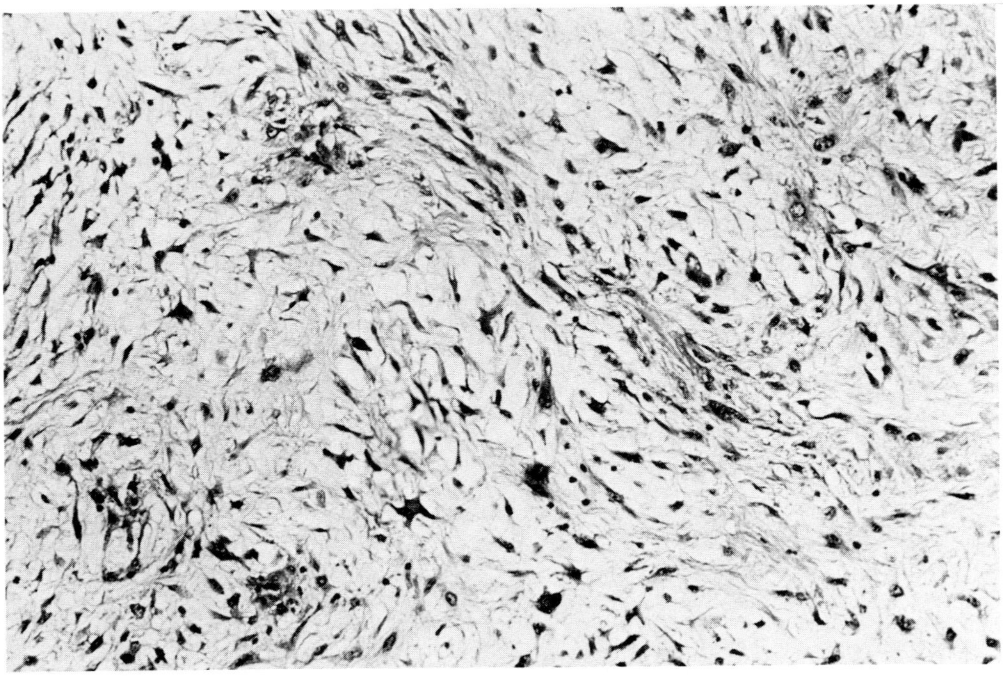

FIGURE 22. Malignant fibrous histiocytoma, myxoid variant. Note aspect of the neoplasm resembling liposarcoma. (H.E.; Magnification × 40.) (From Ferlito, A. et al., *J. Laryngol. Otol.*, 93, 1021, 1979. With permission.)

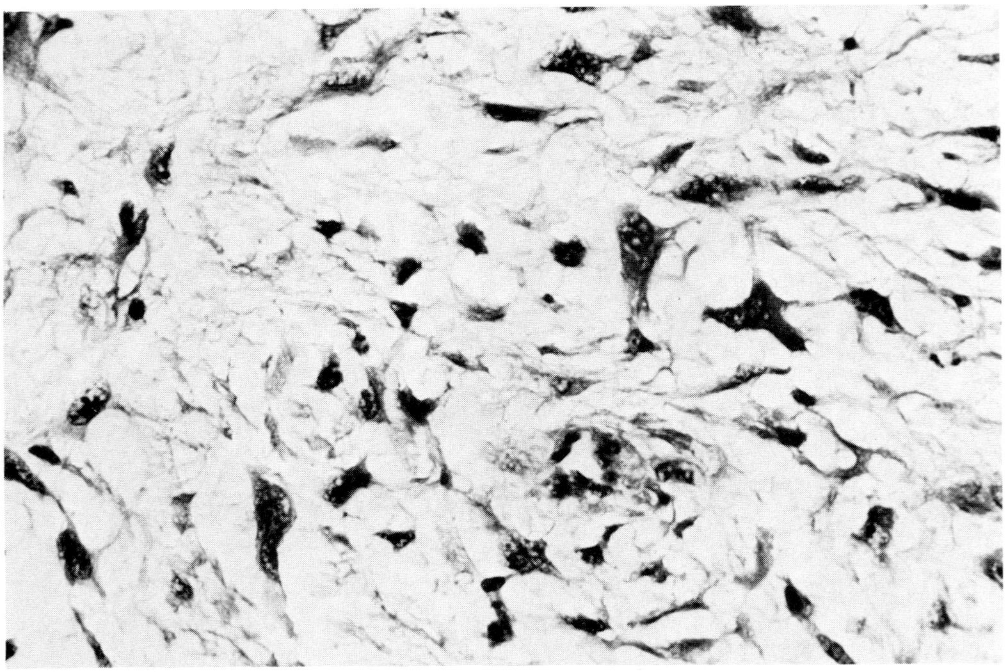

FIGURE 23. Malignant fibrous histiocytoma, myxoid variant. This field shows another area of tumor resembling liposarcoma. Tumor cells are 'lipoblasts-like', but no definite recognizable lipoblasts may be seen. (H.E.; Magnification × 100.) (From Ferlito, A. et al., *J. Laryngol. Otol.*, 93, 1021, 1979. With permission.)

first described by Virchow,[70] who considered this neoplasm as a separate entity. The variegated histological picture has long been recognized and has led to the introduction of several classifications.[71-77] The one proposed by Enzinger and Winslow[73] is mainly used today and distinguishes the following four types of liposarcoma: myxoid, round-cell, well-differentiated, and pleomorphic.

Many liposarcomas have two main components: (1) fat cells of varying maturity, ranging from recognizable adipose tissue of adult type to rounded lipoblasts of assorted sizes, and (2) myxoid tissue composed of stellate and spindle cells in a mucoid background containing acid mucopolysaccharide. The combination of these two components in varying proportions and degrees of maturity constitutes the *myxoid* variant, which is the most common type.

The *round-cell* (or epithelioid) type is composed by a marked proliferation of uniform rounded cells which have a distinctly acidophilic cytoplasm.

The *pleomorphic* type (Figures 24 to 28) is characterized by a marked pleomorphism and bizarre giant cells, many of which are multinucleated with acidophilic cytoplasm.

The *well-differentiated* (adult) type is divided into two forms: (1) the well-differentiated "lipoma-like", often considered as an atypical lipoma, and (2) the sclerosing liposarcoma in which lipoma-like portions alternate with areas of dense fibrosis. These tumors are well-differentiated and frequently indistinguishable from benign lipomas and are believed to be nonmetastasizing variety.

The subdivision of liposarcomas is useful from the point of view of the prognosis, inasmuch as the two subgroups (the well-differentiated and myxoid liposarcoma) almost always remain localized or recur locally after resection, whereas the other forms (the pleomorphic and round-cell types) are more aggressive, recur easily, and metastasize.

Overlap in these classifications undoubtedly occurs and this might imply that such subdivisions are arbitrary and academic, but the exercise nevertheless has a practical justification. Spittle et al.,[75] in a review of 60 cases of general distribution, showed that the 5-year survival rate in the myxoid group was over 80% but in the pleomorphic group it was under 50%; the average for all types was 64%.

Electron microscopy — Krausen et al.[61] reported the first electron microscopic studies of laryngeal liposarcoma. The neoplasm was composed of tumor cells arranged in a perivascular fashion, being surrounded entirely by basement membrane. Numerous lipids were present in the cytoplasm of the tumor cells. Ultrastructural investigations have also shown that liposarcomas are often mixed mesenchymatous neoplasms "composed of fibroblasts, myoblasts, as well as lipoblasts".[9]

I. Diagnosis and Differential Diagnosis

Special histochemical stains and electron microscopic studies may help in establishing the correct diagnosis.[9,78]

Differential diagnosis between lipoma and well-differentiated liposarcoma may be difficult. The absence of the characteristic storiform pattern in liposarcoma and the content of neutral fat in the cells distinguishes it from malignant fibrous histiocytoma, whose cells contain mucopolysaccharides.

J. Behavior and Prognosis

Laryngeal liposarcomas may recur locally after excision. The histological subtypes and site of the neoplasm are important for the prognosis. In the reported cases lymph node metastases were not found.

V. LEIOMYOSARCOMA

A. Definition

Leiomyosarcoma is a malignant mesenchymal neoplasm that arises from smooth muscle cells.

B. Incidence

Leiomyosarcoma of the larynx is rare and the first case was reported by Frank[79] in 1941. Since then, some additional cases have been reported.[80-91]

C. Age and Sex

The tumor occurs mainly in middle-aged males, but any age may be affected. Chizh[89] described a case in an 8-year-old girl.

D. Site

The most affected areas are the glottic and supraglottic regions.

E. Pathology

Gross pathology — The most common appearance of the tumor is polypoid.

Light microscopy (Figures 29 to 32) — Microscopy shows well-defined bundles of spindle-shaped cells. A suggestion of nuclear palisading or a "storiform pattern" may be observed focally, although these are never dominant features. The cytoplasm is abundant, acidophilic, and apparently vacuolated. The cellularity is considerable. There are often vascular areas and some of the irregular vascular channels may be enveloped by tumor cells. Neoplastic cells sometimes are intermingled with lymphocytes, plasma, and mast cells. Special stains, such as phosphotungstic acid hematoxylin and trichrome modifications, or ultrastructural studies reveal the presence of myofibrils. Reticulin stain shows the characteristic arrangement of the fibers parallel to the long axis of the tumor cells. At times, cells, beside displaying a marked pleomorphism, appear to be multinucleated. PAS-positive (non-diastase-resistant) cells containing glycogen may be seen. The surface epithelium may assume a hyperplastic pseudoepitheliomatous aspect.

F. Diagnosis and Differential Diagnosis

The microscopic diagnosis can often be difficult. The presence of myofibrils is conclusive for the diagnosis. Fibrosarcoma, malignant schwannoma, hemangiopericytoma, malignant fibrous histiocytoma, angiosarcoma, spindle cell squamous carcinoma, and spindle cell amelanotic melanoma should be considered in differential diagnosis. The mitotic activity is the most reliable criterion for distinguishing between leiomyoma and leiomyosarcoma.

G. Behavior and Prognosis

The neoplasm is aggressive and both metastases, lymphatic or hematogenous, have been reported,[90] especially in poorly differentiated leiomyosarcoma. Systemic metastases commonly involve the lungs. The prognosis is poor.

VI. RHABDOMYOSARCOMA

A. Terminology

The terms "rhabdomyosarcoma" and "malignant rhabdomyoma" are used synonymously. The old expression "rhabdomyoma sarcomatodes" has been abandoned.

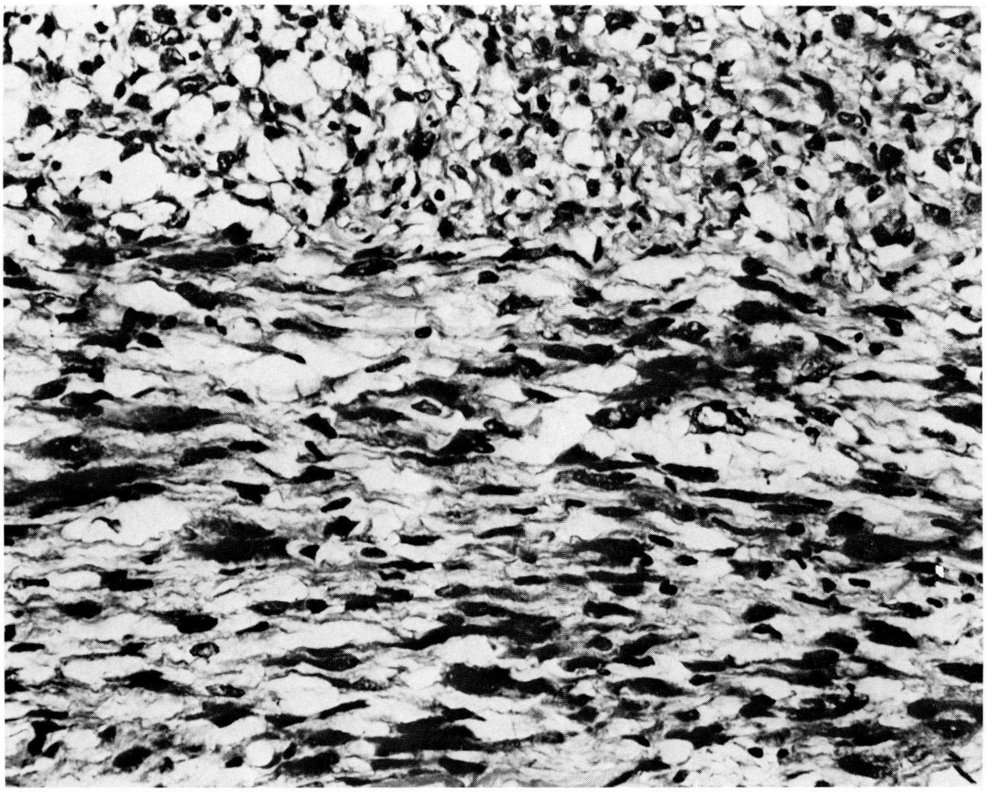

FIGURE 24. Pleomorphic liposarcoma. Neoplasm occurring in a 52-year-old male. Note the spindle cell area. (H.E.; Magnification × 100.)

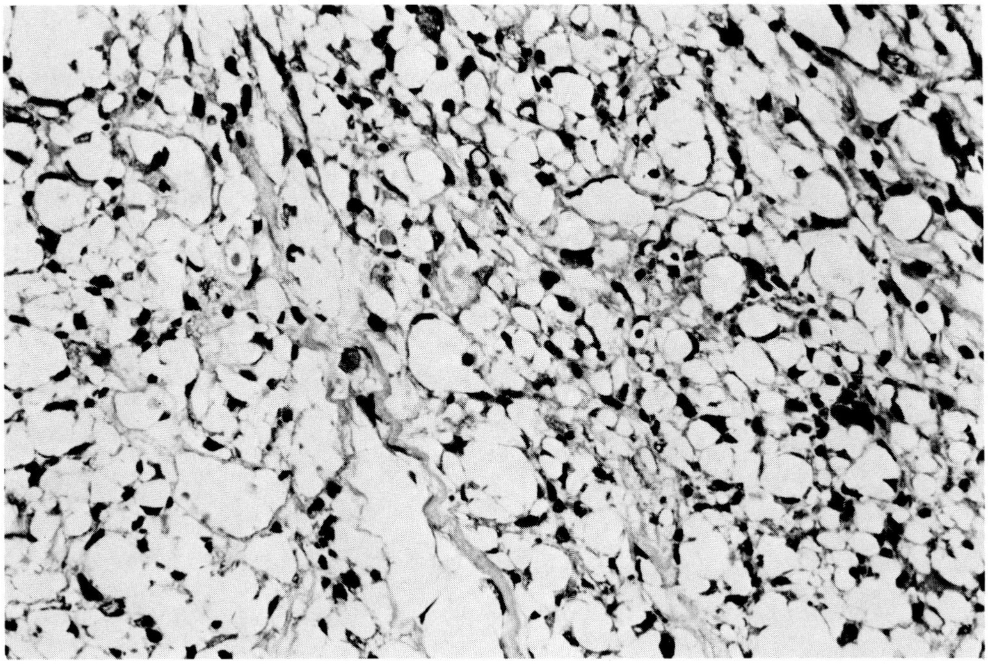

FIGURE 25. Pleomorphic liposarcoma. The neoplasm is composed of cells with vacuolated cytoplasm. (H.E.; Magnification × 100.)

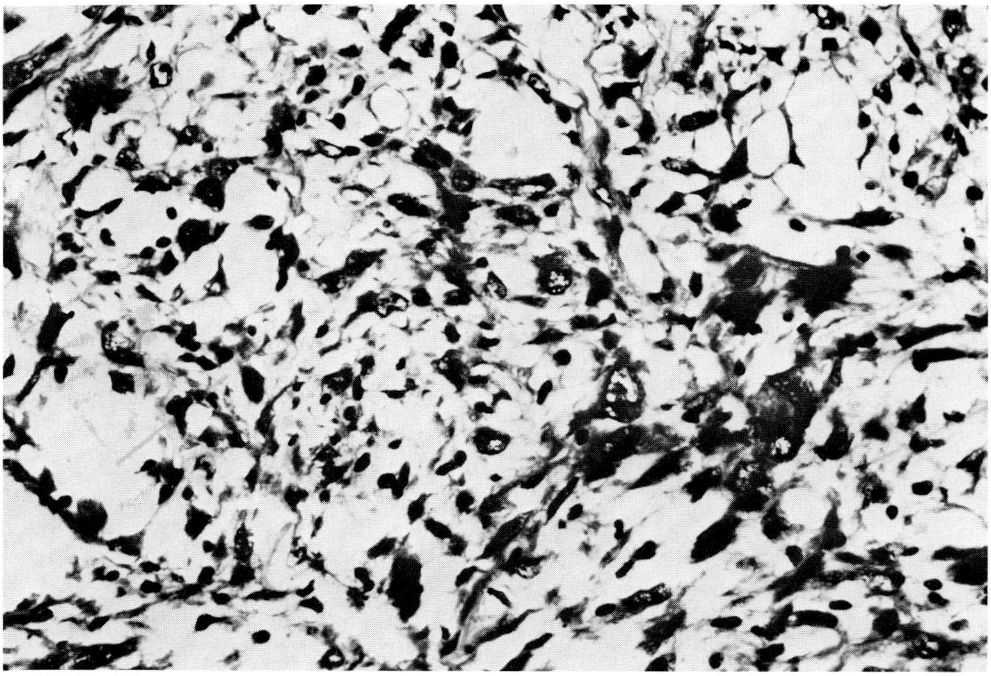

FIGURE 26. Pleomorphic liposarcoma. Same tissue as previous figures, showing atypical lipoblasts. (H.E.; Magnification × 100.)

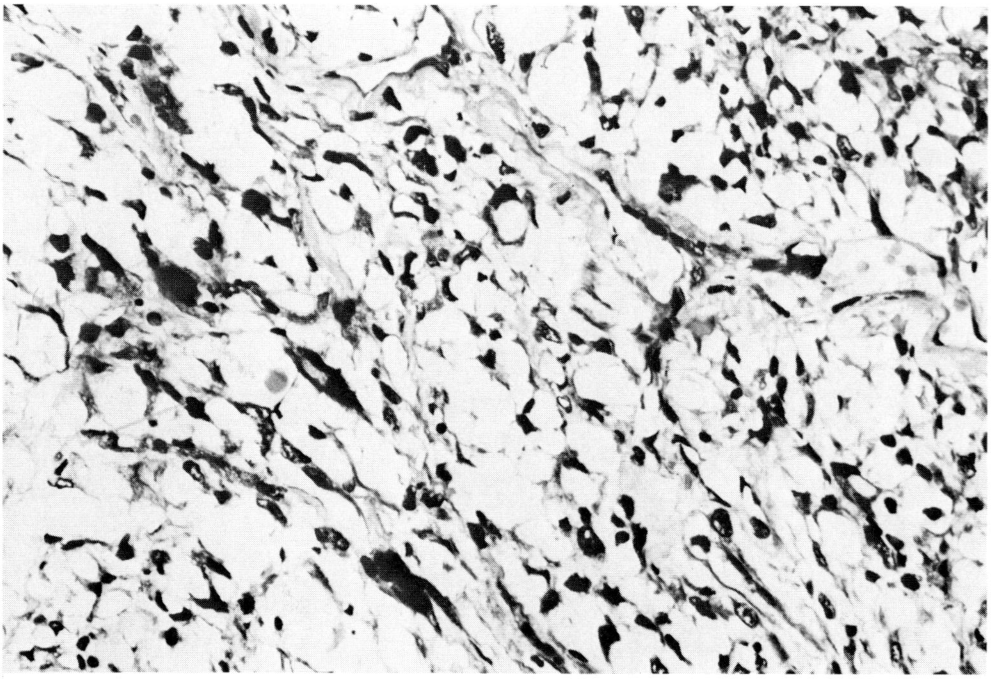

FIGURE 27. Pleomorphic liposarcoma. Note the relationship of the tumor cells to thin-walled vessels. (H.E.; Magnification × 100.)

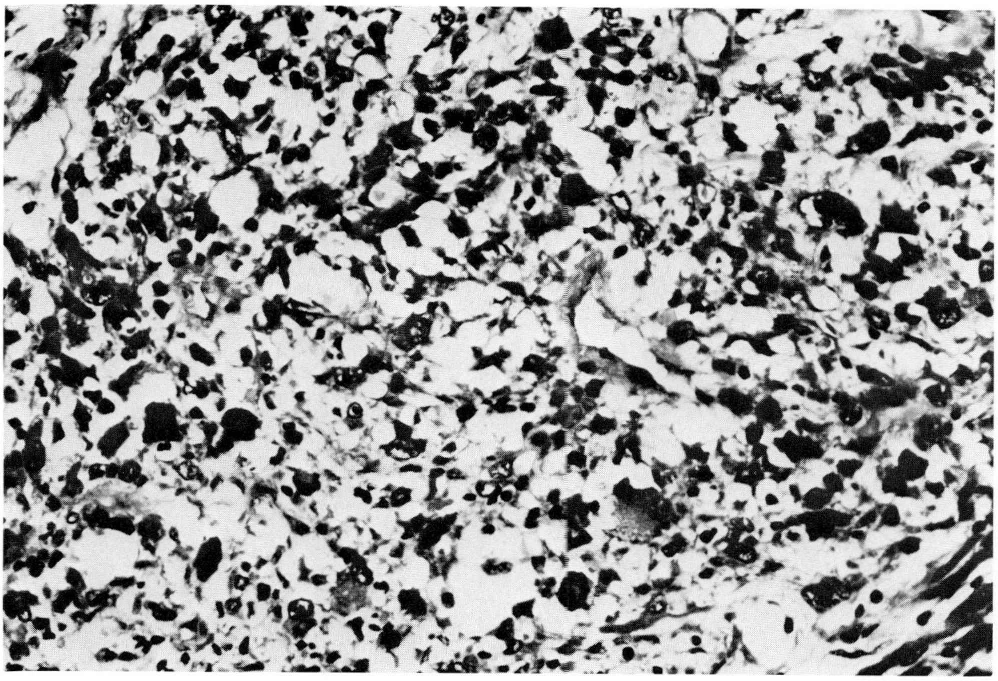

FIGURE 28. Pleomorphic liposarcoma. Marked pleomorphism and bizarre giant cells are present. (H.E.; Magnification × 100.)

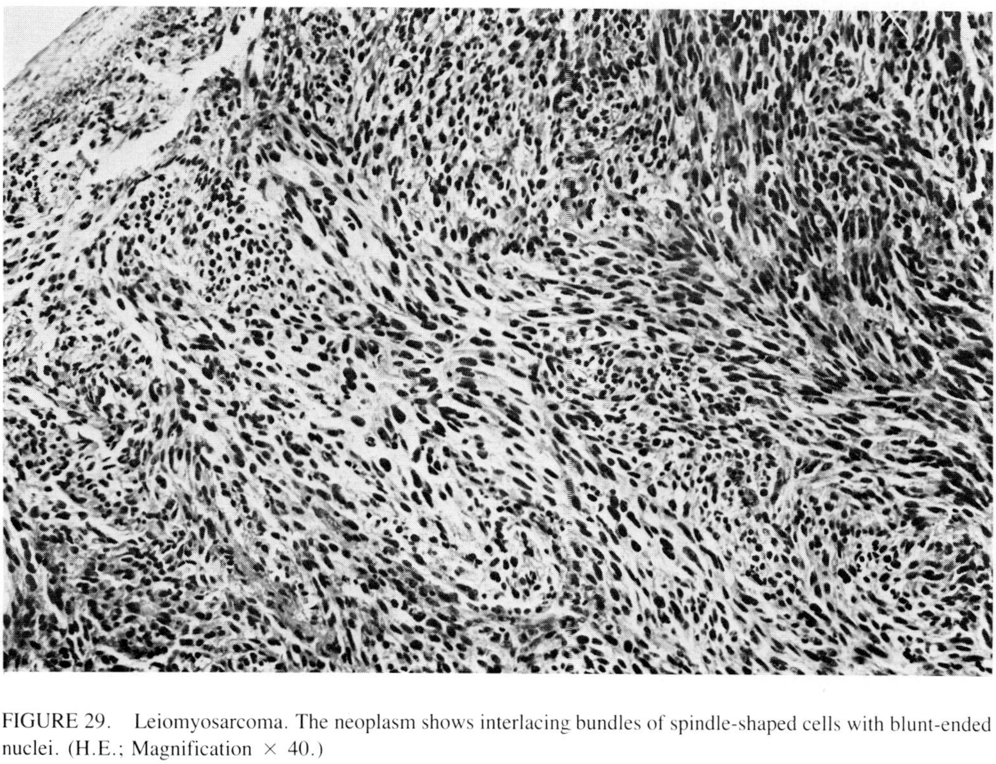

FIGURE 29. Leiomyosarcoma. The neoplasm shows interlacing bundles of spindle-shaped cells with blunt-ended nuclei. (H.E.; Magnification × 40.)

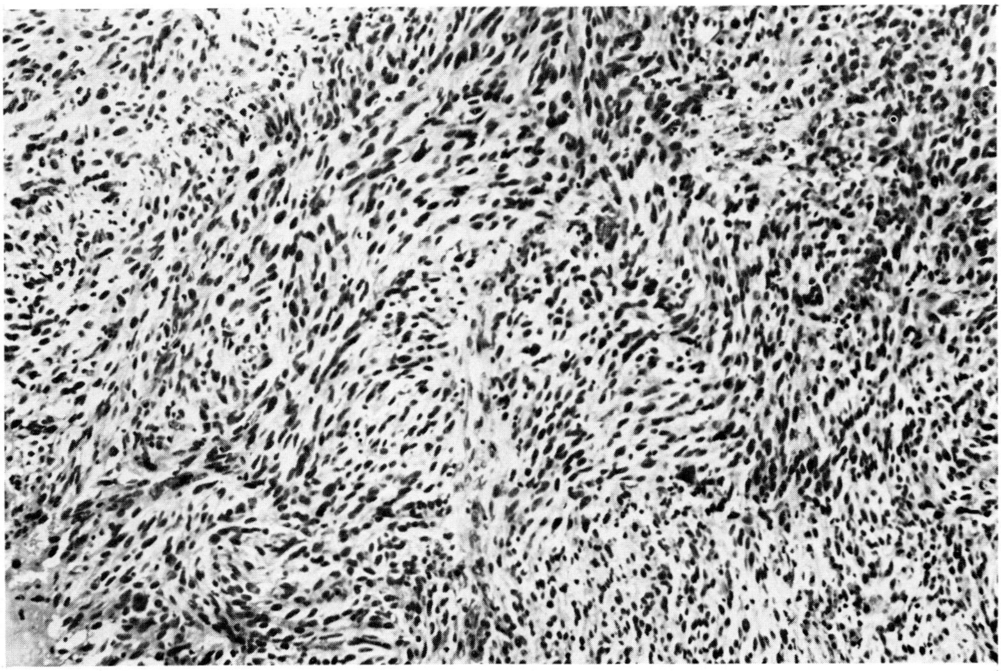

FIGURE 30. Leiomyosarcoma. Another area of the neoplasm. (H.E.; Magnification × 40.)

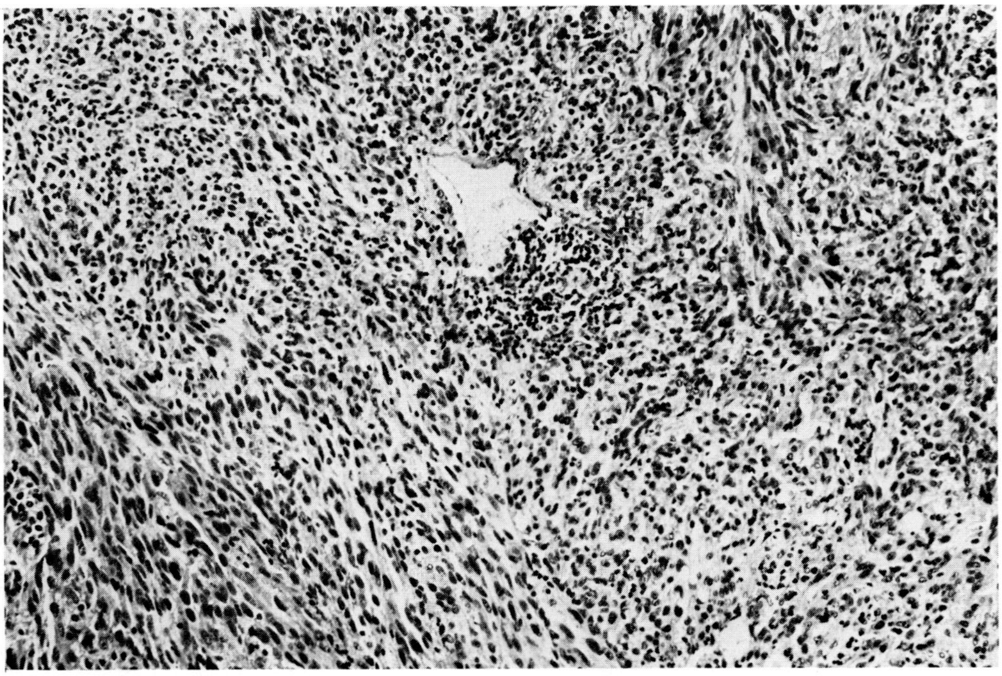

FIGURE 31. Leiomyosarcoma. The tumor shows marked cellularity. (H.E.; Magnification × 40.)

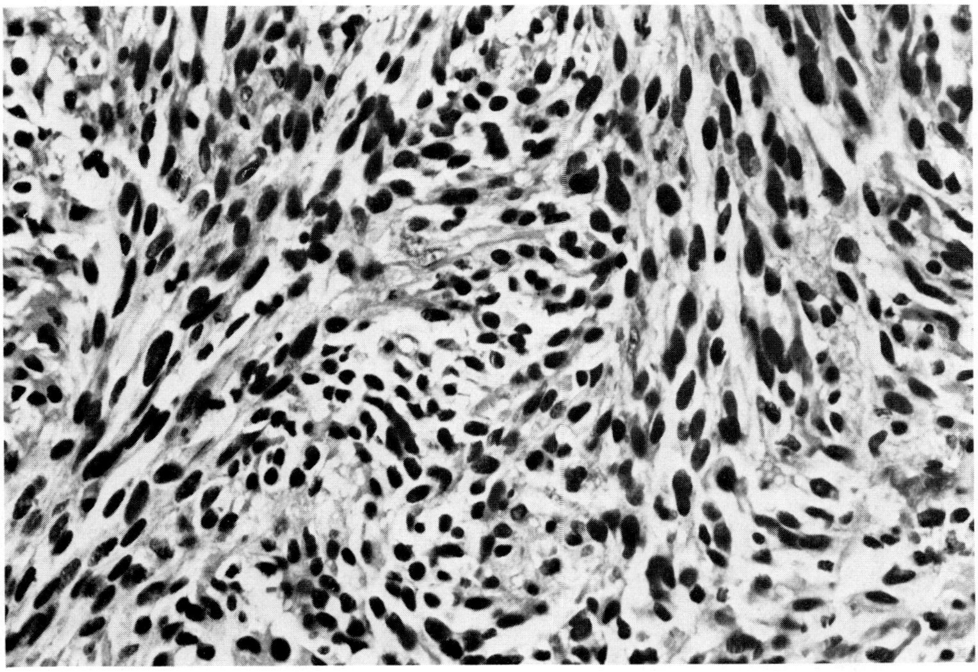

FIGURE 32. Leiomyosarcoma. Note pleomorphic and hyperchromatic nuclei. (H.E.; Magnification × 100.)

B. Definition

Rhabdomyosarcoma is a malignant tumor of rhabdomyoblasts in varying stages of differentiation.

C. Incidence

The literature contains many unconvincing reports, but several well-documented and acceptable cases of laryngeal rhabdomyosarcoma have been reported.[3,90,92-102a]

D. Age and Sex

The laryngeal rhabdomyosarcoma may occur at any age, but most of the reported cases of embryonal variant have been observed in infants and children. In adults, the pleomorphic type is more common, although the embryonal type does occur also. There is a slight male preponderance, but the difference is probably insignificant.

E. Site

The glottic region is the most affected by the tumor, but it is capable of arising anywhere.

F. Histogenesis

According to Willis,[103] most rhabdomyosarcomas of children and adolescents are derived from embryonic tissue and not from muscle, "either from immature prospective muscular tissue or indifferent mesenchymal tissue with the potency for aberrant differentiation of muscle fibres". This would explain the high incidence of rhabdomyosarcoma at the site with only "scraps of muscle".[104]

G. Pathology

Gross pathology — The neoplasm may show a lobulated or polypoid mass and is usually hard, though sometimes it may be soft because of hemorrhagic and necrotic areas. The botryoid variant presents a typical aspect: the neoplasm resembles a cluster of grapes.

Light microscopy and classification — Horn and Enterline[105] have distinguished four basic variants: pleomorphic, embryonal, botryoid, and alveolar. Evans[106] has considered the botryoid variant as a purely macroscopic and not a microscopic feature, and has recognized only three variants of rhabdomyosarcoma.

Enzinger and Shiraki,[107] in accordance with the nomenclature recommended by the World Health Organization, classify rhabdomyosarcomas into four groups: embryonal, alveolar, pleomorphic, and mixed type.

There are probably only two basic groups of rhabdomyosarcomas: the pleomorphic and the embryonal type. The botryoid sarcoma and the alveolar rhabdomyosarcoma are only two subgroups of embryonal rhabdomyosarcoma. The term "juvenile rhabdomyosarcoma" comprises the embryonal, botryoid, and alveolar types.

Ashton and Morgan,[108] considering the degree of cellular differentiation of rhabdomyosarcoma, have proposed the following distinction: (1) embryonal sarcoma, completely undifferentiated, (2) nonstriated embryonal rhabdomyosarcoma (in this variant rhabdomyoblasts are seen, but cross-striations cannot be evidenced), (3) striated embryonal rhabdomyosarcoma, where cross-striations have been demonstrated at some stage and show at electron microscopy well-differentiated, striated myofilaments.

Pleomorphic rhabdomyosarcoma (also known as adult rhabdomyosarcoma, adult pleomorphic rhabdomyosarcoma, differentiated adult pleomorphic rhabdomyosarcoma, or malignant adult rhabdomyoma) — This is the most differentiated form and the easiest to identify microscopically. Histologically (Figures 33 to 36), it is characterized by a marked polymorphism. The cells are of several types, and strap-like, racquet- and spindle-shaped, ovoid, polygonal, multinucleated, and bizarre giant cells are present. Their cytoplasm is highly acidophilic, granular, or homogenous. The nuclei of these cells are hyperchromatic and numerous atypical mitotic figures are seen. The stroma is usually scanty. There are often extensive necrotic areas. The histological pattern is so peculiar that it can hardly be mistaken for any other neoplastic lesion. The numerous types of cells present lead to the correct diagnosis, which can be made simply by means of the conventional hematoxylin-eosin stain. Staining methods making cross-striations evident (phosphotungstic acid hematoxylin-PTAH, Heidenhain hematoxylin) and stains evidencing the high glycogen content of many neoplastic cells (PAS, PAS with diastase predigestion, PAS-hematoxylin) may be useful. To avoid misinterpretations in making a diagnosis of a neoplasm of striated muscle, cross-striations are considered a necessary finding by some investigators while for others, on the contrary, this feature is not essential.[109-112] Experimental studies have shown the absence of cross-striations in rhabdomyosarcoma.[113] This subtype has been described in the larynx by several authors.[3,93,96,98-100,102]

Embryonal rhabdomyosarcoma — This is characteristically a tumor of childhood but has been occasionally observed in adolescents and rarely in adults. This neoplasm develops most commonly in the genitourinary tract, in the head and neck, in the limbs, nasopharynx, retroperitoneum, the ear, and less commonly, in the region of salivary glands and mandible. The neoplasm is therefore located in the regions where striated muscle is not abundant or is lacking altogether. Microscopically, the tumor is composed of a mainly myxoid stroma, including small, roundish, undifferentiated cells with scanty cytoplasm. The giant cells are uncommon, unlike what is usually seen in pleomorphic rhabdomyosarcoma. Mitoses are rare and cross-striations, which are not essential to establish the diagnosis, may be observed only in the largest and most elongated cells. This variant has been described in the larynx by some investigators.[92,94,95,97,97a]

Embryonal botryoid rhabdomyosarcoma (also called botryoid rhabdomyosarcoma or myxoid rhabdomyosarcoma) — This is considered to be a variant of embryonal rhabdomyosarcoma. The tumor is composed of round and short spindle cells contained in a myxoid stroma. The nuclei of the neoplastic cells are well defined but the cytoplasm is minimal and poorly outlined. Areas of cartilaginous tissue and of striated muscle cells may also be noted. This neoplasm may be mistaken for edematous or myxomatous polyps. This variant was observed by some authors.[97a,101,102a]

Embryonal alveolar rhabdomyosarcoma (also called alveolar rhabdomyosarcoma) is a rare variant of embryonal rhabdomyosarcoma. The neoplasm is composed of rounded or oval cells having an eosinophilic cytoplasm and tending to assume a pseudoglandular pattern. The tumor cells are separated by connective tissue trabeculae. In the cytoplasm of many elements a longitudinal or transverse striation of myofibrils or at least a granular cytoplasm may be seen. Stains for glycogen give a more or less marked positive reaction, which is possibly the morphological equivalent of cross-striation. This tumor may also show pleomorphic areas. A case of laryngeal alveolar rhabdomyosarcoma has been reported by Winther and Lorentzen.[99]

H. Diagnosis and Differential Diagnosis

The identification of this neoplasm is difficult, particularly when diagnosis has to be made in biopsy material.

Friedmann and Bird[114] state that electron microscopy may be of diagnostic assistance in certain cases of rhabdomyosarcoma in which cross-striations are not detectable under the light microscope. Williamson et al.[115] also think that the conventional histochemical methods do not always allow the identification of cross-striations, while ultrastructural study makes the myofibrils visible. Recently, the world literature for diagnostic ultrastructural features of rhabdomyosarcomas has been accurately reviewed by Bundtzen and Norback,[116] who considered that a specific feature of the sarcomere within a representative malignant cell is necessary and sufficient for diagnosis of rhabdomyosarcoma by ultrastructure.

The diagnostic value of histochemistry in embryonal rhabdomyosarcoma has been emphasized.[117] Special histochemical stains, such as modified Gomori trichrome method, nicotinamide adenine dinucleotide-tetrazolium reductase, succinate dehydrogenase, and calcium-mediated adenosine triphosphatase may show longitudinal and cross-striations that are not easily seen with hematoxylin and eosin or phosphotungstic acid-hematoxylin stains.[117]

The demonstration of myoglobin, a tumor marker, in neoplastic skeletal muscle cells by the immunoperoxidase method may aid in the diagnosis of well-differentiated neoplasms.[118,119]

Malignant fibrous histiocytoma, myxoid liposarcoma, and leiomyosarcoma have to be distinguished by special staining methods and electron microscopy.

I. Behavior and Prognosis

The biological course of laryngeal rhabdomyosarcoma is less aggressive than that of the head and neck.[93,120] Lymphatic and blood-borne metastases are not uncommon.[101] Batsakis[121] considers the clinical staging according to site and extent of growth convenient for prognostication and of more value than the histological subtyping.

VII. ANGIOSARCOMA

A. Introduction

Angiosarcoma (or malignant hemangioendothelioma) and hemangiopericytoma have been erroneously considered as identical lesions, whereas they represent two distinct entities.[122]

B. Terminology

"Malignant hemangioendothelioma" and "angiosarcoma" are terms used as synonyms. The tumor is also indicated as hemangioendotheliosarcoma.

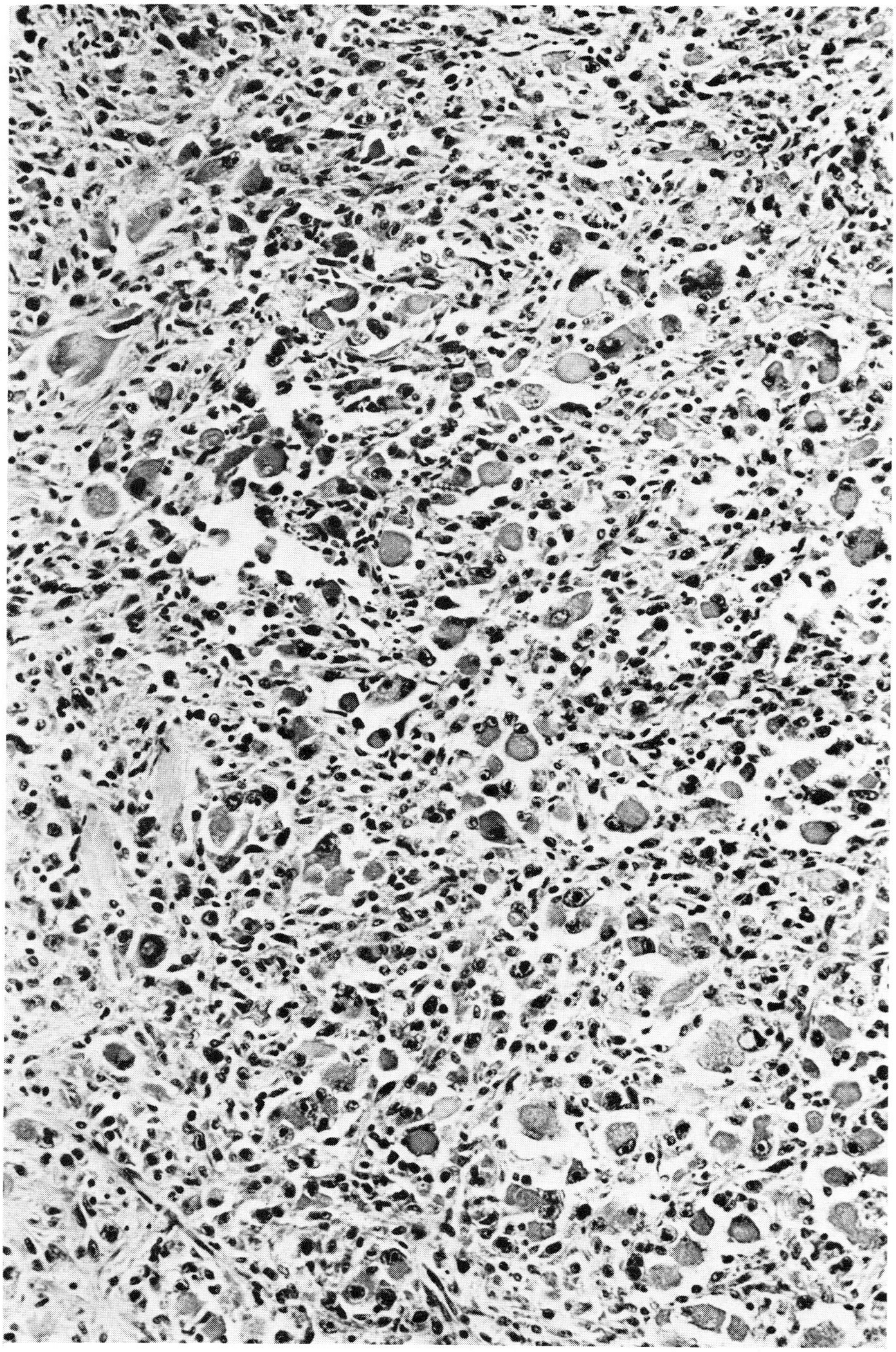

FIGURE 33. Pleomorphic rhabdomyosarcoma. The neoplasm shows a great variety of cells. (H.E.; Magnification × 40.) (From Frugoni, P. and Ferlito, A., *J. Laryngol. Otol.*, 90, 687, 1976. With permission.)

C. Definition

It is a malignant vascular neoplasm characterized by the formation of vessels and capillary-like structures of an anastomosing nature lined by atypical endothelial cells.

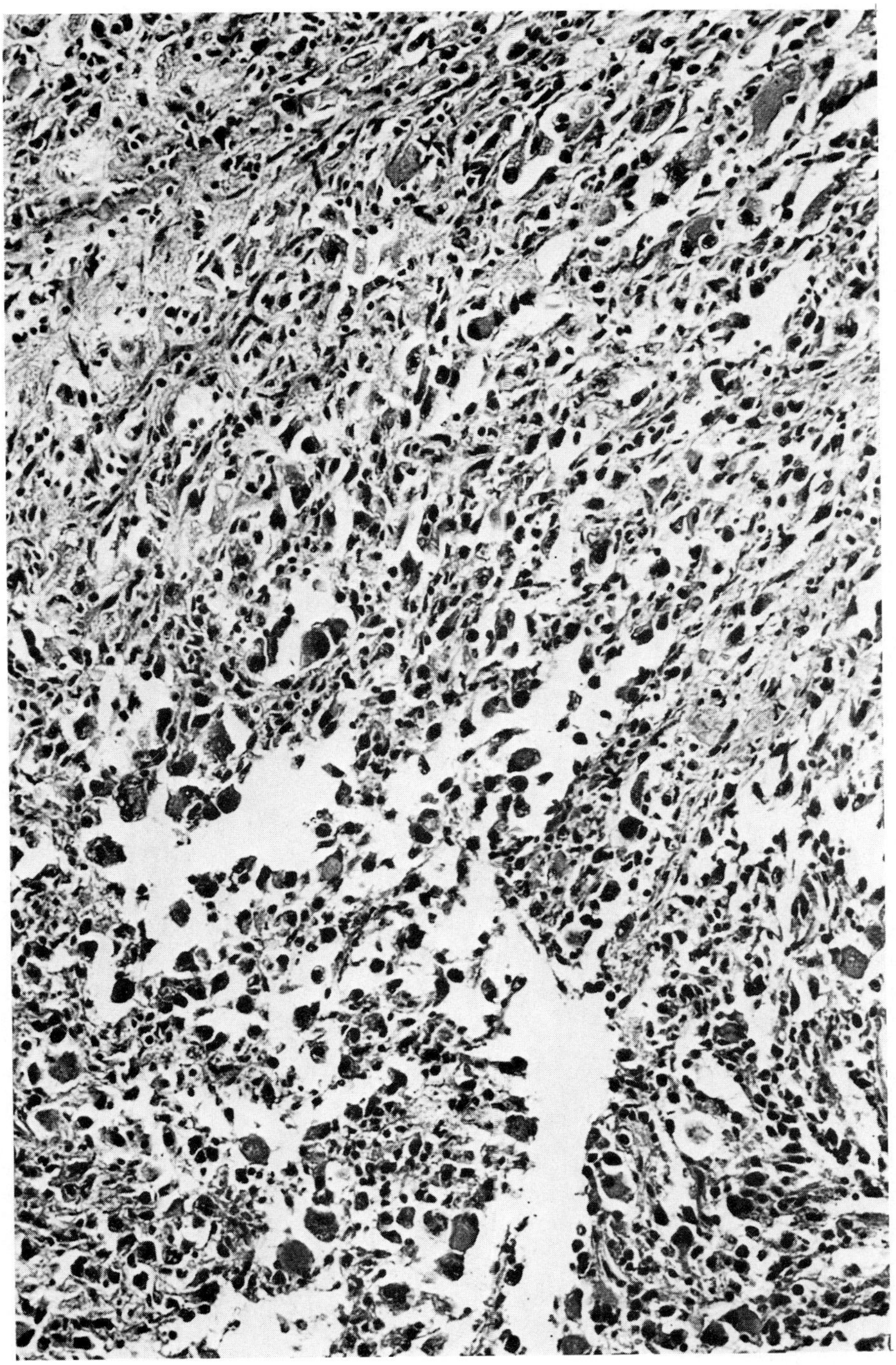

FIGURE 34. Pleomorphic rhabdomyosarcoma. Another area of the same tumor in which extensive cellular pleomorphism is visible. (H.E.; Magnification × 40.) (From Frugoni, P. and Ferlito, A., *J. Laryngol. Otol.*, 90, 687, 1976. With permission.)

D. Incidence

The larynx may be rarely involved by this necplasm but the true incidence is difficult to ascertain because angiosarcoma has been confused with other vascular neoplasms (i.e.,

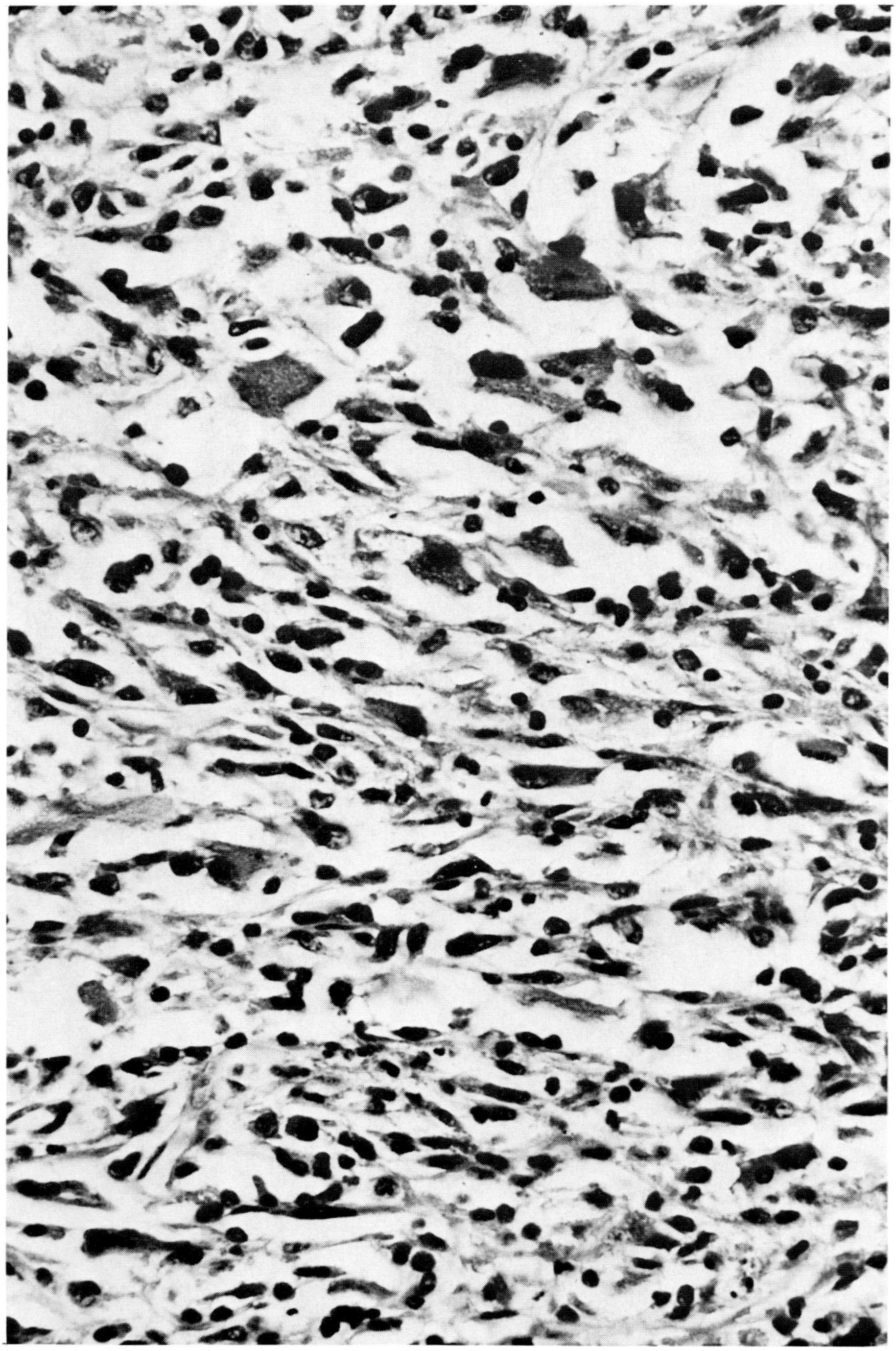

FIGURE 35. Pleomorphic rhabdomyosarcoma. Higher magnification shows many cells varying in size and shape, among which elongated cells and strap-like cells with peripheral nucleus can be noted. (H.E.; Magnification × 100.) (From Frugoni, P. and Ferlito, A., *J. Laryngol. Otol.*, 90, 687, 1976. With permission.)

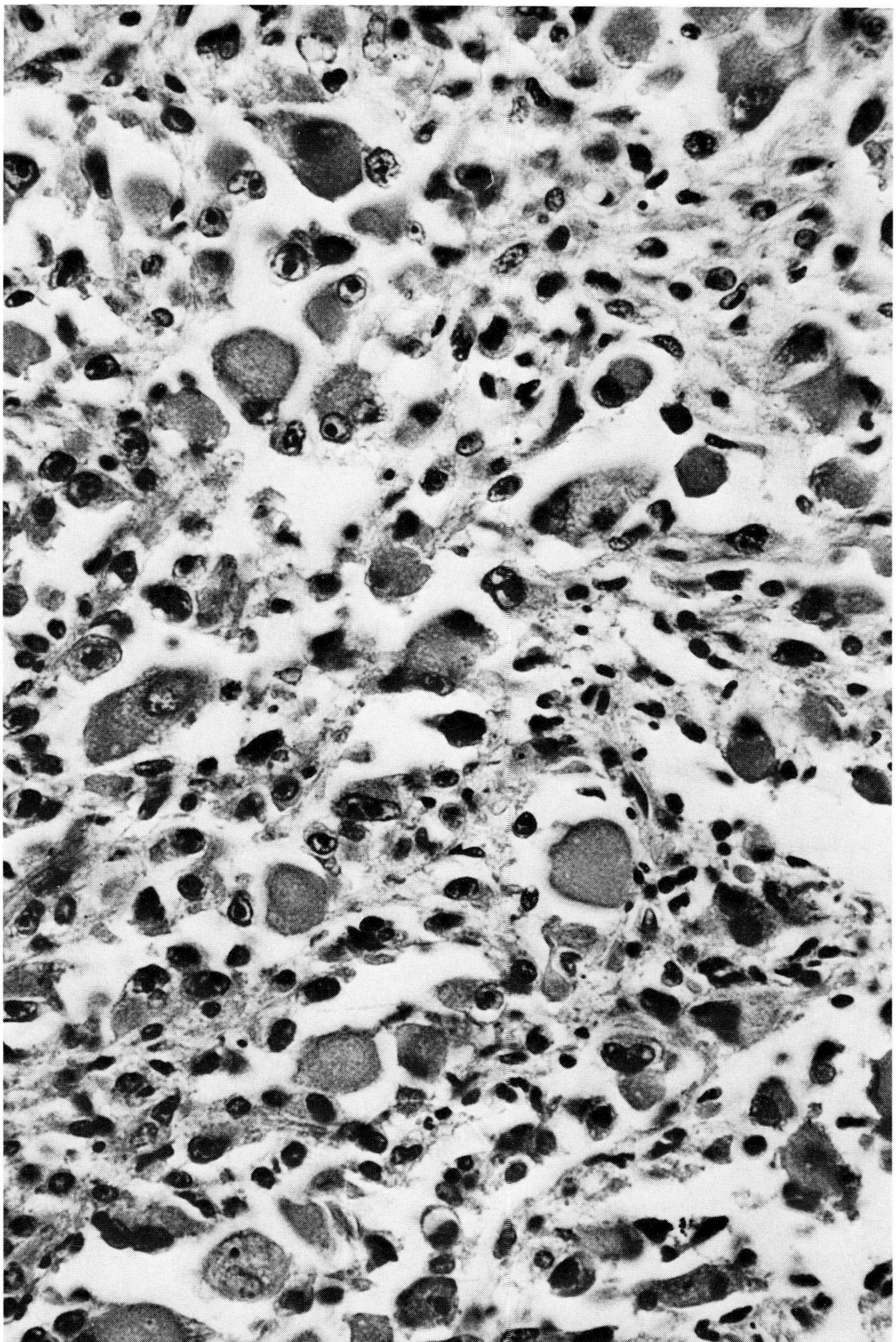

FIGURE 36. Pleomorphic rhabdomyosarcoma. Note giant cells with eccentrically located large nuclei and abundant acidophilic granular cytoplasm. (H.E.; Magnification × 100.) (From Frugoni, P. and Ferlito, A., *J. Laryngol. Otol.*, 90, 687, 1976. With permission.)

hemangiopericytoma, Kaposi's sarcoma, hemangioma) and with non-neoplastic diseases (i.e., intubation granuloma). The first case of laryngeal angiosarcoma reported in the literature dates back to Yankauer.[123] The neoplasm presented as a pedunculated growth implanted on a vocal cord, which was removed at indirect laryngoscopy. Havens and Parkhill[124] reviewed 3 cases of laryngeal hemangioendothelioma and reported 26 cases of malignant laryngeal tumor other than squamous cell carcinoma observed at the Mayo Clinic over a period of 30 years, and 8 of these neoplasms were diagnosed as hemangioendothelioma. Most of these tumors were of low-grade malignancy; six were grade I, one was grade II, and one III.* Pratt and Goodof[126] reported a well-documented case of hemangioendotheliosarcoma of the larynx in which the neoplasm had metastasized to the lung and had spread to the root of the neck and skin of the cheek. These authors have also reviewed the literature and collected only 15 previously reported cases. Nevertheless, Batsakis and Fox[1] think that their discrimination leaves much to be desired and consider the diagnosis inaccurate in many instances. Later, other cases were reported.[63,127-130]

E. Age and Sex

The tumor most often occurs in males between 40 and 70 years of age.

F. Site

Any site of the larynx may be affected.

G. Etiology

It seems that radiotherapy might have a causative role in the occurrence of some of these tumors. In the cases described by Thomas,[129] the patient had been irradiated 11 years earlier (7000R given over a period of 43 days) for a squamous carcinoma of the vocal cord.

H. Histogenesis

The neoplasm arises from neoformed endothelial cells of blood vessels.

I. Pathology

Gross pathology — The tumor appears as a white or pink pedunculated mass of friable consistency and there are often areas of hemorrhage in its substance.

Light microscopy (Figures 37 to 42) — The lesion is composed of poorly cohesive cells forming vascular channels lined by atypical, large, pleomorphic, endothelial cells. Mitoses may be numerous and atypical, and areas of neocrosis may be seen. Reticulin stain shows well-defined sheaths containing tumor cells.

Electron microscopy — Ultrastructural studies have not been reported for laryngeal angiosarcorma, whereas they have been described in other organs.[131-133] Characteristic ultrastructural features of this neoplasm are intracellular lumina and Weibel-Palade bodies.[132-133]

J. Diagnosis and Differential Diagnosis

The histologic diagnosis of angiosarcoma may be difficult, in particular in poorly differentiated neoplasms. Mallory[134] and Stout[135] confirmed that the existence of a reticular network encircling the neoformed endothelial cells is of great importance for its diagnosis.

The differential diagnosis must be made in particular from hemangiopericytoma and Kaposi's sarcoma. As to the differences between angiosarcoma and hemangiopericytoma, in the former, tumor elements grow within the lumen of the vessel, whereas the latter displays a perivascular proliferation of tumor cells. Unlike other vascular neoplasms, in the stromal proliferation of angiosarcoma there is constantly the presence of sulfated acid mucosaccharides. This feature may be of help in differential diagnosis.[136] According to Stout,[135] reticulin stains are important for distinguishing the two neoplasms. However, the two tumors

* Nosaka and Nagata[125] described a case of malignant hemangioendothelioma of the larynx.

are not always easy to distinguish and particularly in the less well-differentiated neoplasms the findings are equivocal.[137] The Kaposi's sarcoma presents, like angiosarcoma, an endothelial endoluminal proliferation, but the vessels are intermingled with spindle-shaped fibroblasts and with a lymphoreticular inflammatory infiltrate. Furthermore, in this disease there are several cutaneous lesions of the lower extremities. Recently, an aid to the diagnosis of angiosarcoma has resulted from the application of the immunoperoxidase technique, which reveals the production of factor VIII-related antigen,[138,139] a protein synthesized primarily by endothelial cells. However, factor VIII-related antigen is not a specific marker of angiosarcoma and may not have as much diagnostic potential as was originally thought.[140] In this connection, Enzinger and Weiss[141] stressed that not only may there be great variation from tumor to tumor in the expression of this antigen, but there is also variation from cell to cell within the same tumor.

K. Behavior and Prognosis

The limited number of reports, not always reliable, do not allow one to draw conclusions, but in some cases the clinical course of the neoplasm is considered very aggressive.[129] The tumor metastasizes preferably via bloodstream, and lung metastases have been reported,[126] as well as subcutaneous metastases.[128]

VIII. HEMANGIOPERICYTOMA

A. Introduction

Hemangiopericytoma was first recognized as a pathological entity by Stout and Murray,[142] who used the term "hemangiopericytoma". The neoplasm derives from elongated and contractile cells (Zimmermann's pericytes), which are usually located outside the basement membrane of capillaries. Ultrastructural studies support the concept of a pericyte origin.[143-145]

B. Definition

It is a vascular neoplasm characterized by a proliferation of rounded and spindle-shaped cells proliferating around endothelial-lined capillaries.

C. Incidence

This tumor is extremely rare in the larynx. Stout[146] had reported 197 cases of hemangiopericytoma recorded at the Laboratory of Surgical Pathology of Columbia University, of which one was located in the larynx, without, however, reporting additional clinicopathological data. Walike and Bailey[147] reported a case of laryngeal hemangiopericytoma occurring in a 64-year-old black woman and considered their report to be the first in literature. Taguchi et al.[148] described another case occurring in a 47-year-old man treated by a surgical operation supplemented by radiation therapy (6120 rads of Co^{60}); 1 year and 3 months after the beginning of treatment the patient developed squamous cell carcinoma of the left inner aspect of the larynx, which was considered to have been induced by previous irradiation. In 1978, Ferlito[149] described a case of malignant hemangiopericytoma occurring in a 50-year-old male patient. Moncade and Demaldent[150] reported a recurrent hemangiopericytoma in a 75-year-old man. This case, however, lacks illustrations. Pesavento and Ferlito[151] described a case of recurrent laryngeal hemangiopericytoma occurring in a 31-year-old male patient (Figure 43), making at the same time a review of the literature. Another case has been reported by Hertzanu et al.[152]

Laryngeal involvement by hemangiopericytoma is also observed in a case of *congenital* hemangiopericytoma of the rhinopharynx,[153] in which the tumor extended from the rhinopharynx down to the level of the cricoid cartilage of the larynx. The infantile or congenital

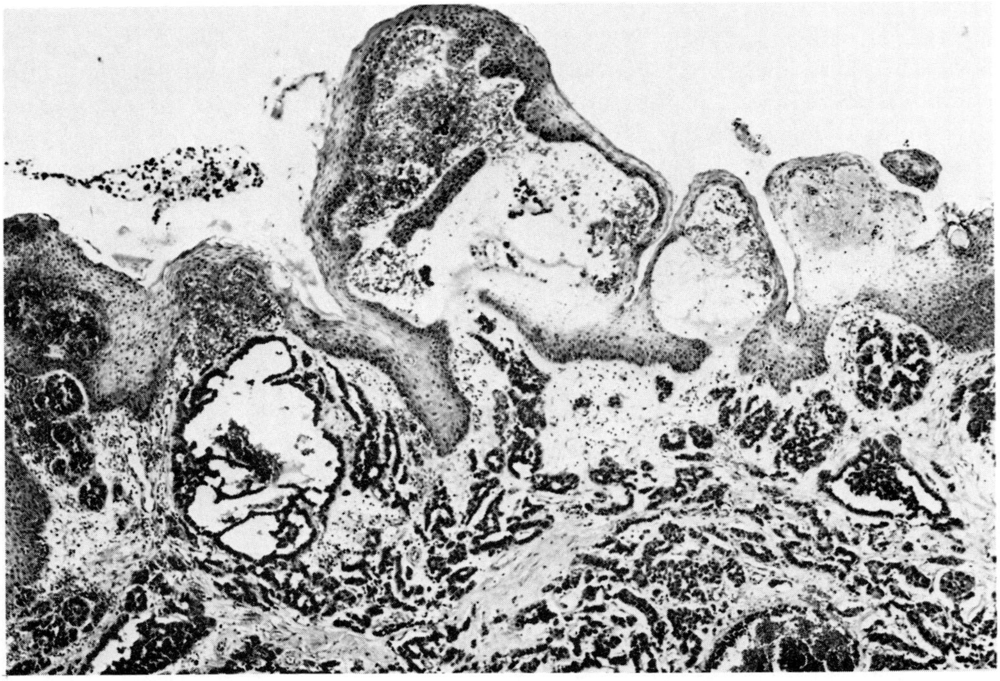

FIGURE 37. Angiosarcoma. The neoplasm is composed of tortuous and anastomosing vascular channels filled with red blood cells and lined by endothelial cells. (H.E.; Magnification × 16.)

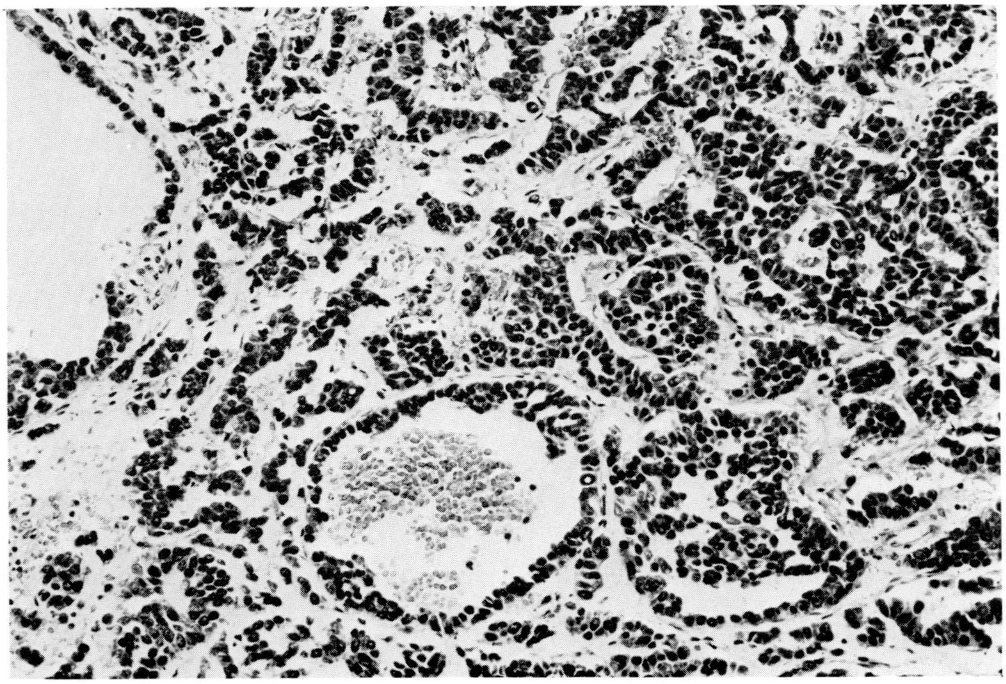

FIGURE 38. Angiosarcoma. The neoplasm shows lumina lined by plump epithelioid endothelial cells. (H.E.; Magnification × 40.)

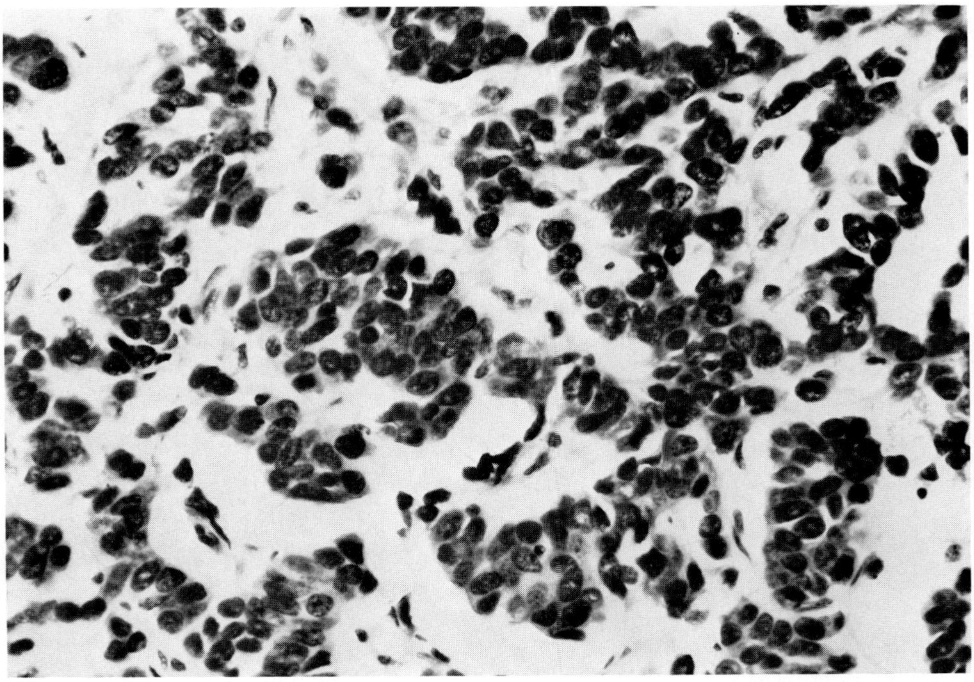

FIGURE 39. Angiosarcoma. Note plump and cuboidal neoplastic cells. (H.E.; Magnification × 100.)

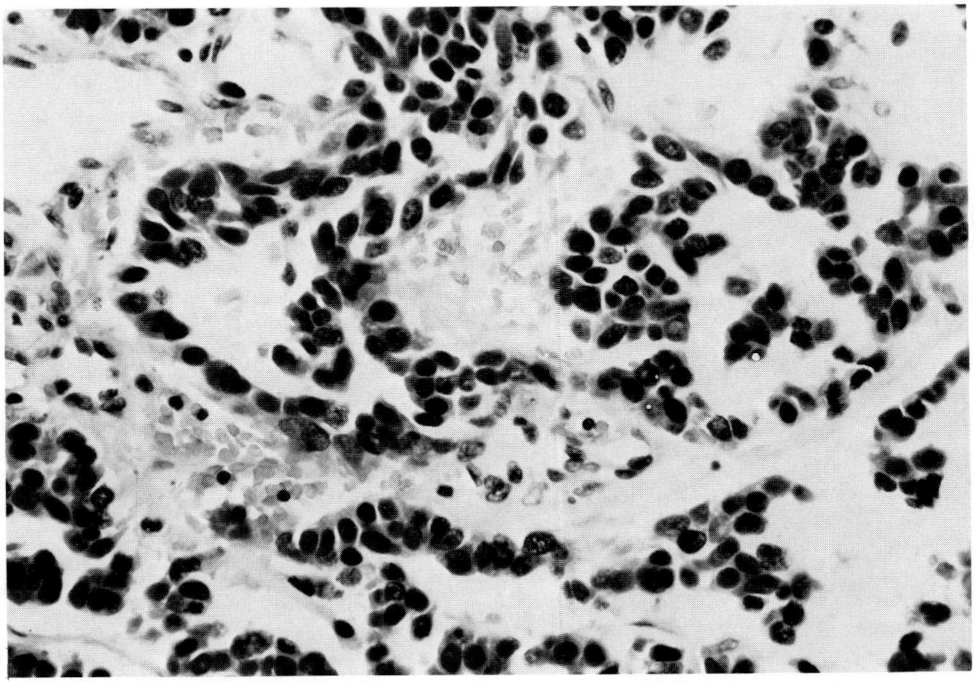

FIGURE 40. Angiosarcoma. Note atypical and hyperchromatic endothelial cells. (H.E.; Magnification × 100.)

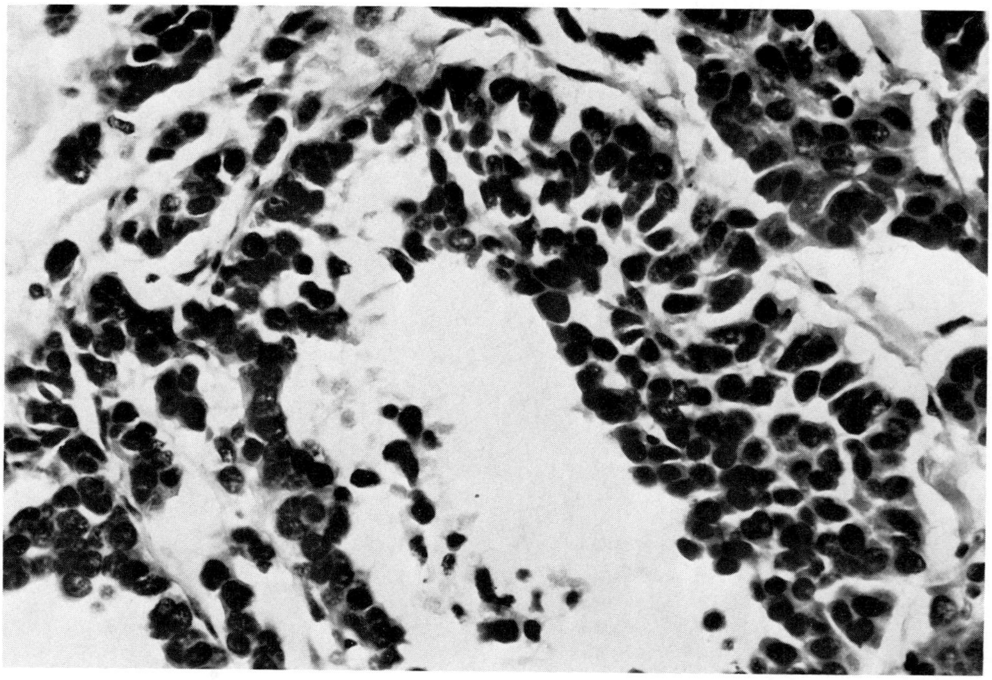

FIGURE 41. Angiosarcoma. Note rounded epithelial-like cells. (H. E.; Magnification × 100.)

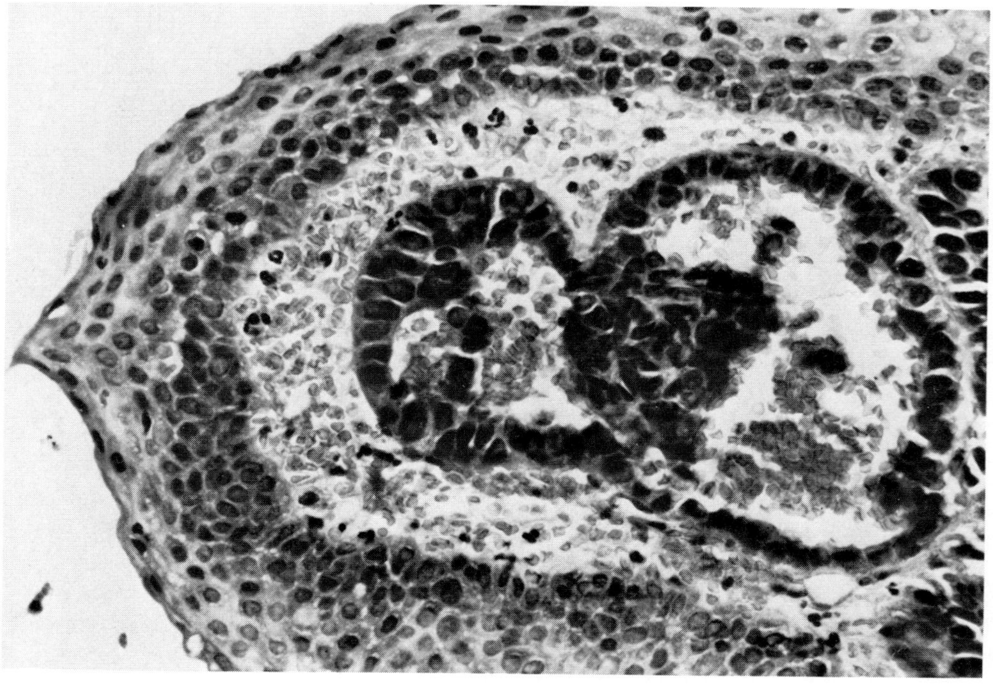

FIGURE 42. Angiosarcoma. Plump and cuboidal neoplastic atypical cells protrude in vascular lumen. (H.E.; Magnification × 100.)(From Ferlito, A. et al., *Ann. Otol. Rhinol. Laryngol.*, 94, 1985. With permission.)

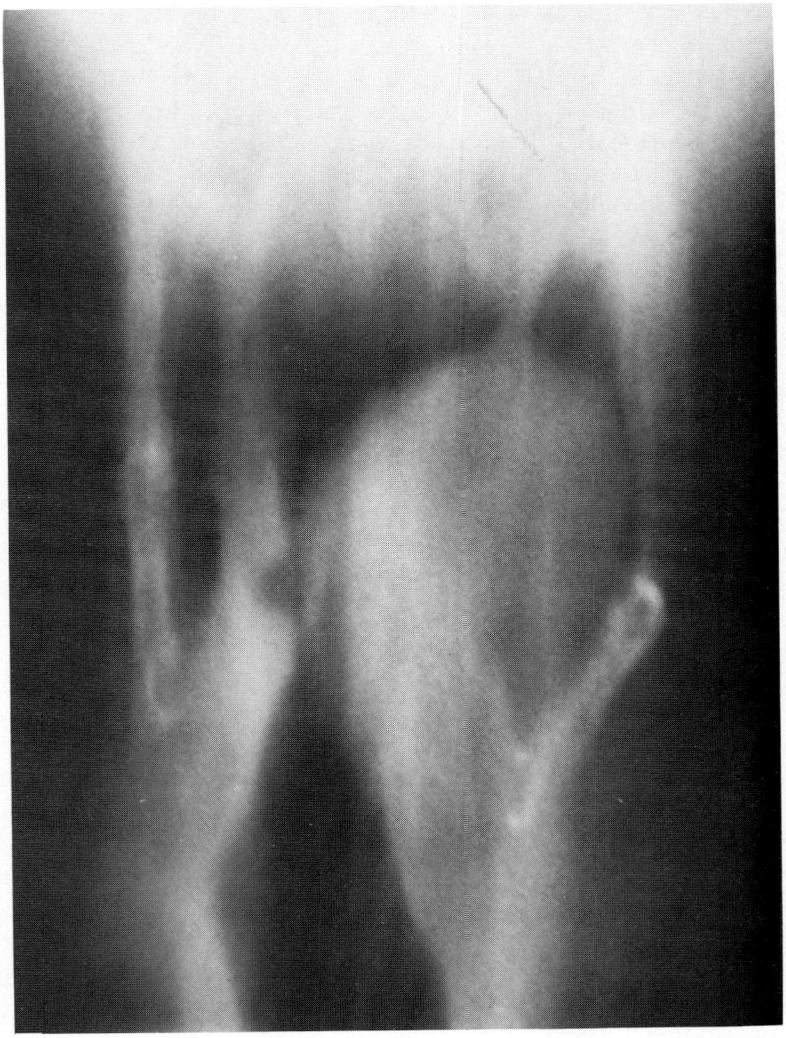

FIGURE 43. Hemangiopericytoma. Antero-posterior laryngeal tomogram revealing an extensive neoplasm.

hemangiopericytoma is now regarded as a separate variant because of its different histological picture and clinical behavior.

D. Age and Sex

The tumor most often occurs in men between 40 and 70 years of age.

E. Etiology

The cause is unknown. Trauma and steroid therapy have occasionally been held responsible for the occurrence of these tumors.[154] It is interesting to mention the case described by Walike and Bailey[147] occurring in a female patient who had been treated with variable doses of prednisone (25 to 100 mg/day) for a period of 20 months because she was suffering from pemphigus vulgaris.

F. Pathology

Gross pathology — The tumor may appear as a well-circumscribed mass of variable size, covered by a thin and vascular pseudocapsule.

Light microscopy (Figures 44 to 49) — The neoplasm is composed of vascular structures from which the neoplastic cells originate. The cells are mainly rounded and fusiform with hyperchromatic nuclei and tend to assume a radial arrangement around the vascular spaces. The cellularity and the number of mitotic figures may vary and in some areas, interstitial fibrosis may be present. Scattered lymphocytes and mast cells may also be seen. Occasional areas of hemorrhage and necrosis may be present. Reticulin stain reveals clearly both the peritheliomatous growth of neoplastic cells and the extensive vascular component. Reticulin also enmeshes individual tumor cells. There are no intracellular myofibrils with the Masson trichrome and the phosphotungstic acid-hematoxylin stains. Interstitial mucoid material may be found.

Electron microscopy — In the larynx there are no well-documented ultrastructural studies available. In the case reported by Hertzanu et al.,[152] the diagnosis was supported by electron microscopy, but the ultrastructural findings have not been described.

G. Diagnosis and Differential Diagnosis

Special histochemical stains and ultrastructural investigations may help in establishing the diagnosis.[145]

Glomangioma and hemangioendothelioma should be considered in differential diagnosis. The glomangioma, unlike hemangiopericytoma, displays a concentric, organoid, perivascular arrangement of tumor cells. These are round and epithelioid in appearance, whereas in hemangiopericytoma the tumor cells are elongated or stellate. Furthermore, axons are never present in hemangiopericytoma, whereas they may be seen in the glomangioma. The vascular spaces are often dilated in hemangiopericytoma, unlike those in the glomangioma, in which these spaces are often collapsed. As to the differences between hemangiopericytoma and angiosarcoma, the former displays a perivascular proliferation of tumor cells, whereas in the latter, tumor elements grow within the lumen of the vessels. In hemangiopericytoma the reticulin stain reveals dense reticulin meshwork surrounding groups of cells or individual tumor cells and vessels, which must be considered the most typical, basic pattern of this neoplasm.

Furthermore, differential diagnosis must be made from poorly differentiated synovial sarcoma, leiomyosarcoma, mesenchymal chondrosarcoma, liposarcoma, and malignant fibrous histiocytoma (in particular with the vascular variant).

H. Behavior and Prognosis

The behavior of hemangiopericytoma is variable and the few cases reported in literature do not allow final conclusions to be drawn. In two of the six cases for which clinical information is available the tumor recurred.[150,151] Lymph node or distant metastases have never been reported.

IX. KAPOSI'S SARCOMA

A. Definition

Kaposi's sarcoma is an uncommon, malignant, neoplastic disease of the skin with usual secondary visceral involvement.

B. Incidence

Kaposi's sarcoma, though uncommon in the larynx, may affect the organ and is usually associated with classical skin changes. The oropharynx and the larynx are areas of predilection for lesions of the mucous membrane in Kaposi's sarcoma.[155,155a]

Abramson and Simons,[156] while reviewing the literature, found 13 cases of localized or extensive laryngeal Kaposi's sarcoma.

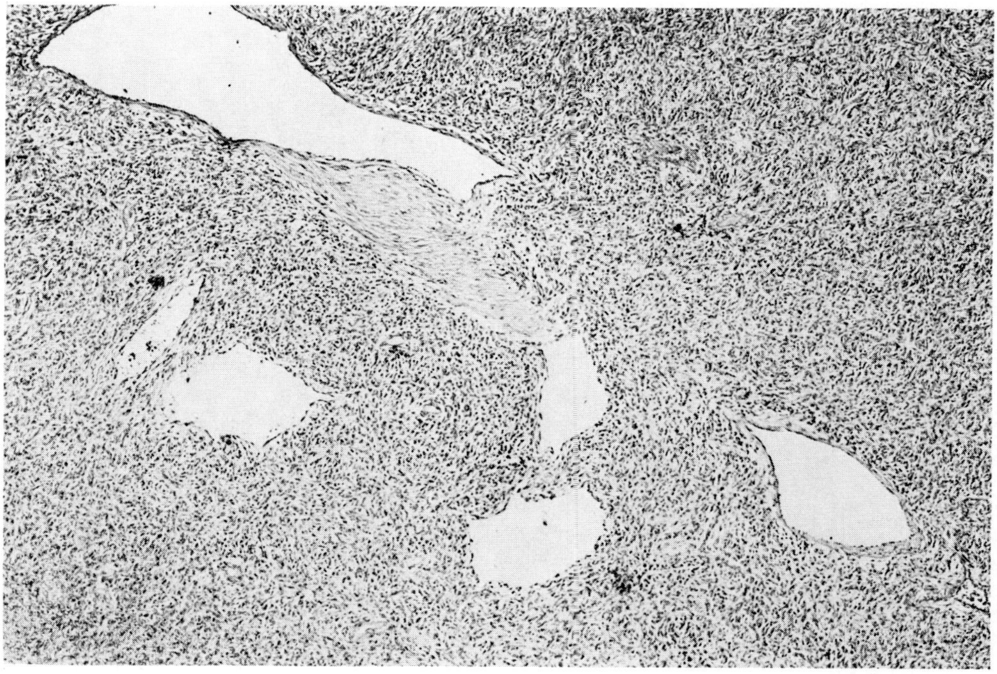

FIGURE 44. Hemangiopericytoma. Low magnification shows several vascular channels and solid areas of the neoplasm. Note the area of fibrosis. (H.E.; Magnification × 16.) (From Pesavento, G. and Ferlito, A., *J. Laryngol. Otol.*, 96, 1065, 1982. With permission.)

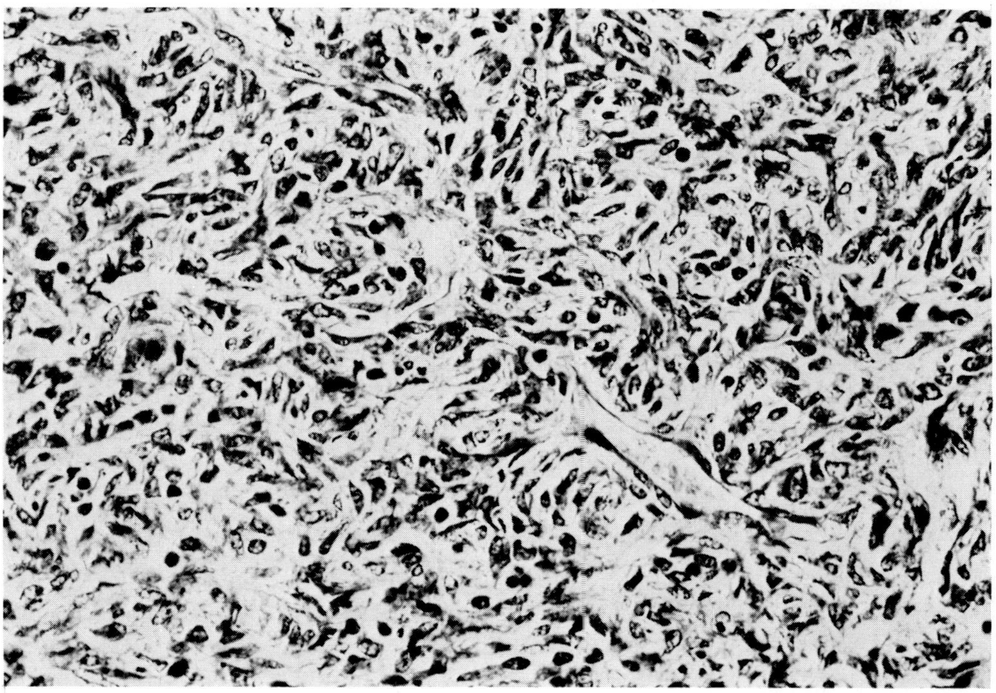

FIGURE 45. Hemangiopericytoma. Typical histologic features of the neoplasm. (H.E.; Magnification × 100.)

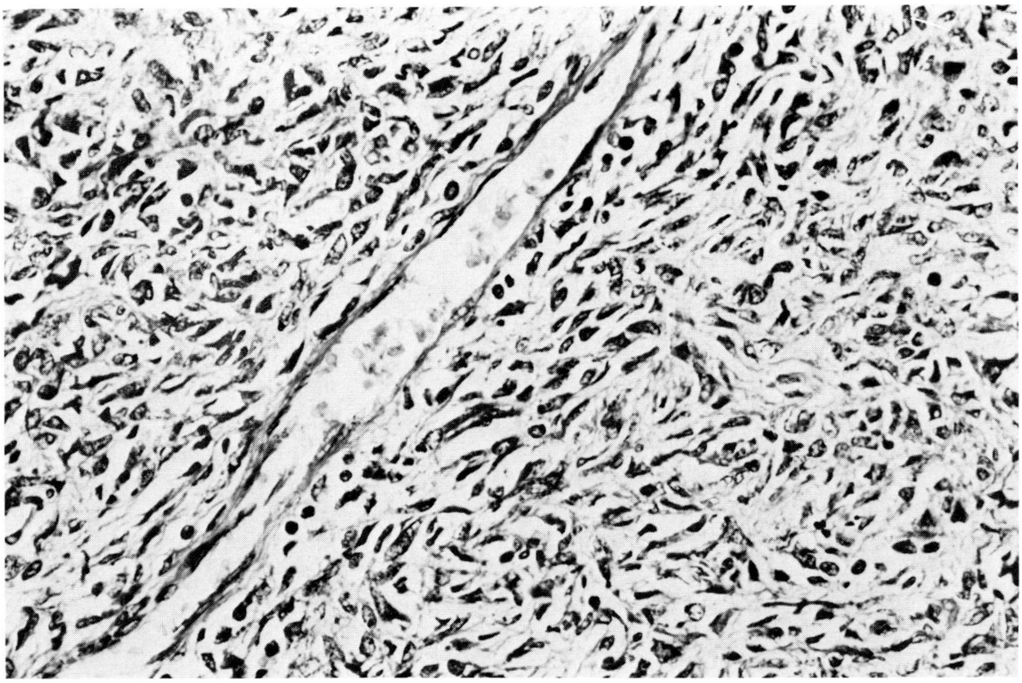

FIGURE 46. Hemangiopericytoma. Another area of the same neoplasm. (H. E.; Magnification × 100.)

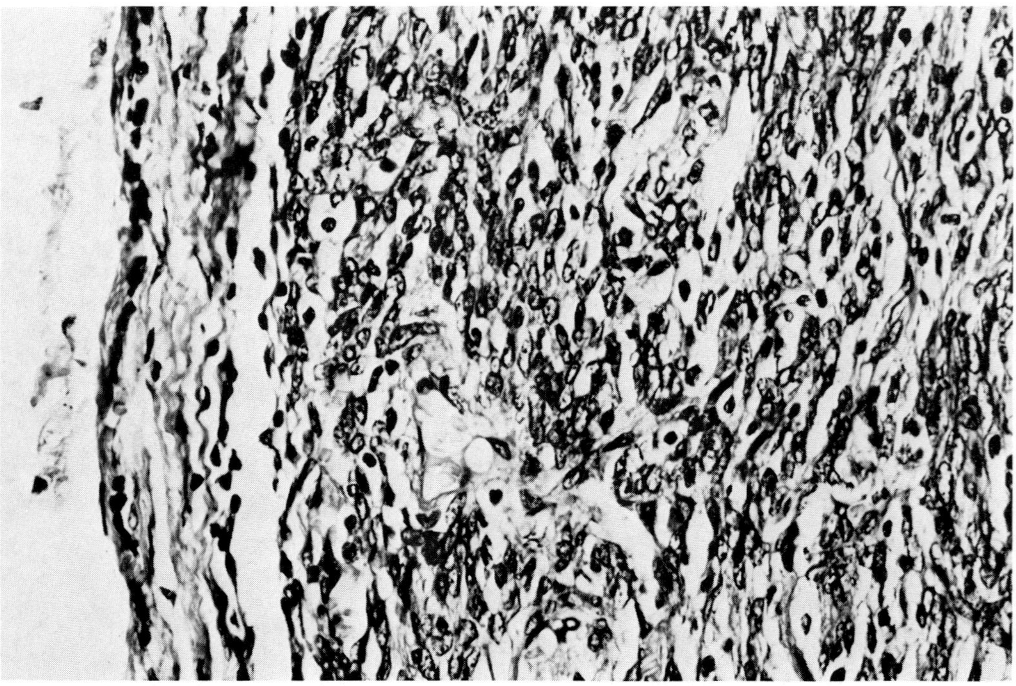

FIGURE 47. Hemangiopericytoma. Note high cellularity of the neoplasm. Cells are hyperchromatic. (H.E.; Magnification × 100.)

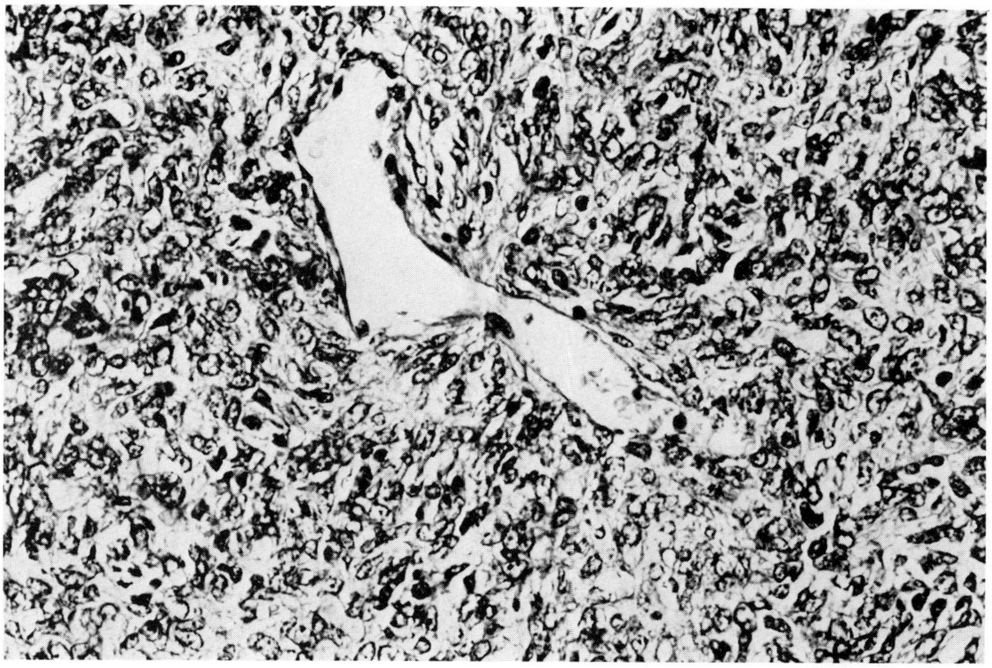

FIGURE 48. Hemangiopericytoma. Note perivascular arrangement of neoplastic cells. (H.E.; Magnification × 100.)

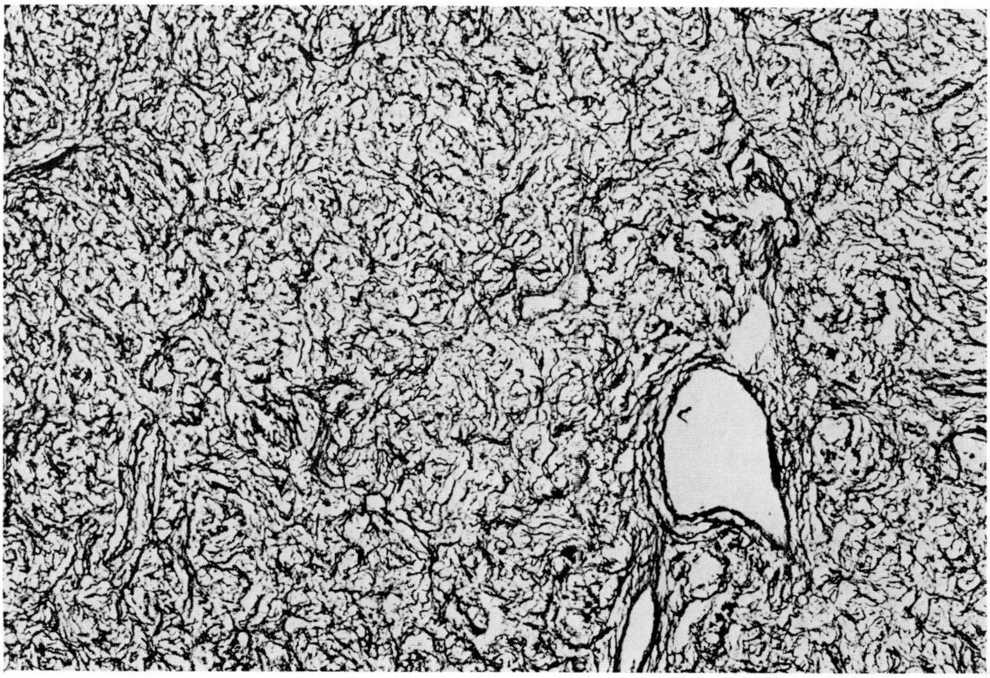

FIGURE 49. Hemangiopericytoma. Reticulin stain reveals dense reticulin meshwork surrounding vessels and tumor cells. (Gomori's stain; Magnification × 100.)

Friedmann[157] mentioned two cases of Kaposi's sarcoma. Moritsch et al.[158] reported a case with pharyngolaryngeal manifestation, in which treatment with Vinblastine sulfate gave satisfactory therapeutic results.

Lothe[159] reported that of the 19 patients with Kaposi's sarcoma who died and for whom autopsy was performed, the larynx and the pharynx were involved in 2 cases, while the tonsil, salivary glands, and trachea were affected in 1 case. Lippi et al.[160] reported a case of Kaposi's sarcoma with endolaryngeal localization. Bottazzi et al.[161] described a case of Kaposi's disease with pharyngolaryngeal secondary localization.

Shanmugaratnam and Sobin[162] believe that in the upper respiratory tract the lesion occurs most frequently in the larynx and only as part of a systemic disease.

Recently, Coyas et al.[163] reported an unusual and interesting example of primary Kaposi's sarcoma of the larynx occurring in a 72-year-old woman.

C. Age and Sex

The lesion affects mostly the male sex between ages 40 and 70.

D. Site

The epiglottis is the most common site of occurrence.

E. Etiology

It is obscure.

F. Histogenesis

The neoplasm seems to originate from vasoformative cells.

G. Pathology

Gross pathology — The neoplasm has a nodular or pedunculated aspect and is covered by an intact or an ulcerated mucosa. The lesions may be solitary or multiple.

Light microscopy — The tumor is composed of a simultaneous proliferation of spindle cells and irregular channels and spaces. Hemosiderin pigment is frequently found. Mitotic figures are visible. In the stroma, nonspecific infiltrate composed of lymphocytes, plasma cells, and histiocytic cells is usually present.

H. Diagnosis and Differential Diagnosis

The presence of multiple lesions occurring in skin, particularly of the lower extremities, as well as in the viscera, together with the histological aspect of the tumor, allow a correct diagnosis.

The differential diagnosis must be made from fibrosarcoma, vascular leiomyosarcoma, angiosarcoma, and pyogenic granuloma.

I. Behavior and Prognosis

The clinical course of Kaposi's sarcoma is variable, but very often patients may live for many years. The prognosis depends upon the clinical patterns of the disease (involvement of the lymph nodes and bone is a poor prognostic sign).

J. Associated Lesions

Kaposi's sarcoma has been found in association with leukemia, multiple myeloma, Hodgkin's disease, non-Hodgkin's lymphomas, mycosis fungoides, thymoma, lymphangioma, autoimmune hemolytic anemia, polymyositis, systemic lupus erythematosus, and hypogammaglobulinemia. Recently there has been an increased incidence of Kaposi's sarcoma in homosexual men.[164]

X. SYNOVIAL SARCOMA

A. Definition

Synovial sarcoma is a highly specialized and rare form of malignant tumor which usually arises in the soft tissues of the extremities.

B. Incidence

Synovial sarcoma of the head and neck is an uncommon neoplasm and only 62 cases have been reported.[165] The exact anatomical site of origin is often difficult to define. The majority of the cases of cervical synovial sarcomas reported in the literature seem to take origin from the paravertebral connective tissue spaces and manifest as solitary retropharyngeal or parapharyngeal masses at the bifurcation of the carotid artery.[141]

Applebaum and Mantravadi[166] reported a case of synovial sarcoma of the hypopharynx and collected only 21 previous reports of this tumor in this site.[167-181] Other cases have been reported.[47a,182-184a] The larynx is usually involved secondarily, but some cases of primary synovial sarcoma of the larynx have been reported.[165,172,184b,c]

C. Age and Sex

The male sex between age 20 and 40 is the most affected by the lesion.

D. Histogenesis

This tumor is thought to arise from undifferentiated mesenchyma that retains the potential for synovioblastic differentiation.

E. Pathology

Gross pathology — The tumor is covered by an intact mucosa and sometimes looks like an encapsulated tumor.

Light microscopy (Figure 50) — The neoplasm shows a distinctive biphasic pattern of pseudoglandular, tubular, and papillary structures, lined by a columnar or cuboidal epithelium. The lumina of these gland-like structures contain mucinous PAS-postive material. Areas of hyaline degeneration and calcification may be seen. At times, the neoplasm is mainly fibrosarcomatous in aspect because of the paucity or absence of the glandular component. There are abundant argyrophilic fibrils in the fibrosarcoma-like stroma.

F. Diagnosis and Differential Diagnosis

When the biphasic histologic pattern is present, diagnosis is not difficult. Ultrastructural investigation (Figures 51 and 52) is helpful to confirm the diagnosis.

The differential diagnosis must be made in particular from fibrosarcoma and angiosarcoma.

G. Behavior and Prognosis

Laryngeal and hypopharyngeal synovial sarcomas usually do not metastasize to cervical lymph nodes. Pulmonary metastases may occur.

XI. CHONDROSARCOMA

A. Incidence

New[185] first used the term "chondrosarcoma" of the larynx. This tumor is the most frequent laryngeal malignant mesenchymal neoplasm but it is very difficult to ascertain its frequency. In a recent review of the literature, Ferlito et al.[186] collected about 150 laryngeal chondrosarcomas and reported 3 personal observations.

B. Age and Sex

The neoplasm occurs most commonly in patients between the ages of 50 to 70. The male to female ratio is 3:1.[186a]

C. Site

Chondrosarcomas are most frequently located in the posterior lamina of the cricoid cartilage.[157,187-192] Only rarely are arytenoids,[193] epiglottis,[186,194,194a] and corniculate cartilages[195] affected. At times, the neoplasm involves both the cricoid and the thyroid cartilages. Chondrosarcoma may also involve the hyoid bone but this is not anatomically part of the larynx.[196]

D. Etiology

Irradiation appears to be a factor in the causation of some of these neoplasms.

E. Pathology

Gross pathology — The tumor presents as a submucosal rounded or oval mass covered by the intact laryngeal mucosa. The neoplasm may be uniformly hard or may have soft and even cystic areas of degeneration.[197]

Light microscopy — These tumors must be distinguished into low-grade (grade I)(Figures 53 to 55), medium-grade (grade II)(Figures 56 to 60), and high-grade chondrosarcoma (grade III).

The histological pattern of low-grade chondrosarcoma is similar to that of a benign chondroma. The neoplasm is composed of abundant basophilic and metachromatic cartilaginous matrixes in which the cells show small densely staining nuclei. Binucleated cells are seen and occasionally, multinucleated cells may be found. Nuclear irregularity and prominence of nucleoli are additional suggestive features of malignancy. Mitoses are usually absent. Calcification and bone formation are frequent.

Medium-grade chondrosarcoma shows an increased cellularity, particularly at the periphery of lobules. The nucleo-cytoplasmic ratio of the chondrocytes is low (cytoplasm is abundant relative to nuclear size). Plump binucleated cells may be frequent and multinucleated cells are also seen. Mitoses are sparse if present.

High-grade chondrosarcoma shows pronounced cellularity, and plump binucleated and multinucleated cells are often seen. The chondrocytes have large nuclei with nucleoli and delicate chromatin, and the nucleo-cytoplasmic ratio is relatively high. Mitoses are frequently seen. At times, spindle cell tissue with features resembling fibrosarcoma may be present.

Electron microscopy — Erlandson and Huvos[197a] reported the first electron microscopic studies of laryngeal chondrosarcoma. Another case was investigated by Ferlito et al.[186] The cells of the neoplasm show cytoplasmatic accumulation of glycogen, lipid droplets (Figure 61), and dilated cisternae of granular endoplasmic reticulum.

F. Diagnosis and Differential Diagnosis

Laryngograms and anteroposterior tomograms help in delineating the lesion, the diagnosis of which can only be done histologically. Radiologically, coarse macroscopic calcifications are pathognomonic and occur in 75% of patients.[198] Fish et al.[199] believe that CT scan is a valuable investigation to establish the origin and extension of the tumor and the presence of calcifications. By this study, even the smallest calcifications, unidentifiable by means of conventional radiology, may be detected.

Due to the firm consistency of the neoplastic tissues, biopsy may be difficult, and more than one biopsy or exploratory thyrotomy is often necessary to reach the diagnosis.[200]

The distinction between benign and malignant varieties of cartilaginous neoplasms of the larynx, though widely recognized, is often difficult. Furthermore, cases reported in the literature as benign chondromas, which actually were laryngeal chondrosarcomas, are not uncommon, and the correct diagnosis could not be established until recurrence or metastases developed. In this connection, Thomas[129] states that there is no evidence of transformation of chondroma into chondrosarcoma.

Photometric investigation of the DNA content of cells may provide an aid in the differential diagnosis between chondroma and highly differentiated chondrosarcoma.[201] The differential diagnosis of chondroblastic osteosarcoma may be assisted by the examination of alkaline phosphatase in smears or cryostat sections. All osteosarcomas (osteoblastic, chondroblastic, fibroblastic, or anaplastic) produce abundant alkaline phosphatase, whereas this enzyme is absent in high-grade chondrosarcoma.[202] Areas of calcification and non-neoplastic bone may be present in chondrosarcoma, but in contrast to osteosarcoma, bone formation by the tumor cells is not seen.

Differential diagnosis also includes fibrosarcoma, myxoid liposarcoma, spindle cell squamous carcinoma with cartilaginous metaplasia, chondrometaplasia,[202a] and tracheopathia osteoplastica.

G. Behavior and Prognosis

Recurrences are not uncommon and are most often seen in patients with high-grade chondrosarcoma. They are not catastrophic[188,203] because they are surgically treatable[204] and occur after reasonably long intervals (from 2 to 20 years).

Local and distant metastases are rare. Cervical lymph node metastases have been reported.[190,195,205-207] In the case by Sirota,[206] later reported also by Hyams and Rabuzzi,[187] metastases were found in cervical lymph nodes, lung, and renal artery at autopsy. In the other case of laryngeal chondrosarcoma with metastases reported by Hyams and Rabuzzi,[187] these were scattered as subcutaneous nodules in the thoracic and abdominal walls. Distant metastases were also reported by several investigators.[187,190,194a,195,201,208-211a]

In our material there are three cases of laryngeal chondrosarcoma, and one of these occurred in a 74-year-old male patient who developed bilateral lung metastases 1 year after total laryngectomy. Death occurred $2^1/_2$ years after surgery.[186]

Summing up, this tumor metastasizes preferably via the bloodstream, and lungs are the most frequently affected organs. At times, though lung metastases are present, cervical lymph nodes do not appear to be involved.[194a,201,210-211a]

Laryngeal chondrosarcomas are much less aggressive lesions than chondrosarcomas originating in extralaryngeal areas.[212] Prognosis is particularly connected with the degree of cellular differentiation of the tumor,[197a,213,215] Low-grade chondrosarcoma is locally invasive and does not metastasize; medium-grade chondrosarcoma is more aggressive but its metastatic risk is nevertheless still low, while high-grade chondrosarcoma recurs more easily and has a greater ability to metastasize, even though only rarely do metastases occur. Chondrosarcomas occasionally invade the thyroid gland.[207,211,216]

Considering the low aggressiveness of this tumor, even when it recurs, and the low ability to metastasize to cervical lymph nodes and to distant organs, the prognosis is better than that of osteosarcoma.

Careful follow-up is mandatory; 5 year survival is not valid for these patients, who have to be followed-up for the rest of their lives.

XII. OSTEOSARCOMA

A. Incidence

Osteosarcoma or osteogenic sarcoma is one of the rarest malignant mesenchymal neoplasms of the larynx. It was first described by Jackson and Jackson,[217] but the histopathology was not illustrated. Clerf[218] reported eight cases of sarcoma of the larynx, of which one was

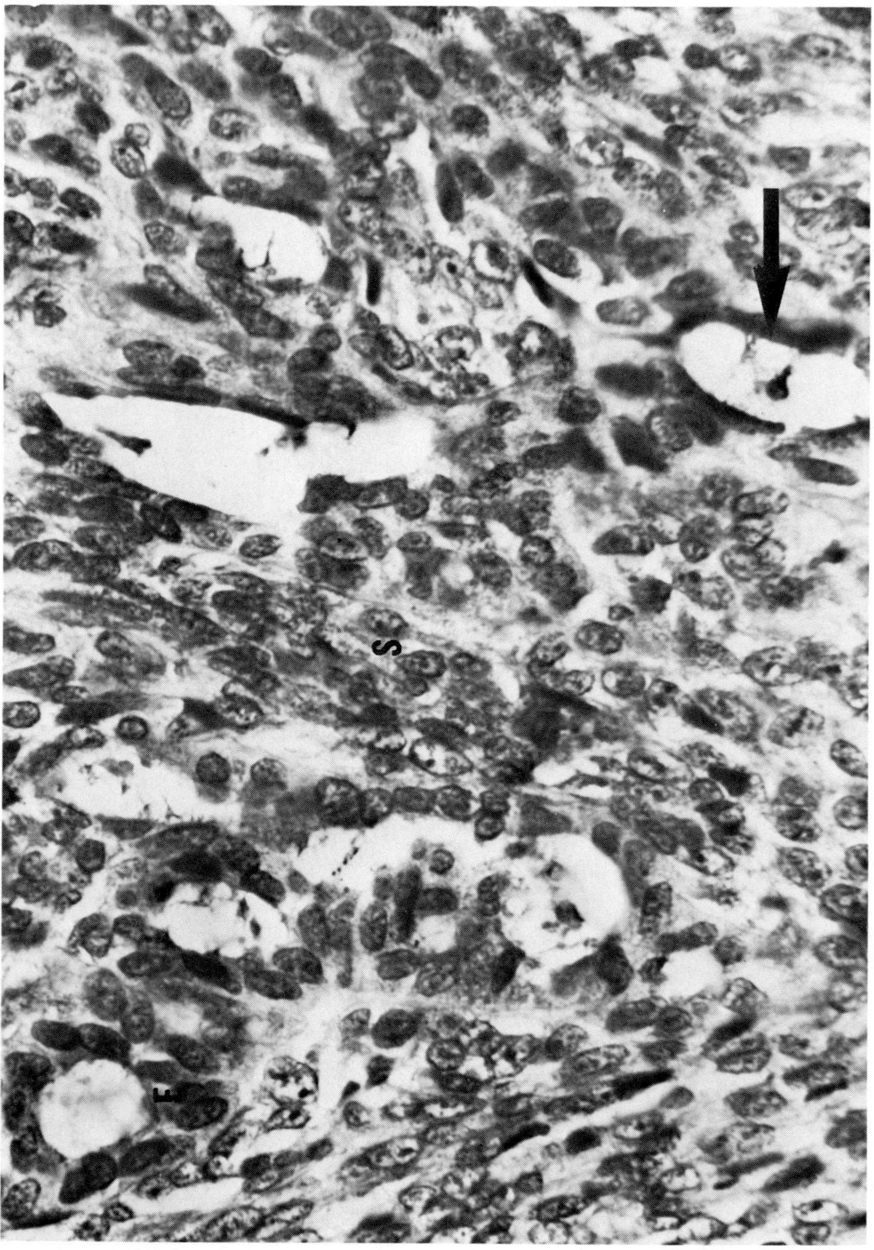

FIGURE 50. Synovial sarcoma. Note the biphasic pattern of the neoplasm with epithelioid cells (E), spindle cells (S), and pseudogland space lined by flattened cells (arrow). (H.E.; Magnification × 200.) (By courtesy of Dr. E. L. Applebaum.)

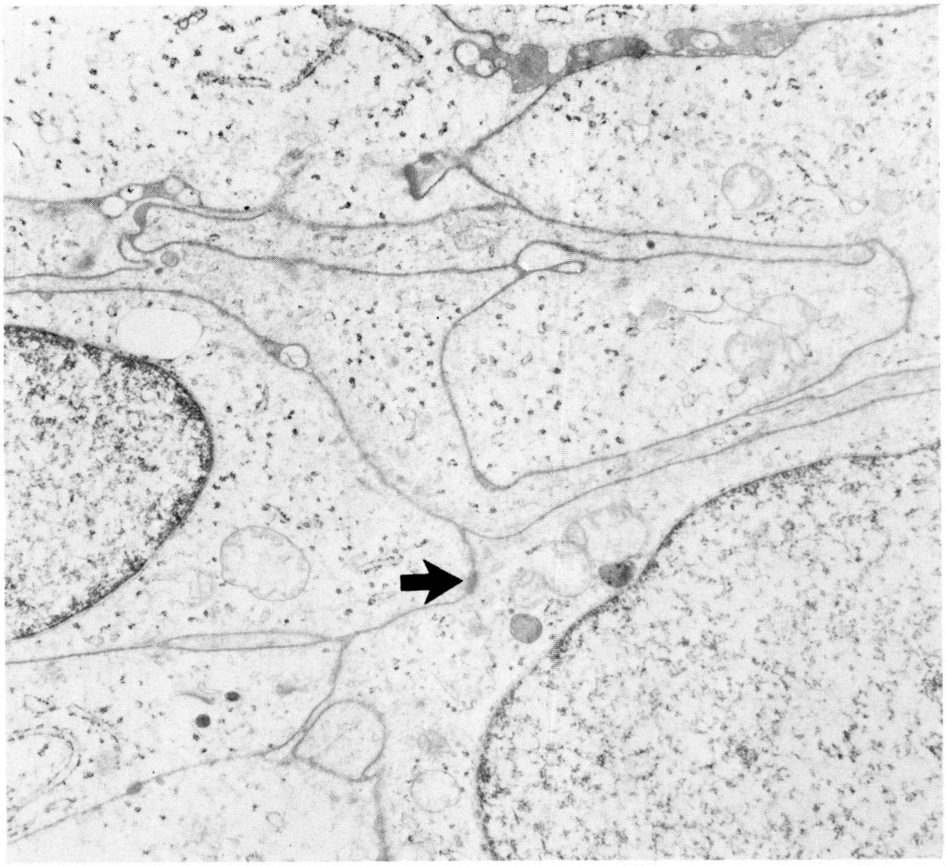

FIGURE 51. Synovial sarcoma. Electron micrograph showing desmosomes (arrows) joining epithelioid cells. (Magnification × 8000.) (By courtesy of Dr. E. L. Applebaum.)

histologically classified as fibroosteosarcoma, but might have been a primary osteosarcoma.

Sprinkle et al.[219] reported a case of osteosarcoma of the larynx diagnosed at first as fibrosarcoma. Other cases were reported in the literature.[220-223a] The case reported by Haar et al.[221] belongs to the chondroblastic variant.

B. Age and Sex

The tumor has a predilection for elderly people of the male sex.

C. Site

The most common locations are the vocal cords and cricoid cartilage.

D. Etiology

Even though trauma and radiation therapy have been implicated as causative agents, the etiology of extraskeletal osteosarcoma is unknown.

E. Histogenesis

The histogenesis of extraskeletal osteosarcoma is not yet established.

F. Pathology

Gross pathology — The neoplasm is mainly polypoid or exophytic in appearance. The

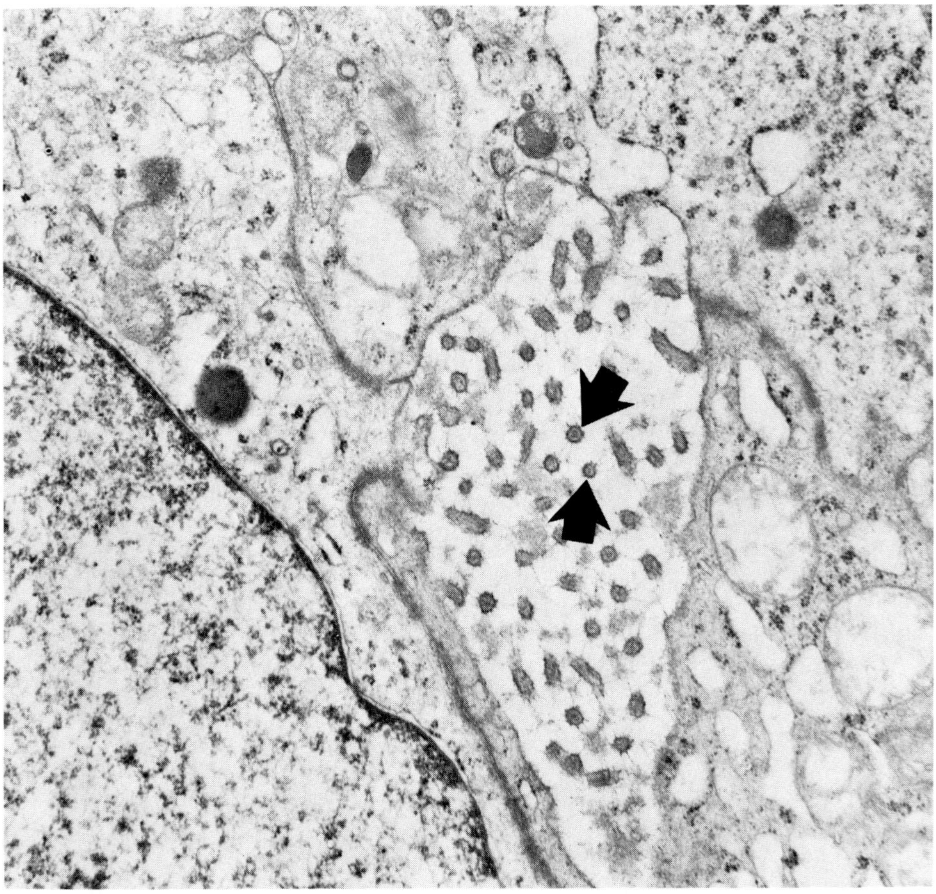

FIGURE 52. Synovial sarcoma. Electron micrograph showing microvilli (arrows) projecting into lumen of pseudogland. (Magnification × 11,000.) (By courtesy of Dr. E. L. Applebaum.)

consistency of the lesion depends on the degree of osteoblastic, fibroblastic, or chondroblastic proliferation.

Light microscopy — The neoplasm essentially consists of a malignant stroma and malignant neoplastic osteoid substance and bone. According to the predominant component — bony, stromal, or cartilaginous— the tumor may be divided into *osteoblastic*, *fibroblastic*, and *chondroblastic* variants. Usually, mitoses are numerous, and atypical and bizarre giant cells are present. Occasionally, the tumor displays islands of multinucleated giant cells. Areas characterized by the presence of homogenous eosinophilic refractile hyaline material (osteoid) may be seen.

Electron microscopy — Electron microscopic studies[222,223] show cells resembling osteoblasts with pleomorphic nuclei and nucleoli of variable size. The abundant cytoplasm contains rough endoplasmic reticulum. The cells are surrounded by a felt-work of interlacing collagen fibrils.

G. Diagnosis and Differential Diagnosis

Because of the variability of the histological appearance in different parts of a tumor, a large incisional biopsy is necessary to provide adequate material for diagnosis.

Differential diagnosis must be made in particular from chondrosarcoma, fibrosarcoma,

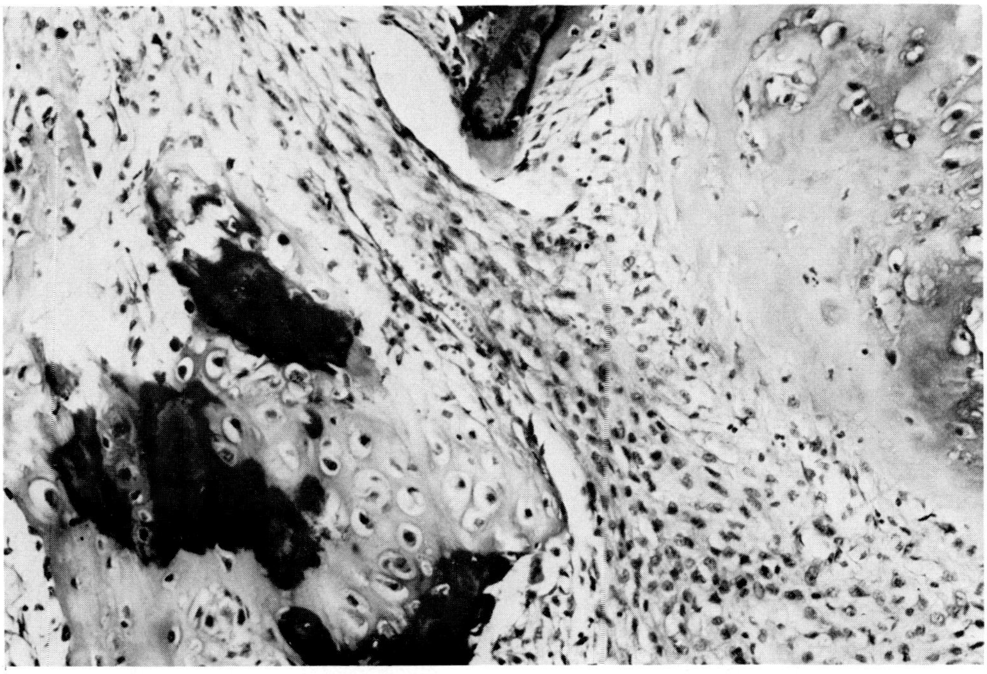

FIGURE 53. Chondrosarcoma (grade I). Ossification in cartilaginous island is present. (H.E.; Magnification × 40.)

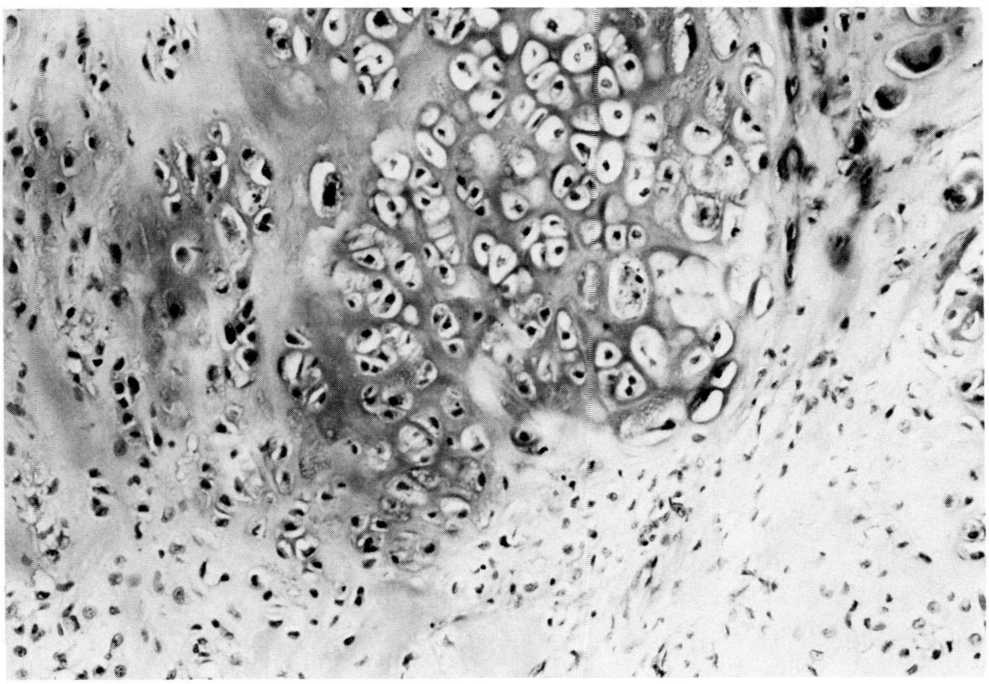

FIGURE 54. Chondrosarcoma (grade I). Lacunae contain plump irregular cells which are occasionally binucleated. (H.E.; Magnification × 40.)

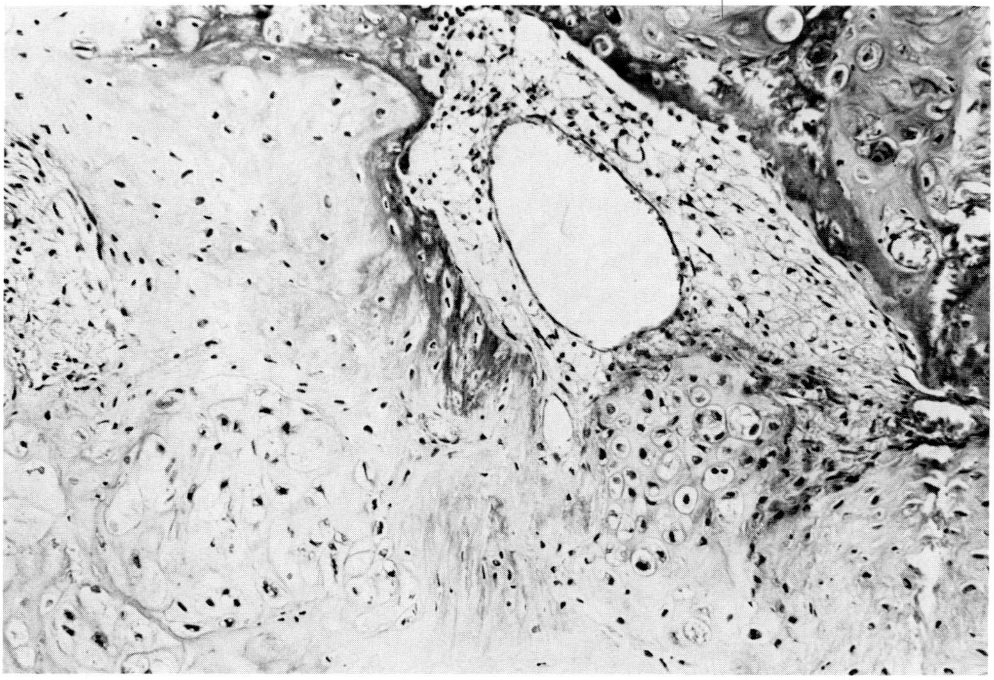

FIGURE 55. Chondrosarcoma (grade I). Note the lobulated character of the tumor. (H.E.; Magnification × 40.)

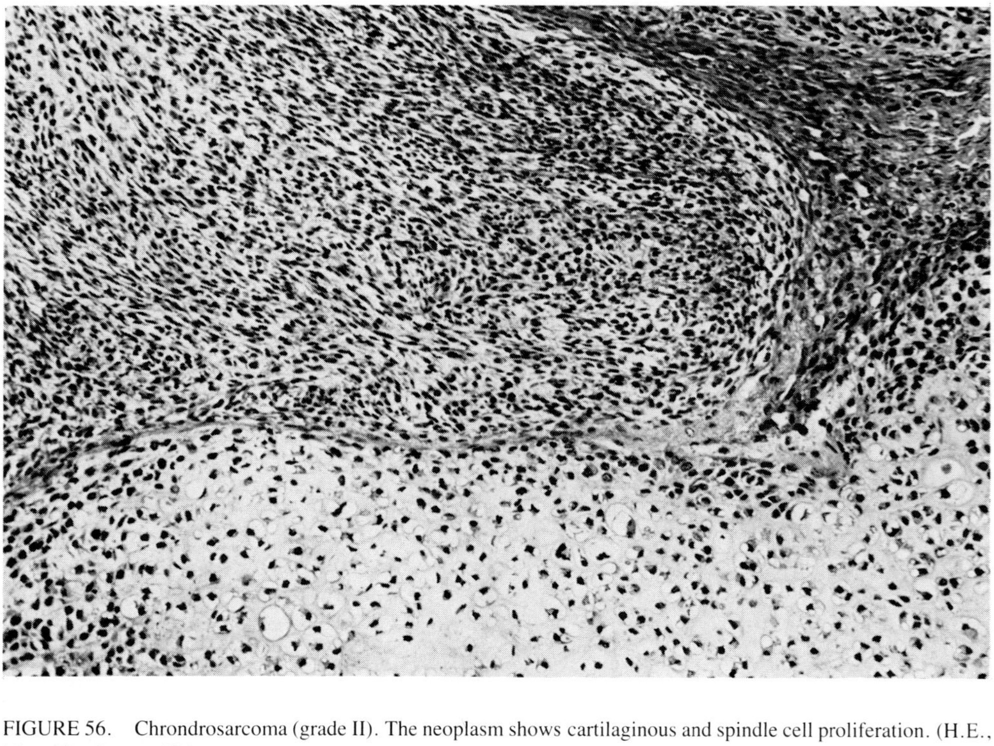

FIGURE 56. Chrondrosarcoma (grade II). The neoplasm shows cartilaginous and spindle cell proliferation. (H.E., Magnification × 40.)

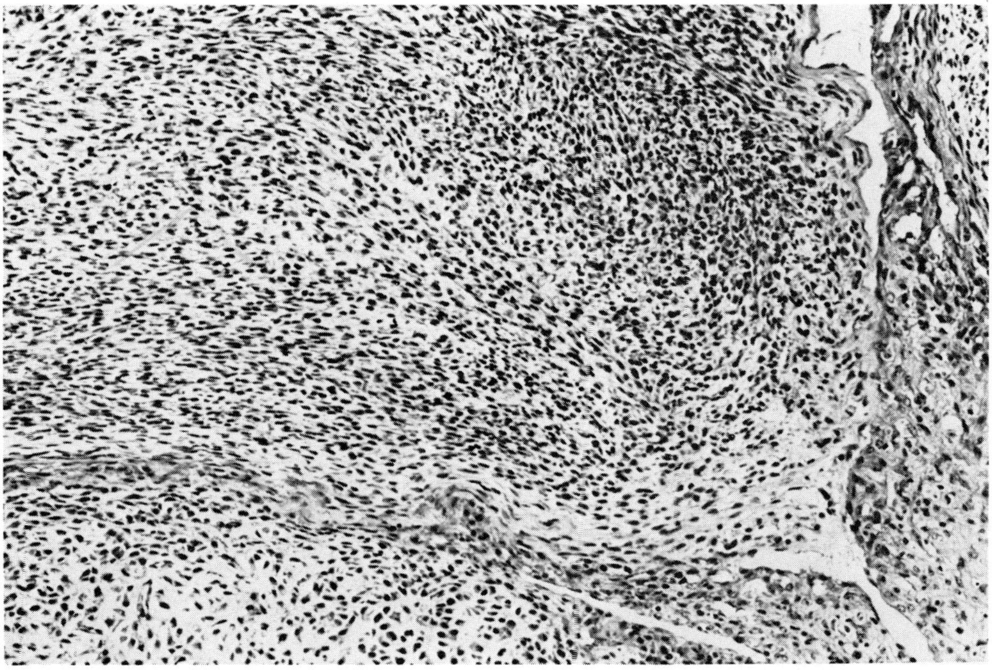

FIGURE 57. Chondrosarcoma (grade II). The neoplasm shows fibrosarcomatous pattern. (H.E.; Magnification × 40.)

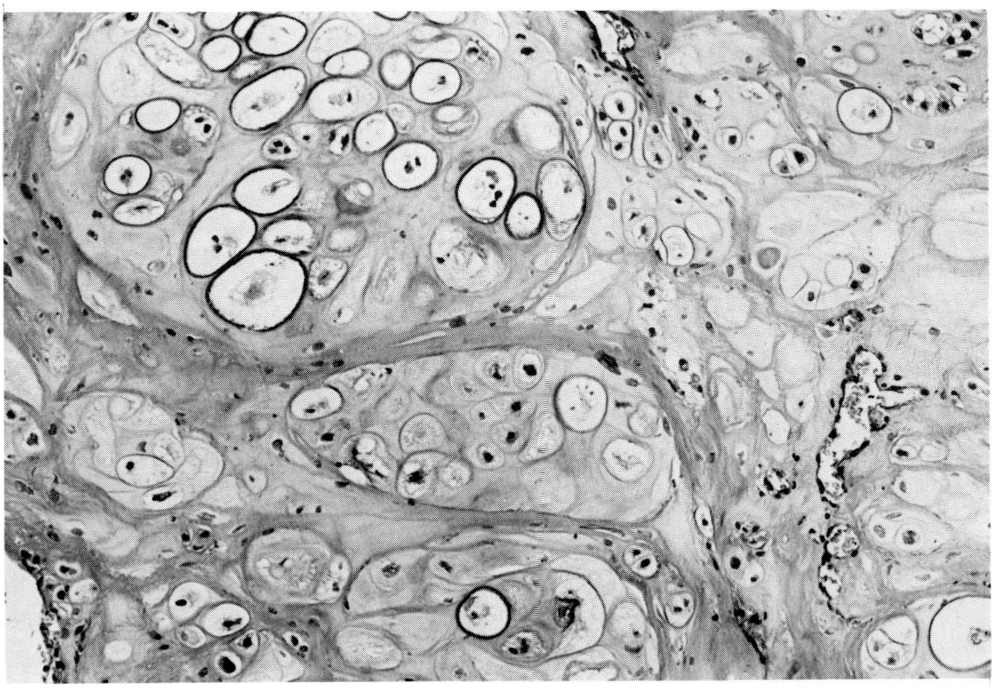

FIGURE 58. Chondrosarcoma (grade II). Another area of the same tumor showing lobulated cartilaginous tissues. (H.E.; Magnification × 40.)

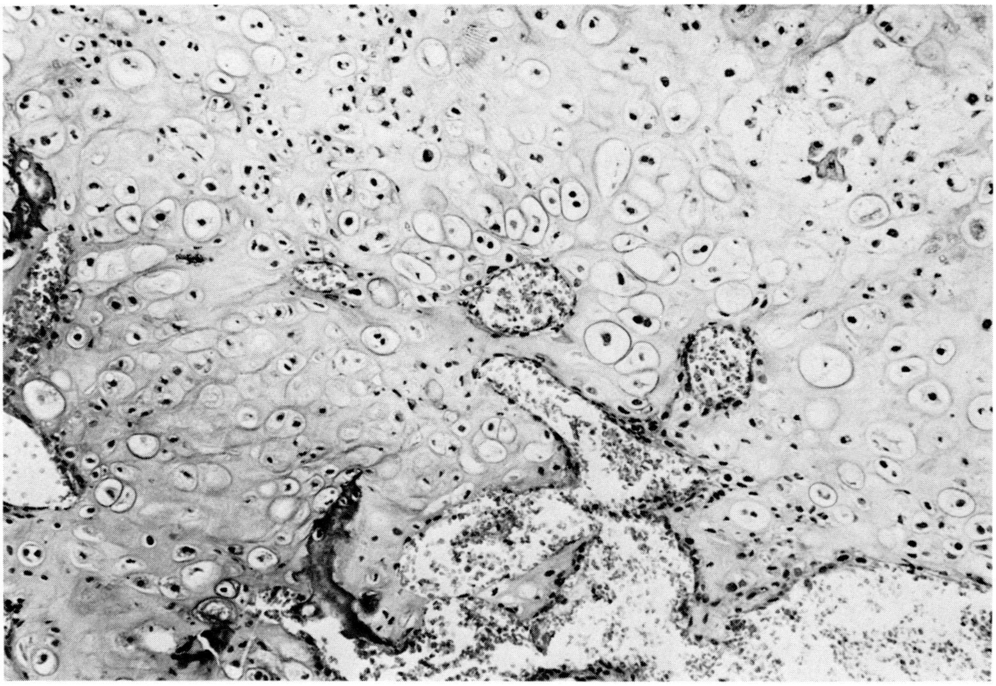

FIGURE 59. Chondrosarcoma (grade II). The neoplasm shows a vascular component. (H.E.; Magnification × 40.)

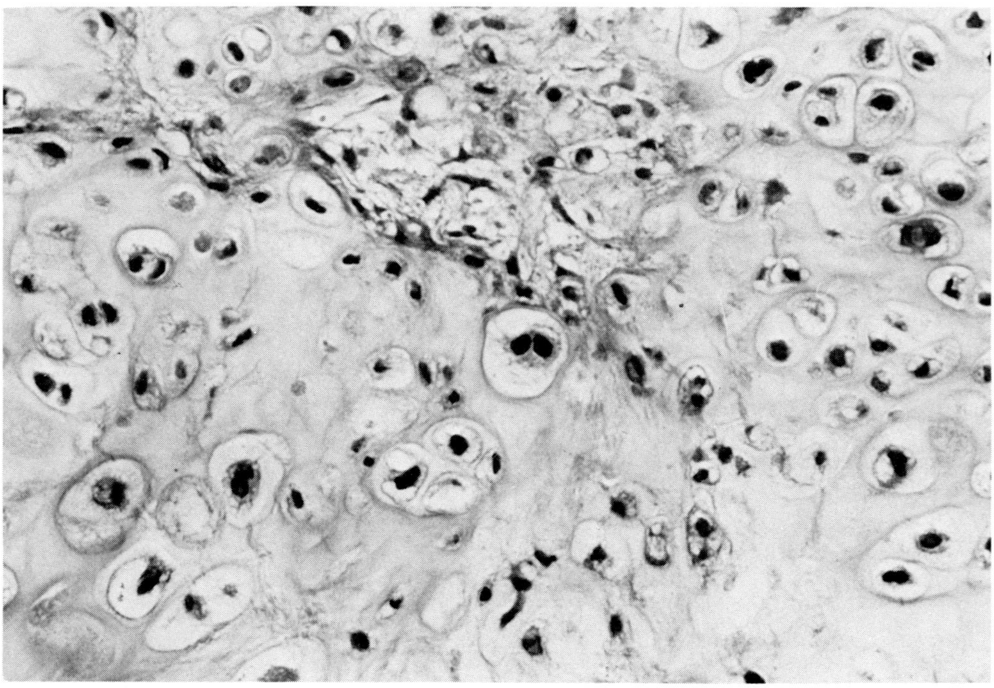

FIGURE 60. Chondrosarcoma (grade II). Enlarged hyperchromatic nuclei and several double-nucleated cells are present. (H.E.; Magnification × 100.)

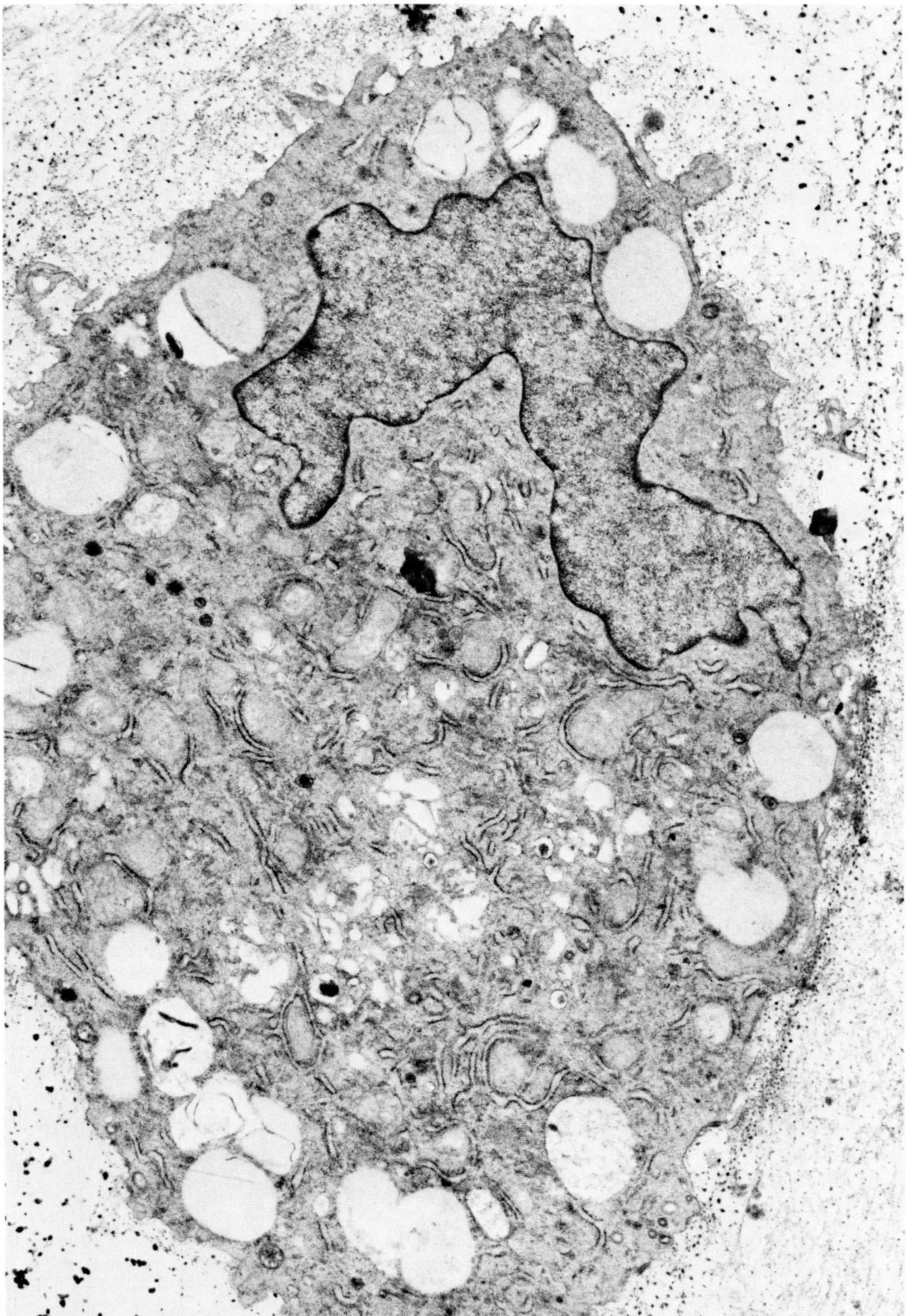

FIGURE 61. Chondrosarcoma (grade II). Cartilaginous cell showing a very irregular nucleus, numerous short RER profiles, and large lipid droplets. Pericellular matrix contains proteoglycan granules and fine filaments. (Magnification × 42,000.)

and spindle cell squamous carcinoma with osteoid differentiation. The presence of osteoid excludes undifferentiated fibrosarcoma,[222] while the presence of islands of carcinoma *in situ* or microinfiltrating carcinoma excludes osteosarcoma. The neoplasm should also be differentiated from myositis ossificans,[224,225] which may affect the larynx.

In the osteogenic sarcoma, clearly sarcomatous areas are present and the "zonal phenomenon" (characterized by a central cellular area, an intermediate zone of osteoid formation, and a peripheral shell of highly organized bone) is absent.[226] The phenomenon of formation of mature bone is most prominent in the periphery of the lesion, and is an important criterion for differentiating myositis ossificans from osteogenic sarcoma (in this latter lesion mature osteoids are located in the center of neoplasm, and neoplastic mesenchymal cells that are forming osteoids are in the periphery).

H. Behavior and Prognosis

Local recurrence is frequent.[220,222] The lung is the usual site of distant metastases.[218,221,222] Cervical lymph node metastases have also been reported.[3,220]

Even though the number of reports is too small to draw final conclusions, it may be said that prognosis for patients with laryngeal osteogenic sarcoma is unfavorable.

XIII. MALIGNANT SCHWANNOMA

A. Terminology

The nomenclature for malignant tumors of nerve sheaths origin is not uniform and various terms have been used. These include malignant neurinoma, neurofibrosarcoma, neurosarcoma, neurogenic sarcoma, neurogenous sarcoma, malignant neurogenous neoplasm, malignant neurofibroma, malignant spindle cell tumor of Schwann cell origin, malignant Triton tumor, and sarcomatous neurofibroma, but the term "malignant schwannoma" is the most common.

B. Incidence

The majority of the neurogenic neoplasms of the larynx are solitary schwannomas,[227,228] and the finding of malignant schwannoma in this organ is extremely rare.

The first well-documented malignant schwannoma of the larynx was reported by Norris and Peale[229] and occurred in a 59-year-old male patient. Iwaszkiewicz and Kamieniec[230] described a case of sarcomatous neurofibroma of the larynx. Gorenstein et al.[3] reported on 17 patients with laryngeal sarcoma treated at the Mayo Clinic from 1949 to 1974, of which 1 was neurofibrosarcoma; the case lacks histological documentation.

DeLozier[231] published a case of intrinsic laryngeal malignant schwannoma occurring in a 46-year-old male patient. The histological diagnosis was also confirmed by Batsakis.

Cummings et al.[232] mentioned the malignant transformation of only one case of neurofibroma and schwannoma (or neurilemmoma) that had been described in the larynx by Pearlman et al.[233] and Stricker,[234] but the photomicrographs are not convincing.

C. Histogenesis

The neoplasm originates from the Schwann cell, which is ultimately of neuroectodermal derivation, and as such, it may differentiate in both ectodermal and mesodermal directions. In the larynx, in the case reported by DeLozier,[231] the tumor most likely derived from the peripheral branch of the superior laryngeal nerve.

D. Pathology

Gross pathology — The neoplasm may be pedunculated or infiltrating.

Light microscopy (Figures 62 to 68) — The tumor consists of spindle-shaped or ovoid cells with nuclei arranged from oval and blunted with finely stippled chromatin. The cells of this neoplasm can produce reticulin and collagen. A myxoid pattern is often found. A suggestion of palisading or organoid areas is a specific feature of this lesion. Mitoses are numerous. Cartilaginous, osteoid, osseous, lipomatous, and rhabdomyomatous tissue, as well as epithelial areas with gland formations and melanin granules have not so far been observed in the laryngeal malignant schwannomas, in spite of the fact that this neoplasm may have a wide spectrum of histologic appearances.

Electron microscopy — Even though DeLozier[231] says that in his case electron microscopy was of no help in establishing the diagnosis, so far, accurate investigations of the ultrastructure of the laryngeal malignant schwannoma have not been reported.

E. Diagnosis and Differential Diagnosis

The diagnosis can be problematic, in particular when the tumor shows evidence of differentiation towards liposarcoma, chondrosarcoma, osteogenic sarcoma, and rhabdomyosarcoma. The presence of nuclear palisading or organoid foci is a typical feature of this neoplasm. Special stains are helpful. Electron microscopy can support the diagnosis.[235]

Benign schwannoma, fibrosarcoma, leiomyosarcoma, monophasic synovial sarcoma, embryonal rhabdomyosarcoma, and spindle cell squamous carcinoma should all be considered in differential diagnosis.

F. Behavior and Prognosis

The limited number of reports does not allow one to draw conclusions on the biological behavior of the neoplasm, but the prognosis seems to be poor.[3,229,231]

XIV. MALIGNANT GRANULAR CELL TUMOR

A. Introduction

Malignant variants of granular cell tumor do rarely occur.[236,237] Robertson et al.[238] collected 25 cases of malignant granular cell tumor (in 20 of which there was evidence of metastatic spread) from various sites and reported one personal case.

B. Terminology

The controversial terminology includes malignant granular cell myoblastoma, malignant myoblastoma, and malignant non-organoid granular cell myoblastoma, but "malignant granular cell tumor" seems to be gaining wider acceptance.

C. Definition

It is the malignant counterpart of the granular cell tumor.[238a]

D. Incidence

This neoplasm is exceptional in the larynx and was first described by Glasunow[239] and Carnevale Ricci.[240] Later, Busanny-Caspari and Hammar[241] reported a case of malignant granular cell tumor in the larynx occurring in a 40-year-old man, in which the neoplasm had metastasized to the cervical lymph nodes. The patient died 2 years after diagnosis. Faleg[242] reported 2 cases of granular cell tumor of the larynx, one benign and the other malignant, the latter occurring in a 39-year-old man and being located in the right vocal cord.

E. Site

The neoplasm develops primarily in the middle or posterior third of the vocal cords.

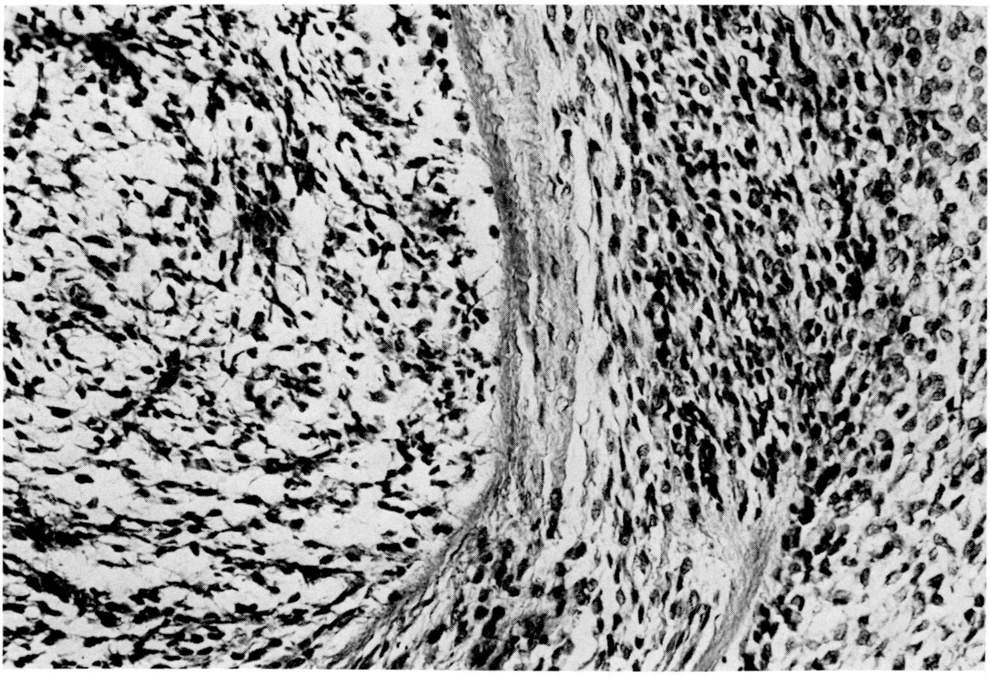

FIGURE 62. Malignant schwannoma. Note the abundant cellularity and the myxoid stroma. (H.E.; Magnification × 40.) (Specimen given by Dr. T. D. Trainer.)

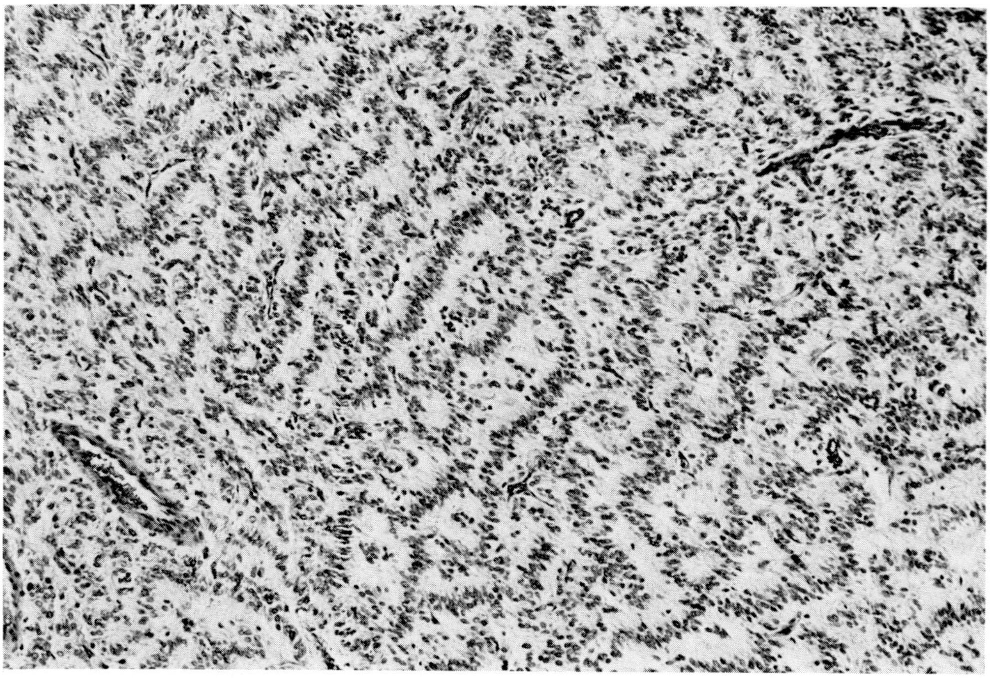

FIGURE 63. Malignant schwannoma. Another area of the neoplasm with well-developed nuclear ''palisading''. (H.E.; Magnification × 16.) (Specimen given by Dr. T. D. Trainer.)

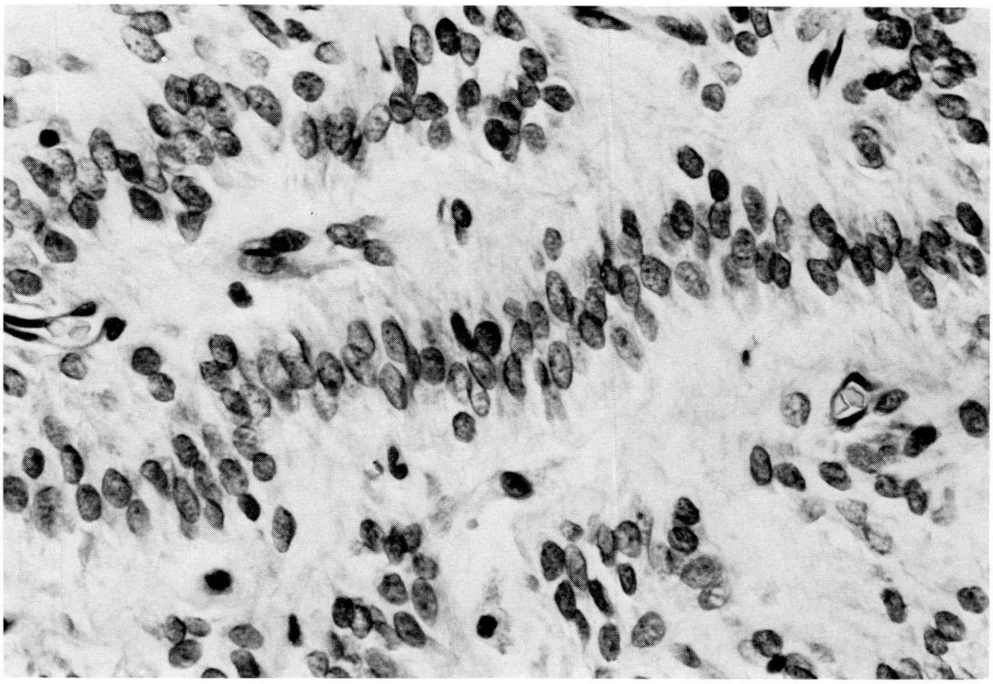

FIGURE 64. Malignant schwannoma. Higher power view shows better the marked palisading of the nuclei. (H.E.; Magnification × 100.) (Specimen given by Dr. T. D. Trainer.)

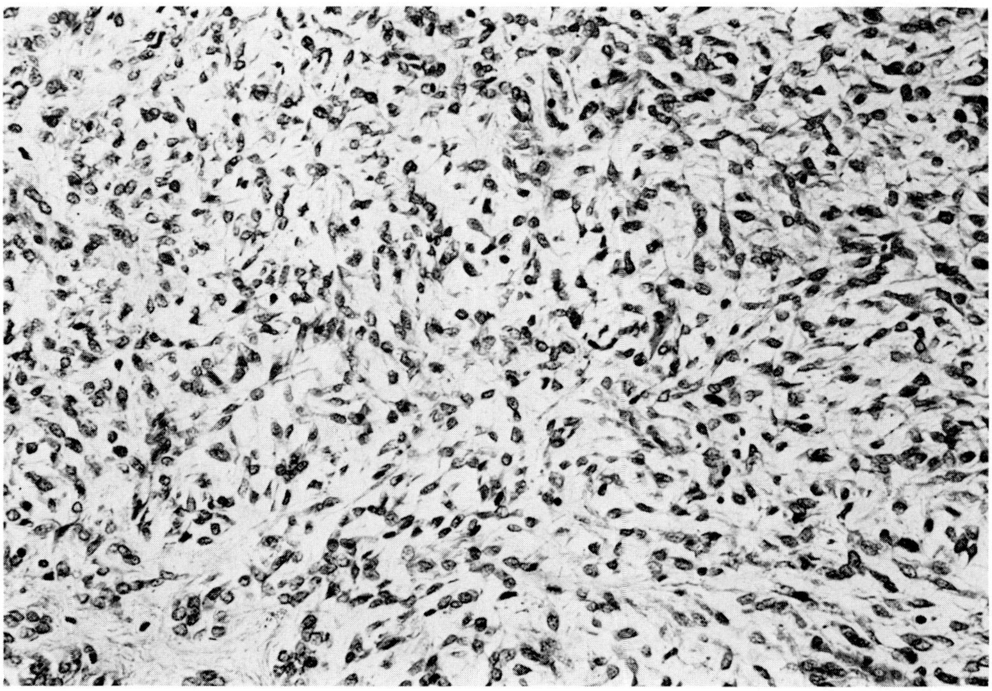

FIGURE 65. Malignant schwannoma. Myxoid change is seen in neoplasm. (H.E.; Magnification × 40.) (Specimen given by Dr. T. D. Trainer.)

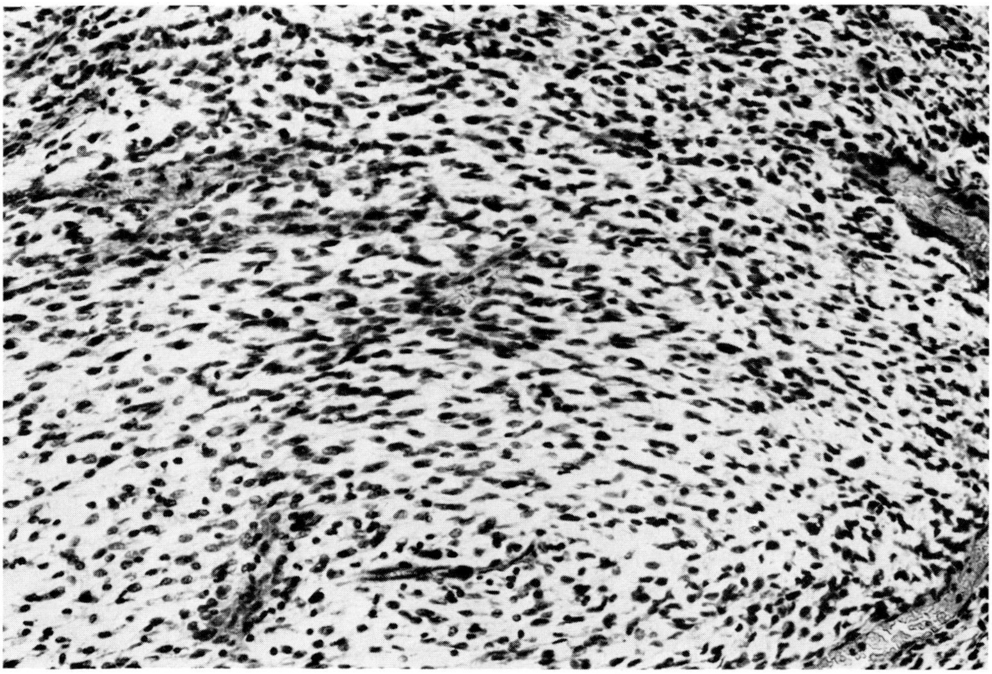

FIGURE 66. Malignant schwannoma. A densely cellular area composed of spindle cells. (H.E.; Magnification × 40.) (Specimen given by Dr. T. D. Trainer.)

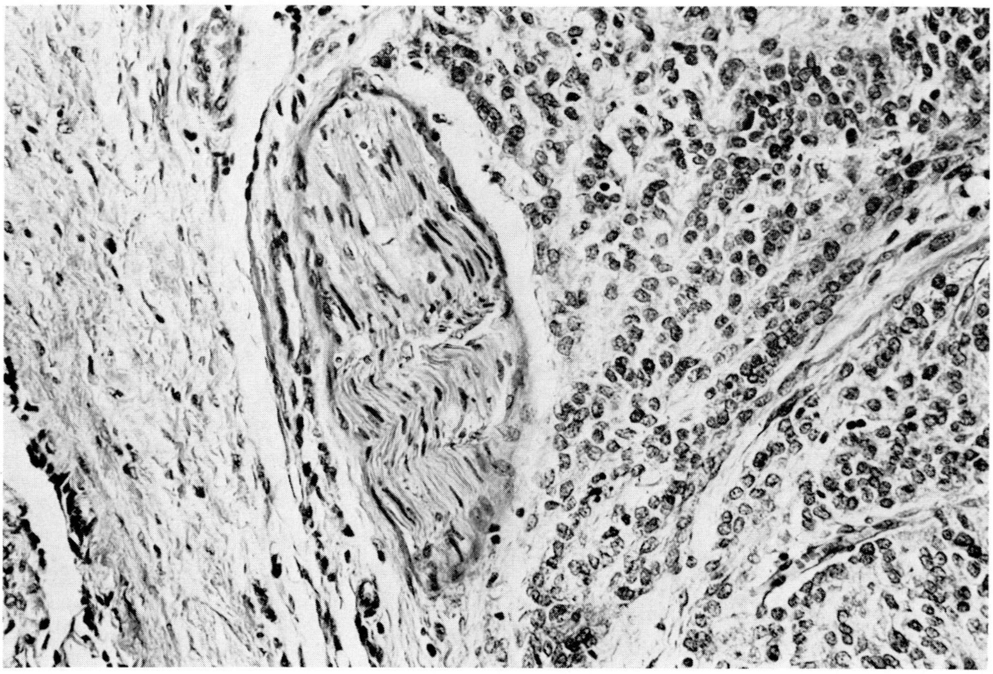

FIGURE 67. Malignant schwannoma. Dense aggregates of round cells invade a nerve trunk. (H.E.; Magnification × 40.) (Specimen given by Dr. T. D. Trainer.)

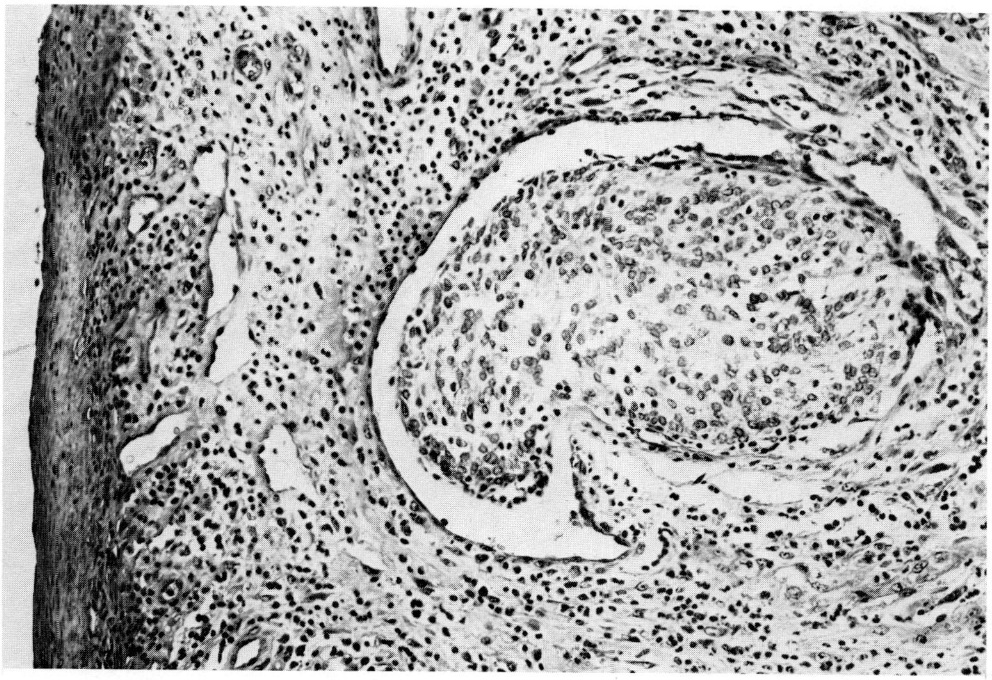

FIGURE 68. Malignant schwannoma. Note the lymphatic infiltration. (H.E.; Magnification × 40.) (Specimen given by Dr. T. D. Trainer.)

F. Histogenesis

The histogenesis of this tumor has remained the subject of great controversy, but probably the lesion is of neurogenic origin, based on ultrastructural[243,244] and immunohistochemical findings.[245,246]

G. Pathology

Gross pathology — Macroscopically, the neoplasm may present as a nodular or polypoid structure.

Light microscopy — The neoplasm is composed of nests of large, round, or polygonal cells with voluminous cytoplasm filled with acidophilic granules, which are diastase resistant and PAS positive. The nuclei are irregular, relatively large, and have prominent nucleoli. Cellular pleomorphism is present. Necrosis may be found.

Electron microscopy — Ultrastructural studies show many cytoplasmic granules which are identified as membrane-bound, round lysosome-like structures.[237,238,243,244,247,248]

Immunohistochemical studies — Recent studies have shown that granular cell tumors stain strongly for CEA (carcinoembryonic antigen) using the immunoperoxidase technique.[238,249]

H. Diagnosis and Differential Diagnosis

The diagnosis may be difficult. The nature of the malignant granular cell tumor may be confirmed by electron microscopy on the basis of the numerous, characteristic, intracytoplasmic, membrane-bound lysosomes. The presence of carcinoembryonic antigen in the cells of this tumor may help in making the diagnosis.[238]

The tumor must be differentiated from rhabdomyoma, paraganglioma, alveolar rhabdomyosarcoma, granular variant of leiomyosarcoma, alveolar soft part sarcoma, melanoma, and squamous cell carcinoma.

I. Behavior and Prognosis

The small number of cases reported does not allow final considerations. However, in the case described by Carnevale-Ricci,[240] the tumor recurred four times and also in that by Caspari and Hammar,[241] the patient died.

REFERENCES

1. **Batsakis, J. G. and Fox, J. E.,** Supporting tissue neoplasms of the larynx, *Surg.Gynecol.Obstet.*, 131, 989, 1970.
2. **Krajina, Z.,** Laryngeal sarcoma, *Can.J.Otolaryngol.*, 4, 303, 1975.
3. **Gorenstein, A., Neel, H. B., III, Weiland, L. H., and Devine, K. D.,** Sarcomas of the larynx, *Arch.Otolaryngol.*, 106, 8, 1980.
4. **Enterline, H. T.,** Histopathology of sarcomas, *Semin.Oncol.*, 8, 133, 1981.
5. **Davies, D. G.,** Fibrosarcoma and pseudosarcoma of the larynx, *J.Laryngol.Otol.*, 83, 423, 1969.
6. **Flanagan, P., Cross, R. M., and Libcke, J. H.,** Fibrosarcoma of the larynx, *J.Laryngol.Otol.*, 79, 1049, 1965.

6a. **Rosenberg, H. S., Vogler, C., Close, L. G., and Warshaw, H. E.,** Laryngeal fibromatosis in the neonate, *Arch.Otolaryngol.*, 107, 513, 1981.

7. **Shin, W. Y. and Abramson, A. L.** The value of electron microscopy in the diagnosis of fibrosarcoma of the larynx, *Trans.Am. Acad.Ophthalmol.Otolaryngol.*, 82, 582, 1976.
8. **Donaldson, I.,** Fibrosarcoma in a previously irradiated larynx, *J.Laryngol.Otol.*, 92, 425, 1978.
9. **Tobey, D. N., Wheelis, R. F., and Yarington, C. T., Jr.,** Electron microscopy in the diagnosis of liposarcoma and fibrosarcoma of the larynx, *Ann.Otol.Rhinol.Laryngol.*, 88, 867, 1979.
10. **Ghadially, F. N.,** *Diagnostic Electron Microscopy of Tumours*, Butterworths, London, 1980.
11. **Johnston, K. C.,** Fibrosarcoma of the larynx, *Laryngoscope*, 67, 1194, 1957.
12. **Prasad, J. N.,** Fibrosarcoma of the larynx, *J.Laryngol.Otol.*, 86, 267, 1972.
13. **Guerrier, Y. and Perdigou, J. B.,** Tumeurs mesenchimateuses du larynx, *Cah.Otorhinolaryngol.*, 15, 569, 1980.
14. **Ferlito, A., Nicolai, P., and Barion, U.,** Critical comments on laryngeal fibrosarcoma, *Acta Otorhino-laryngol.Belg.*, 37, 918, 1983.
15. **Cady, B., Rippey, J. H., and Frazell, E. L.,** Non-epidermoid cancer of the larynx, *Ann. Surg.*, 167, 116, 1968.
16. **Shaw, H.,** Tumours of the larynx, in *Scott-Brown's Diseases of the Ear, Nose and Throat*, Ballantyne, J. and Groves, J. Eds., 4th ed., Butterworths, London, 1979.
17. **Batsakis, J. G., Rice, D. H., and Howard, D. R.,** The pathology of head and neck tumors: spindle cell lesions (sarcomatoid carcinomas, nodular fasciitis, and fibrosarcoma) of the aerodigestive tracts, part 14, *Head Neck Surg.*, 4, 499, 1982.
18. **Crocker, D. J. and Murad, T. M.,** Ultrastructure of fibrosarcoma in a male breast, *Cancer*, 23, 891, 1969.
19. **Churg, A. M., and Kahn, L. B.,** Myofibroblasts and related cells in malignant fibrous and fibrohistiocytic tumors, *Hum.Pathol.*, 8, 205, 1977.
20. **Vasudev, K. S. and Harris, M.,** A sarcoma of myofibroblasts. An ultrastructural study, *Arch.Pathol. Lab.Med.*, 102, 185, 1978.
21. **Guber, S. and Rudolph, R.,** The myofibroblast, *Surg.Gynecol.Obstet.*, 146, 641, 1978.
22. **Harris, M.,** Differential diagnosis of spindle cell tumours by electron microscopy — personal experience and a review, *Histopathology*, 5, 81, 1981.
23. **Fu, Y. S., and Perzin, K. H.,** Nonepithelial tumors of the nasal cavity, paranasal sinuses, and nasopharynx. A clinicopathologic study. VI. Fibrous tissue tumors (fibroma, fibromatosis, fibrosarcoma), *Cancer*, 37, 2912, 1976.
24. **Pritchard, D. J., Soule, E. H., Taylor, W. F., and Ivins, J. C.,** Fibrosarcoma — a clinicopathologic and statistical study of 199 tumors of the soft tissues of the extremities and trunk, *Cancer*, 33, 888, 1974.
25. **Ozzello, L., Stout, A. P., and Murray, M. R.,** Cultural characteristics of malignant histiocytomas and fibrous xanthomas, *Cancer*, 16, 331, 1963.
26. **O'Brien, J. E., and Stout, A. P.,** Malignant fibrous xanthomas, *Cancer*, 17, 1445, 1964.
27. **Stout, A. P. and Lattes, R.,** Tumors of the Soft Tissues, Fascicle 1, Second Series, Atlas of Tumor Pathology, Armed Forces Institute of Pathology, Washington D.C., 1967.

28. **Kempson, R. L., and Kyriakos, M.,** Fibroxanthosarcoma of the soft tissues. A type of malignant fibrous histiocytoma, *Cancer,* 29, 961, 1972.
29. **Weiss, S. W. and Enzinger, F. M.,** Malignant fibrous histiocytoma: an analysis of 200 cases, *Cancer,* 41, 2250, 1978.
30. **Kearney, M. M., Soule, E. H., and Ivins, J. C.,** Malignant fibrous histiocytoma. A retrospective study of 167 cases, *Cancer,* 45, 167, 1980.
31. **Blitzer, A., Lawson, W., Zak, F. G., Biller, H. F., and Som, M. L.,** Clinical-pathological determinants in prognosis of fibrous histiocytomas of head and neck, *Laryngoscope,* 91, 2053, 1981.
32. **Rolander, T., Kim, O. J., and Shumrick, D. A.,** Fibrous xanthoma of the larynx, *Arch.Otolaryngol.,* 96, 168, 1972.
33. **Ferlito, A.,** Histiocytic tumors of the larynx. A clinicopathological study with review of the literature, *Cancer,* 42, 611, 1978.
34. **Canalis, R. F., Green, M., Konard, H. R., Hirose, F. M., and Cooper, S.,** Malignant fibrous xanthoma (xanthofibrosarcoma) of the larynx, *Arch.Otolaryngol.,* 101, 135, 1975.
35. **Ferlito, A.,** Simultaneous malignant pleomorphic fibrous histiocytoma and squamous cell carcinoma "in situ" of the larynx, *Acta Otorhinolaryngol.Belg.,* 30, 390, 1976.
36. **Johnson, J. T. and Poushter, D. L.,** Fibrous histiocytoma of the subglottic larynx, *Ann.Otol.Rhinol.Laryngol.,* 86, 243, 1977.
37. **Ferlito, A., Recher, G., Polidoro, F., and Rossi,M.,** Malignant pleomorphic fibrous histiocytoma of the larynx. Further observations, *J.Laryngol.Otol.,* 93, 1021, 1979.
38. **Keenan, J. P., Snyder, G. G., and Toomey, J. M.,** Malignant fibrous histiocytoma of the larynx, *Otolaryngol.Head Neck Surg.,* 87, 599, 1979.
39. **Ogura, J. H., Toomey, J. M., Setzen, M., and Sobol, S.,** Malignant fibrous histiocytoma of the head and neck, *Laryngoscope,* 90, 1429, 1980.
40. **Neblett, L. M. and Coller, F. C.,** Malignant fibrous histiocytoma of the larynx, *Am.J.Otolaryngol.,* 2, 163, 1981.
41. **Ferlito, A., Nicolai, P., Recher, G., and Narne, S.,** Primary laryngeal malignant fibrous histiocytoma. Review of the literature and report of seven cases, *Laryngoscope,* 93, 1351, 1983.
42. **Hall-Jones, J.,** Giant cell tumour of the larynx, *J.Laryngol.Otol.,* 86, 371, 1972.
43. **Ribari, O., Elemer, G., and Balint, A.,** Laryngeal giant cell tumour, *J.Laryngol.Otol.,* 89, 857, 1975.
44. **Goyas, A., Anastassiades, O. T., and Kyriakos, I.,** Malignant giant cell tumour of the larynx, *J.Laryngol.Otol.,* 88, 799, 1974.
45. **Alguacil-Garcia, A., Unni, K. K., and Goellner, J. R.,** Malignant giant cell tumor of soft parts. An ultrastructural study of four cases, *Cancer,* 40, 244, 1977.
46. **Lattes, R.,** Malignant fibrous histiocytoma. A review article, *Am.J.Surg.Pathol.,* 6, 761, 1982.
47. **Weiss, S. W.,** Malignant fibrous histiocytoma. A reaffirmation, *Am.J.Surg.Pathol,* 6, 773, 1982.
47a. **Kleinsasser, O.,** Pathologie and Klinik besonderer Formen maligner Tumoren des Kehlkopfes und des Hypopharynx, Hals-Nasen-Ohren-Heilkunde in *Praxis und Klinik,* Berendes, J., Link, R., and Zöllner, F., Eds., 2nd ed., Vol. IV/2, Verlag, Stuttgart, 1983.
47b. **Rivas, S., Peris, J. L., Mayayo, E., and Tortosa, V.,** Histiocitoma fibroso maligno de laringe, *Acta Otorrinolaringol., Esp.,* 33, 637, 1982.
47c. **Ramadass, T., Balasubramaniam, V. C., and Annamalai, L.,** Malignant pleomorphic fibrous histiocytoma of the larynx. A case report with review of literature, *J.Laryngol.Otol.,* 98, 93, 1984.
47d. **Löbe, L. P. and Katenkamp, D.,** Malignes fibröses Histiozytom des Larynx, *Laryngol.Rhinol.Otol.,* 63, 257, 1984.
48. **Kauffman, S. L. and Stout, A. P.,** Histiocytic tumors (fibrous xanthoma and histiocytoma) in children, *Cancer,* 14, 469, 1961.
49. **Merkow, L. P., Frich, J. C., Sliekin, M., Kyreages, C. G., and Pardo, M.,** Ultrastructure of a fibroxanthosarcoma (malignant fibroxanthoma), *Cancer,* 28, 372, 1971.
50. **Fu, Y. S., Gabbiani, G., Kaye, G. I., and Lattes, R.,** Malignant soft tissue tumors of probably histiocytic origin (malignant fibrous histiocytomas): general considerations and electron microscopic and tissue culture studies, *Cancer,* 35, 176, 1975.
51. **Enzinger, F. M.,** Recent developments in the classification of soft tissue sarcomas, in *Management of Primary Bone and Soft Tissue Sarcomas,* Year Book, Chicago, 1977.
52. **Alguacil-Garcia, A., Unni, K. K., and Goellner, J. R.,** Malignant fibrous histiocytoma: an ultrastructural analysis of six cases, *Am.J.Clin.Pathol.,* 69, 121, 1978.
53. **Guccion, J. G. and Enzinger, F. M.,** Malignant giant cell tumor of soft parts. An analysis of 32 cases, *Cancer,* 29, 1518, 1972.
54. **Enzinger, F. M.,** Angiomatoid malignant fibrous histiocytoma: a distinct fibrohistiocytic tumor of children and young adults simulating a vascular neoplasm, *Cancer,* 44 2147, 1979.

55. **Weiss, S. W. and Enzinger, F. M.,** Myxoid variant of malignant fibrous histiocytoma, *Cancer,* 39, 1672, 1977.
56. **Kyriakos, M. and Kempson, R. L.,** Inflammatory fibrous histiocytoma: an aggressive and lethal lesion, *Cancer,* 37, 1584, 1976.
57. **von Urfer, F.,** Myxolipom des Kehlkopfes, *Pract.Otorhinolaryngol.,* 8, 545, 1946.
58. **Kapur, T. R.,** Recurrent lipomata of the larynx and the pharynx with late malignant change, *J.Laryngol.Otol.,* 82, 761, 1968.
59. **Miller, D., Goodman, M., Weber, A., and Goldstein, A.,** Primary liposarcoma of the larynx, *Trans.Am.Acad.Ophthalmol.Otolaryngol.,* 80, 444, 1975.
60. **Velek, J. P.,** Liposarcoma of the larynx, *Trans.Am.Acad.Ophthalmol.Otolaryngol.,* 82, 569, 1976.
61. **Krausen, A. S., Gall, A. M., Garza, R., Spector, G. J., and Ansel, D. G.,** Liposarcoma of the larynx: a multicentric or a metastatic malignancy, *Laryngoscope,* 87, 1116, 1977.
62. **Ferlito, A.,** Primary pleomorphic liposarcoma of the larynx, *J.Otolaryngol.,* 7, 161, 1978.
63. **Setzen, M., Sobol, S., and Toomey, J. M.,** Clinical course of unusual malignant sarcomas of the head and neck, *Ann.Otol.Rhinol.Laryngol.,* 88, 486, 1979.
63a. **Dockerty, M. B., Parkhill, E. M., Dahlin, D. C., Woolner, L. B., Soule, E. H., and Harrison, E. G.,** Tumors of the Oral Cavity and Pharynx, Atlas of Tumor Pathology, Armed Forces Institute of Pathology, Washington D.C., 1968.
64. **Frey-Schlottmann, M. L., and Stiens, R.,** Liposarkom in Hypopharynxbereich, *Arch.Otorhinolaryngol.,* 223, 419, 1979.
65. **Wheelis, R. F., Hammer, S. P., and Yarington, C. T.,** Ultrastructural diagnosis of tumors of the head and neck, *Laryngoscope,* 89, 234, 1979.
65a. **Gaynor, E. B., Raghausan, U., and Weisbrot, I. M.,** Primary myxoid liposarcoma of the larynx, *Otolaryngol.Head Neck Surg.,* 92, 476, 1984.
66. **Baden, E. and Newman, R.,** Liposarcoma of the oropharyngeal region. Review of the literature and report of two cases, *Oral Surg.,* 44, 889, 1977.
67. **Morton, D. L., Hall, W. T., and Malurgren, R. A.,** Human liposarcoma. Tissue cultures containing foci of transformed cells with viral particles, *Science,* 165, 813, 1969.
68. **Györkey, F., Sinkovics, L. G., and Györkey, P.,** Electron microscopy observations on structures resembling myxovirus in human sarcomas, *Cancer,* 27, 1449, 1971.
69. **Eilber, F. R. and Morton, D. L.,** Immunologic studies of human sarcomas: additional evidence suggesting an associated sarcoma virus, *Cancer,* 26, 588, 1970.
70. **Virchow, R.,** Ein Fall von Bosartigen, zun Theil in der Form des Neuromas auftretenden Fellgeschwulsten, *Virchows Arch. (Pathol.Anat.),* 11, 281, 1857.
71. **Stout, A. P.,** Liposarcoma — malignant tumor of lipoblasts, *Ann.Surg.,* 119, 86, 1944.
72. **Enterline, H. T., Culbertson, J. D., Rochlin, D. B., and Brady, L. W.,** Liposarcoma. A clinical and pathological study of 53 cases, *Cancer,* 13, 932, 1960.
73. **Enzinger, F. M. and Winslow, D. J.,** Liposarcoma: a study of 103 cases, *Virchows Arch. (Pathol.Anat.),* 335, 367, 1962.
74. **Enzinger, F. M., Lattes, R., and Torloni, H.,** Histological Typing of Soft Tissue Tumours, International Histological Classification of Tumours, No. 3, World Health Organization, Geneva, 1969.
75. **Spittle, M. F., Newton, K. A., and Mackenzie, D. H.,** Liposarcoma: a review of 60 cases, *Br.J.Cancer,* 24, 696, 1970.
76. **Kindblom, L. G., Angerwall, L., and Svendsen, P.,** Liposarcoma: a clinicopathologic, radiographic and prognostic study, *Acta Pathol.Microbiol.Scand. A,* Suppl. 253, 1975.
77. **Evans, H. L., Soule, E. H., and Winkelmann, R. K.,** Atypical lipoma, atypical intramuscular lipoma, and well differentiated retroperitoneal liposarcoma. A reappraisal of 30 cases formerly classified as well differentiated liposarcoma, *Cancer,* 43, 574, 1979.
78. **Friedmann, I.,** Electron microscopy in head and neck oncology, *Acta Otolaryngol.,* 71, 115, 1971.
79. **Frank, D. L.,** Leiomyosarcoma of the larynx, *Arch.Otolaryngol.,* 34, 493, 1941.
80. **Eggston, A. A. and Wolff, D.,** *Histopathology of the Ear, Nose and Throat,* Williams & Wilkins, Baltimore, 1947.
81. **Stewart and Watson,** Quoted by **Eggston, A. A. and Wolff, D.,** *Histopathology of the Ear, Nose and Throat,* Williams & Wilkins, Baltimore, 1947.
82. **Manara, E.,** I tumori mesenchimali maligni della laringe. Considerazioni su di un raro caso di leiomiosarcoma, *Otorinolaringol.Ital.,* 28, 167, 1959.
83. **Pennelli, N. and Mazzilli, G.,** Leiomiosarcoma del laringe, *Arch.Ital.Laringol.,* 70, 343, 1962.
84. **Kawabe, Y. and Kondo, T.,** A laryngeal leiomyosarcoma. Evaluation of the authors case and observation of the literature. *Otolaryngology,* 39, 427, 1967.
85. **Amendolea, L.,** Leiomiosarcoma della laringe, *Valsalva,* 44, 268, 1969.

86. **Talavera Sanchez, J., Segura Coronado, E., and Sanchez Hidalgo, A.,** Asociacion laringocele-leiomiosarcoma de la cuerda vocal, *Acta Otorrinolaringol.Esp.*, 20. 74, 1969.
87. **Gryczynski, M.,** Leiomyosarcoma krtani, *Otolaryngol.Pol.*, 25, 545, 1971.
88. **Wolfowitz, B. L. and Schmaman, A.,** Smooth-muscle tumours of the upper respiratory tract, *S.Afr.Med.J.*, 47, 1189, 1973.
89. **Chizh, G. I.,** Leiomyosarcoma of the larynx in an 8-year-old girl, *Vestn.Otorinolaringol.*, 5, 104, 1976.
90. **Kleinsasser, O. and Glanz, H.,** Myogenic tumours of the larynx, *Arch.Otorhinolaryngol.*, 225, 107, 1979.
91. **Lehmann, W., Pidoux, J. M., and Widmann, J. J.,** *Larynx. Microlaryngoscopy and Histopathology*, Inpharzam, Cadempino. 1981.
92. **Canalis, R. F., Platz, C. E., and Cohn, A. M.,** Laryngeal rhabdomyosarcoma, *Arch.Otolaryngol.*, 102, 104, 1976.
93. **Frugoni, P. and Ferlito, A.,** Pleomorphic rhabdomyosarcoma of the larynx. A case report and review of the literature, *J.Laryngol.Otol.*, 90, 687, 1976.
94. **Glick, H. N.,** An unusual neoplasm in the larynx of a child (rhabdomyosarcoma), *Ann.Otol.Rhinol.Laryngol.*, 53, 699, 1944.
95. **Harris, H. H.,** Rhabdomyosarcoma of the larynx, *Arch.Otolaryngol.*, 74, 205, 1961.
96. **Filipo, D. and Crifò, S.,** Il sarcoma muscolare primitivo della laringe, *Boll.Mal.Orecch.Gola Naso*, 87, 599, 1964.
97. **Batsakis, J. G. and Fox, J. E.,** Rhabdomyosarcoma of the larynx. Report of a case, *Arch.Otolaryngol.*, 91, 136, 1970.
97a. **Diehn, K. W., Hyams, V. J., and Harris, A. E.,** Rhabdomyosarcoma of the larynx: a case report and review of the literature, *Laryngoscope*, 94, 201, 1984.
98. **Rodriguez, L. A. and Ziskind, J.,** Rhabdomyosarcoma of the larynx, *Laryngoscope*, 80, 1733, 1970.
99. **Winther, L. K., and Lorentzen, M.,** Rhabdomyosarcoma of the larynx: report of two cases and a review of the literature, *J.Laryngol.Otol.*, 92, 417, 1978.
100. **Franz, B.,** Beitrag zur Zytopathologie des pleomorphen Rhabdomyosarkoms des Kehlkopfes, *Laryngol.Rhinol.Otol.*, 58, 920, 1979.
101. **DeGroot, T. R., Frazer, J. T., and Wood, B. P.,** Combination therapy for laryngeal rhabdomyosarcoma, *Am.J.Otolaryngol.*, 1, 456, 1980.
102. **Lamendola, M. G. and Buonocore, U.,** Il rabdomiosarcoma della laringe (Studio anatomopatologico di un caso e revisione della letteratura), *Riv.Anat.Patol.Oncol.*, 17, 111, 1977.
102a. **Hacihanefioglu, U. and Öztürk, A. S.,** Sarcomas of the larynx. Report of ten cases, *Ann.Otol.Rhinol.Laryngol.*, 92, 81, 1983.
103. **Willis, R.A.,** *Pathology of Tumours*, Butterworths, London, 1960.
104. **Miller, R.W. and Dalage, N.A.,** U.S.childhood cancer deaths by cell type 1960-68, *J. Pediatr.*, 85, 664, 1974.
105. **Horn, R.C., Jr. and Enterline, H.T.,** Rhabdomyosarcoma: a clinicopathological study and classification of 39 cases, *Cancer*, 11, 181, 1958.
106. **Evans, R.W.,** *Histological Appearance of Tumours*, Churchill Livingstone, Edinburgh, 1968.
107. **Enzinger, F.M. and Shiraki, M.,** Alveolar rhabdomyosarcoma. An analysis of 110 cases, *Cancer*, 24,18,1969.
108. **Ashton, N. and Morgan, G.,** Orbital rhabdomyosarcoma, *J. Clin. Pathol.*, 18, 699, 1965.
109. **Nanavati, A.D.N.,** Rhabdomyosarcoma. A clinico-pathologic study of 18 cases, *Indian J.Med.Sci.*, 6, 775, 1952.
110. **Batsakis, J. G.,** *Tumors of the Head and Neck. Clinical and Pathological Considerations*, 2nd ed., Williams & Wilkins, Baltimore, 1979.
111. **Feldman, B. A.,** Rhabdomyosarcoma of the head and neck, *Laryngoscope*, 92, 424, 1982.
112. **Horn, R. C., Jr. and Enterline, H. T.,** Rhabdomyosarcoma. A clinicopathological study and classification of 39 cases, *Cancer*, 11, 181, 1958.
113. **Haran Ghera, N., Trainin, N., Fiore Donati, L., and Berenblum, I.,** A possible two-stage mechanism in rhabdomyosarcoma induction in rats, *Br.J.Cancer*, 16, 653, 1962.
114. **Friedmann, I. and Bird, E. S.,** Electron-microscope investigation of experimental rhabdomyosarcoma, *J.Pathol.*, 97, 375, 1969.
115. **Williamson, M. E., Leestma, J. E., Black, W. C., and King, D. W.,** *Histologic Patterns in Tumor Pathology*, Hoeber, N.Y., 1968.
116. **Bundtzen, J. L. and Norback, D. H.,** The ultrastructure of poorly differentiated rhabdomyosarcomas: a case report and literature review, *Hum.Pathol.*, 13, 301, 1982.
117. **Sarnat, H. B., De Mello, D. E., and Siddiqui, S. Y.,** Diagnostic value of histochemistry in embryonal rhabdomyosarcoma, *Am.J.Surg.Pathol.*, 3, 177, 1979.

118. **Mukai, K., Rosai, J., and Hallaway, B. E.,** Localization of myoglobin in normal and neoplastic human skeletal muscle cells using an immunoperoxidase method, *Am.J.Surg.Pathol.,* 3, 373, 1979.
119. **Lloyd, R. V., Hajdu, S. I., and Knapper, W. A.,** Embryonal rhabdomyosarcoma in adults, *Cancer,* 51, 557, 1983.
120. **Batsakis, J. G., Regezi, J. A., and Rice, D. H.,** The pathology of head and neck tumors: fibroadipose tissue and skeletal muscle, Part 8, *Head Neck Surg.,* 3, 145, 1980.
121. **Batsakis, J. G.,** *Tumors of the Head and Neck. Clinical and Pathological Considerations,* Williams & Wilkins, Baltimore, 1974.
122. **Unni, K., Ivins, J. C., Beabout, J. W., and Dahlin, D. C.,** Hemangioma, hemangiopericytoma, and hemangioendothelioma (angiosarcoma) of bone, *Cancer,* 27, 1403, 1971.
123. **Yankauer, S.,** Angiosarcoma of the larynx removed by indirect laryngoscopy, *Laryngoscope,* 34, 488, 1924.
124. **Havens, F. Z. and Parkhill, E. M.,** Tumors of the larynx other than squamous cell epithelioma, *Arch.Otolaryngol.,* 34, 1113, 1941.
125. **Nosaka, Y. and Nagata, K.,** Rare case of malignant hemangioendothelioma of the larynx, *Otolaryngology (Tokyo),* 39, 495, 1967.
126. **Pratt, L. W. and Goodof, I. I.,** Hemangioendotheliosarcoma of the larynx, *Arch.Otolaryngol.,* 87, 484, 1968.
127. **Alvarez Vicent, J. J.,** Sobre un caso de hemangiotelioma maligno de subglottis, *Acta Otorrinolaringol.Esp.,* 20, 1, 1969.
128. **Triplet, I, Vankemmel, B., and Madelain, M.,** Hémangioendothéliome malin du larynx avec métastases sous-cutanées, *Lille Méd.,* 19, 743, 1974.
129. **Thomas, R. L.,** Non-epithelial tumours of the larynx, *J.Laryngol.Otol.,* 93, 1131, 1979.
130. **Ferlito, A., Nicolai, P., and Caruso, G.,** Angiosarcoma of the larynx. Case report, *Ann.Otol. Rhinol.Laryngol.,* 94, 1985.
131. **Steiner, G. C. and Dorfman, H. D.,** Ultrastructure of hemangioendothelial sarcoma of bone, *Cancer,* 29, 122, 1972.
132. **Rosai, J., Summer, H. W., Kostianovsky, M., Perez-Mesa, C.,** Angiosarcoma of the skin, A clinicopathologic and fine structural study, *Hum. Pathol.,* 1, 83, 1976.
133. **Llombart-Bosch, A., Peydro-Olaya, A., and Paris-Romeu, F.,** Fine structure of malignant hemangioendothelioma of the esophagus, *Virchows Arch. (Pathol.Anat.),* 391, 107, 1981.
134. **Mallory, F. B.,** The results of the application of special histological methods to the study of tumors, *J.Exp.Med.,* 10, 575, 1908.
135. **Stout, A. P.,** Haemangio-endothelioma: a tumor of blood vessels featuring vascular endothelial cells, *Ann.Surg.,* 118, 445, 1943.
136. **Girard, C., Johnson, W. C., and Graham, J. H.,** Cutaneous angiosarcoma, *Cancer,* 26, 868, 1970.
137. **Friedmann, I. and Osborn, D. A.,** The larynx, in *Systemic Pathology,* 2nd ed., Symmers, W. St. C., Ed., Churchill Livingstone, Edinburgh, 1976.
138. **Burgdorf, W. H. C., Mukai, K., and Rosai, J.,** Immunohistochemical identification of factor VIII-related antigen in endothelial cells of cutaneous lesion of alleged vascular nature, *Am.J.Clin.Pathol.,* 75, 167, 1981.
139. **Guarda, L. A., Ordonez, N. J., Smith, J. L., Jr., and Hanssen, G.,** Immunoperoxidase localization of factor VIII in angiosarcomas, *Arch.Pathol.Lab.Med.,* 106, 515, 1982.
140. **Brooks, J. J.,** Immunohistochemistry of soft tissue tumors, *Hum.Pathol.,* 13, 969, 1982.
141. **Enzinger, F. M. and Weiss, S. W.,** *Soft Tissue Tumors,* C. V. Mosby, St.Louis, 1983.
142. **Stout, A. P. and Murray, M. R.,** Hemangiopericytoma: vascular tumor featuring Zimmermann's pericytes, *Ann.Surg.,* 116, 26, 1942.
143. **Ramsey, H. J.,** Fine structure of hemangiopericytoma and hemangioendothelioma, *Cancer,* 19, 2005, 1966.
144. **Battifora, H.,** Hemangiopericytoma: ultrastructural study of five cases, *Cancer,* 31, 1418, 1973.
145. **Nunnery, E. W., Kahn, L. B., Reddick, R. L., and Lipper, S.,** Hemangiopericytoma. A light microscopic and ultrastructural study, *Cancer,* 47, 906, 1981.
146. **Stout, A. P.,** Tumors featuring pericytes. Glomus tumor and hemangiopericytoma, *Lab.Invest.,* 5, 217, 1956.
147. **Walike, J. W. and Bailey, B. J.,** Head and neck hemangiopericytoma, *Arch.Otolaryngol.,* 93, 345, 1971.
148. **Taguchi, K. et al.,** Hemangiopericytoma of the larynx. A case report, *Otolaryngology,* 46, 21, 1974.
149. **Ferlito, A.,** Primary malignant haemangiopericytoma of the larynx (a case report with autopsy), *J.Laryngol.Otol.,* 92, 511, 1978.
150. **Moncade, J. and Demaldent, J. E.,** A propos de deux cas d'hémangiopéricytomes O.R.L., *Ann. Otolaryngol.Chir.Cervicofac.,* 96, 789, 1979.

151. **Pesavento, G. and Ferlito, A.,** Haemangiopericytoma of the larynx. A clinico-pathological study with review of the literature, *J.Laryngol.Otol.*, 96, 1065, 1982.
152. **Hertzanu, Y., Mendelsohn, D. B., Kassner, G., and Hockman, M.,** Haemangiopericytoma of the larynx, *Br.J.Rad.*, 55, 870, 1982.
153. **Abdalla, A. M.,** Congenital hemangiopericytoma of the nasopharynx, *Can.J.Otolaryngol.*, 2, 357, 1973.
154. **Güdrün, R.,** Haemangiopericytoma in otolaryngology, *J.Laryngol.Otol.*, 93, 477, 1979.
155. **Batsakis, J. G. and Rice, D. H.,** The pathology of head and neck tumors: vasoformative tumors, Part 9B, *Head Neck Surg.*, 3, 326, 1981.
155a. **Abemayor, E. and Calcaterra, T. C.,** Kaposi's sarcoma and community-acquired immune deficiency syndrome. An update with emphasis on its head and neck manifestations, *Arch.Otolaryngol.*, 109, 536, 1983.
156. **Abramson, A. L. and Simons, R. L.,** Kaposi's sarcoma of the head and neck, *Arch. Otolaryngol.*, 92, 505, 1970.
157. **Friedmann, I.,** Sarcomas of the larynx, *Can.J.Otolaryngol.*, 4, 297, 1975.
158. **Moritsch, E., Jarisch, R., and Konrad, K.,** Morbus Kaposi. Pharyngolaryngeale Manifestation, Therapie, *Laryngol.Rhinol.Otol.*, 57, 792, 1978.
159. **Lothe, F.,** 1960, Quoted by **Lippi, L., Brizzi, G., and Polli, G.,** Su di un caso di manifestazione laringea di morbo di Kaposi, *Boll.Mal.Orecchio Gola Naso.*, 93, 137, 1975.
160. **Lippi, L., Brizzi, G., and Polli, G.,** Su di un caso di manifestazione laringea di morbo di Kaposi, *Boll.Mal.Orecchio Gola Naso*, 93, 137, 1975.
161. **Bottazzi, D., Collini, M., and Pelizza, A.,** Morbo di Kaposi. Manifestazione secondaria faringo-laringea, *Ann.Laringol.Otol.Rinol.Faringol.*, 78, 261, 1980.
162. **Shanmugaratnam, K. and Sobin, L. H.,** Histological Typing of Upper Respiratory Tract Tumours, in International Histological Classification of Tumours, No. 19, World Health Organization, Geneva, 1978.
163. **Coyas, A., Eliadellis, E., and Anastassiades, O.,** Kaposi's sarcoma of the larynx, *J.Laryngol.Otol.*, 97, 647, 1983.
164. **Hymes, K. B., Greene, J. B., Marcus, A., William, D. L., Cheung. T., Prose, N., Ballard, H., and Canbestein, L.,** Kaposi's sarcoma in homosexual men. A report of 8 cases, *Lancet*, 2, 598, 1981.
165. **Geahchan, N. E., Lambert, J., Micheau, C., and Richard, J. M.,** Synovialome malin du larynx, *Ann.Otolaryngol.Chir.Cervicofac.*, 100, 61, 1983.
166. **Applebaum, E. L. and Mantravadi, R. P.,** Synovial sarcoma of the hypopharynx, *Otolaryngol.Head Neck Surg.*, 91, 452, 1983.
167. **Jernström, P.,** Synovial sarcoma of the pharynx: report of a case, *Am.J.Clin.Pathol.*, 24, 957, 1954.
168. **Martens, V. E.,** Unusual synovial tumors, *JAMA*, 1547, 888, 1955.
169. **Pricolo, V. and Cenci, N.,** Sinovioma maligno dell'ipofaringe, *Minerva Otorinolaringol.*, 7, 218, 1957.
170. **Cachin, Y., Gérard-Marchant, R., Schweitsguth, O., Richard, J., and Varret, D.,** Les synovialomes malins parapharyngés. Revue générale et présentation d'une observation, *Ann.Otolaryngol.*, 83, 41, 1966.
171. **Vande Weghe, J. P. and Kluyskens, P.,** Un cas de synovialome du pharynx, *Acta Otorhinolaryngol.Belg.*, 22, 658, 1968.
172. **Gatti, W.M., Strom, G., and Orfei, E.,** Synovial sarcoma of the laryngopharynx, *Arch.Otolaryngol.*, 101, 633, 1975.
173. **Minnigerode, B.,** Le synovialo-sarcoma de l'hypopharynx, *J. Fr.Otorhinolaryngol.*, 23, 861, 1974
174. **Roth, J. A., Enzinger, F. M., and Tannenbaum, M.,** Synovial sarcoma of the neck: a followup study of 24 cases, *Cancer*, 35, 1243, 1975.
175. **Lockey, M. W.,** Rare tumors of the ear, nose and throat: synovial sarcoma of the head and neck. *S. Med.J.*, 69, 316, 1976.
176. **Panh, M. H., Aftimos, G., Pasquier, B., Courdec, P., and Mazabraud, A.,** Les synovialosarcomes cervicaux extraarticulaires. Revue de la littérature à propos de deux observations, *Bull.Cancer*, 63, 309, 1976.
177. **Chelloul, N. and Labayle, J.,** Les synovialoblastomes extraarticulaires parapharyngés. A propos d'une observation, *Semin.Hôp.Paris*, 53, 707, 1977.
178. **Gapany-Gapanavicius, B., Behar, A.J., and Chisin, R.** Synovial sarcoma of the hypopharynx, *Ann.Otol.Rhinol.Laryngol.*, 87, 356, 1978.
179. **Choux, R., Jaquemier, J., Chrestian, M. A., Andrac, L., Vague, D., Lieutaud, R., and Cannoni, M.,** Synovialosarcoma pharyngé. Etude ultrastructurale d'un cas, *Bull.Cancer*, 65, 3, 1978.
180. **Martin, F., Behbehani, A., and Wiebecke, B.,** Zervikale Synovialsarkome im Kindesalter, *Laryngol.Rhinol.Otol.*, 58, 871, 1979.
181. **Hirokawa, R. H., Stucker, F. J., and Bryarly, R. C.,** Synovial cell sarcoma, *Otolaryngol.Head Neck Surg.*, 88, 227, 1980.

182. **Junien-Lavillauroy, C., Roux, O., Pasquier, R., and Charachon, R.,** Synovialosarcome du sinus périforme chez l'enfant, *Ann.Otolaryngol.Chir.Cervicofac.*, 95, 336, 1978.
182a. **Palmer, B. V., Levene, A., and Shaw, H. J.,** Synovial sarcoma of the pharynx and oesophagus, *J.Laryngol.Otol.*, 97, 1173, 1983.
183. **Labayle, J., Brocheriou, C., Paraire, F., Dumaine, A., Dahan, S., and Cuzin, O.,** A propos de 2 cas de synovialosarcome cervical extra-articulaire, *Ann.Otolaryngol.Chir.Cervicofac.*, 97, 461, 1980.
184. **Wilhelm, H. J., Dietz, R., and Schöndorf, J.,** Diagnostik und Therapie seltener Tumoren im Larynx-Pharynx-Bereich, *Laryngol.Rhinol.Otol.*, 59, 137, 1980.
184a. **Mohr, W. and Pirsig, W.,** Synoviales Sarkom des Larynx. Fallbeschreibung und kurze Literaturübersicht, *Laryngol.Rhinol.Otol.*, 63, 453, 1984.
184b. **Miller, L. H., Santaella-Latimer, L., and Miller, T.,** Synovialsarcoma of the larynx, *Trans.Am. Acad.Ophthalmol.Otolaryngol.*, 80, 448, 1975.
184c. **Quinn, H. J., Jr.,** Synovial sarcoma of the larynx treated by partial laryngectomy, *Laryngoscope*, 94, 1158, 1984.
185. **New, G. B.,** Sarcoma of the larynx: report of two cases. *Arch.Otolaryngol.*, 21, 648, 1935.
186. **Ferlito, A., Nicolai, P., Montaguti, A., Cecchetto, A., and Pennelli, N.,** Chondrosarcoma of the larynx. Review of the literature and report of 3 cases, *Am. J. Otolaryngol.*, 5, 350, 1984.
186a. **Kramer, D. S., Brown, G. P., and Schuller, D. E.,** Proximal airway obstruction presenting as dyspnea. A case of chondrosarcoma of the larynx, *Postgrad.Med.*, 73, 133, 1983.
187. **Hyams, V. J. and Rabuzzi, D. D.,** Cartilaginous tumors of the larynx, *Laryngoscope*, 80, 755, 1970.
188. **Goethals, P. L., Dahlin, D. C., and Devine, K. D.,** Cartilaginous tumors of the larynx, *Surg.Gynecol.Obstet.*, 117, 77, 1963.
189. **Putney, F. J. and Moran, J. J.,** Cartilaginous tumors of the larynx, *Ann.Otol.Rhinol.Laryngol.*, 73, 370, 1964.
190. **Huizenga, C. and Balogh, K.,** Cartilaginous tumors of the larynx. A clinicopathologic study of 10 new cases and a review of the literature, *Cancer*, 26, 201, 1970.
191. **Chambers, R. G. and Friedel, W.,** Chondrosarcoma of the larynx, *Laryngoscope*, 86, 713, 1976.
192. **Cantrell, R. W., Reibel, J. F., Jahrsdoerfer, R. A., and Johns, M. E.,** Conservative surgical treatment of chondrosarcoma of the larynx, *Ann.Otol.Rhinol.Laryngol.*, 89, 567, 1980.
193. **Milanesi, I.,** Considerazioni istopatogenetiche su un caso di condrosarcoma laringeo, *Ann.Laringol. Otol.Rinol.Faringol.*, 67, 767, 1968.
194. **Rethi, A.,** 1921, Quoted by **Milanesi, I.,** Considerazioni istopatogenetiche su un caso di condrosarcoma laringeo, *Ann.Laringol. Otol.Rinol.Faringol.*, 67, 767, 1968.
194a. **Gray, S. D., Blanke, S. B., Babin, R. W., and Robinson, R. A.,** Chondrosarcoma of the epiglottis with pulmonary metastases, Annual Meeting Am.Ac.Otolaryngol.Head Neck Surg., Inc., Las Vegas, Nevada, 1984.
195. **Bronzini, E.,** Condrosarcoma della laringe, *Ann.Laringol.Otol.Rhinol.Faringol.*, 58, 497, 1959.
196. **Greer, J. A. Jr., Devine, K. D., and Dahlin, D. C.,** Gardner's syndrome and chondrosarcoma of the hyoid bone, *Arch.Otolaryngol.*, 103, 425, 1977.
197. **Lawson, V.G., Bryce, D. P., and Briant, T. D. R.,** Chondroma and chondrosarcoma of the larynx, *Can.J.Otolaryngol.*, 1, 213, 1972.
197a. **Erlandson, R. A. and Huvos, A. G.,** Chondrosarcoma: a light and electron microscopic study, *Cancer*, 34, 1642, 1974.
198. **Zizmor, J., Noyek, A. M., and Lewis, J. S.,** Radiologic diagnosis of chondroma and chondrosarcoma of the larynx, *Arch.Otolaryngol.*, 101, 232, 1975.
199. **Fish, B., Nussbaum, M., and Smulewicz J. J.,** Chondrosarcoma of the larynx. Computerized tomographic study, *N.Y. State J. Med.*, 82, 216, 1982.
200. **Jones, H. M.,** Cartilaginous tumours of the head and neck, *J.Laryngol.Otol.*, 87, 135, 1973.
201. **Hellquist, H., Olofsson, J., and Gröntoft, O.,** Chondrosarcoma of the larynx, *J.Laryngol.Otol.*, 93, 1037, 1979.
202. **Sanerkin, N. G.,** Definitions of osteosarcoma, chondrosarcoma, and fibrosarcoma of bone, *Cancer*, 46, 178, 1980.
202a. **Ferlito, A. and Recher, G.,** Chondrometaplasia of the larynx, in press.
203. **Barsocchini, L. M. and McCoy, G.,** Cartilaginous tumors of the larynx. A review of the literature and a report of four cases, *Ann.Otol.Rhinol.Laryngol.*, 77, 146, 1968.
204. **LeJeune, F. E., Jr., Van Horn, H. W., III, and Farr, G. H.,** Chondrosarcoma of the larynx: excision of massive recurrence, *Ann.Otol.Rhinol.Laryngol.*, 91, 392, 1982.
205. **Frenzel, H.,** Kehlkopfekondrome und ihr Charakteristisches, *Mschr.Ohrenheilk.*, 87, 281, 1953.
206. **Sirota, H. H.,** 1958, Quoted by **Hyams, V. J. and Rabuzzi, D. D.,** Cartilaginous tumors of the larynx, *Laryngoscope*, 80, 755, 1970.
207. **Al-Saleem, T., Tucker, G. F., Jr., Peale, A. R., and Norris, C. M.,** Cartilaginous tumors of the larynx. Clinical-pathologic study of ten cases, *Ann.Otol.Rhinol.Laryngol.*, 79, 33, 1970.

208. **Harwood, A. R., Krajbich, J. I., and Fornasier, V.L.,** Radiotherapy of chondrosarcoma of the bone, *Cancer,* 45, 2769, 1980.
209. **Neel, H. B. III and Unni, K. K.,** Cartilaginous tumors of the larynx: a series of 33 patients, *Otolaryngol.Head Neck Surg.,* 90, 201, 1982.
210. **Ungerecht, K.,** Multiple Chondrome und Chondrosarkome des Larynx und der Trachea mit chondromyxosarkomatösen Rezidiven, *Arch.Klin.Ohren Nasen Kehlkopfheilkd.,* 160, 158, 1951.
211. **Ghalib, S. H., Warner, E. D., and DeGowin, E. L.,** Laryngeal chondrosarcoma after thyroid irradiation, *JAMA,* 210, 1762, 1969.
211a. **Escher, A., Escher, F., and Zimmermann, A.,** Zur Klinik und Pathologie chondromatöser Tumoren des Larynx, *HNO,* 32, 269, 1984.
212. **Östberg, Y., Boquist, L., and Diamant, H.,** Laryngeal chondrosarcoma in Sweden, *Acta Otolaryngol.,* 88, 142, 1979.
213. **Evans, H. L., Ayala, A. G., and Romsdahl, M. M.,** Prognostic factors in chondrosarcoma of bone. A clinicopathological analysis with emphasis on histological grade, *Cancer,* 40, 818, 1977.
214. **Pritchard, D. J., Lunke, R. J., Taylor, W. F., Dahlin, D. C., and Medley, B. E.,** Chondrosarcoma: a clinicopathologic and statistical analysis, *Cancer,* 45, 149, 1980.
215. **Fu, Y. and Perzin, K. H.,** Non-epithelial tumors of the nasal cavity, paranasal sinuses, and nasopharynx: a clinicopathologic study. III. Cartilaginous tumors (chondroma, chondrosarcoma), *Cancer,* 34, 453, 1974.
216. **Ross, D. E.,** Chondrosarcoma of the larynx invading the thyroid gland, *Laryngoscope,* 81, 379, 1971.
217. **Jackson, C. and Jackson, C. L.,** *Diseases and Injuries of the Larynx,* Macmillian, N.Y., 1942.
218. **Clerf, L. H.,** Sarcoma of the larynx: report of eight cases, *Arch. Otolaryngol.,* 44, 517, 1946.
219. **Sprinkle, P. M., Allan, M.S., and Brookshire, P. F.,** Osteosarcoma of the larynx (a true primary sarcoma of the larynx), *Laryngoscope,* 76, 325, 1966.
220. **Morley, A. R., Cameron, D. S., and Watson, A. J.,** Osteosarcoma of the larynx, *J. Laryngol. Otol.,* 87, 997, 1973.
221. **Haar, J. G., Chaudhry, A. P., Karanjia, M. D., and Milley, P. S.,** Chondroblastic osteosarcoma of the larynx, *Arch. Otolaryngol.,* 104, 477, 1978.
222. **Dahm, L. J., Schaefer, S. D., Carder, H. M., and Vellios, F.,** Osteosarcoma of the soft tissue of the larynx. Report of a case with light and electron microscopic studies, *Cancer,* 42, 2343, 1978.
223. **Suchatlampong, V., Sriumpai, S., and Khawcharoenporn, V.,** Osteosarcoma of the larynx. The first case report in Thailand with ultrastructural study, *J.Med.Assoc.Thai.,* 64, 301, 1981.
223a. **Remagen, W., Löhr, J., and von Westernhagen, B.,** Osteosarkom des Kehlkopfes, *HNO,* 31, 366, 1983.
224. **Pappas, D. J. and Johnson, L. A.,** Laryngeal myositis ossificans, *Arch.Otolaryngol.,* 81, 227, 1965.
225. **Ferlito, A., Barion, U., and Nicolai, P.,** Myositis ossificans of the head and neck. Review of the literature and report of a case, *Arch. Otorhinolaryngol.,* 237, 103, 1983.
226. **Ackerman, L. V.,** Extra-osseous localized non-neoplastic bone and cartilage formation (so-called myositis ossificans), *J. Bone J. Surg. (Am.),* 40, 279, 1958.
227. **Chang-Lo, M.,** Laryngeal involvement in von Recklinghausen's disease: a case report and review of the literature, *Laryngoscope,* 87, 435, 1977.
228. **Nanson, E. M.,** Neurilemoma of the larynx: a case study, *Head Neck Surg.,* 1, 69, 1978.
229. **Norris, C. M. and Peale, A. R.,** Sarcoma of the larynx, *Ann. Otol. Rhinol. Laryngol.,* 70, 892, 1961.
230. **Iwaszkiewicz, J. and Kamieniec, M.,** Sarcomatous neurofibroma of the larynx, *Otolaryngol. Pol.,* 20, 541, 1966.
231. **DeLozier, H. L.,** Intrinsic malignant schwannoma of the larynx. A case report, *Ann. Otol. Rhinol. Laryngol.,* 91, 336, 1982.
232. **Cummings, C. W., Montgomery, W. W., and Balogh, K., Jr.,** Neurogenic tumors of the larynx, *Ann. Otol. Rhinol. Laryngol.,* 78, 76, 1969.
233. **Pearlman, S. J., Friedman, E. A., and Appel, M.,** Neurofibroma of the larynx, *Arch.Otolaryngol.,* 52, 8, 1950.
234. **Stricker, F. J.,** Neurinom und Spindelzellssarkom des Kehlkopfes, *HNO,* 1, 554, 1949.
235. **Taxy, J. B., Battifora, H., Trujillo, Y., and Dorfman, H. D.,** Electron microscopy in the diagnosis of malignant schwannoma, *Cancer,* 48, 1381, 1981.
236. **Hajdu, S. I.,** *Pathology of the Soft Tissue Tumors,* Lea & Febiger, Philadelphia, 1979.
237. **Wetzel, W., Leipzig, B., Grunow, W., Kenna, M., Kalderon, A., and Morgan, B.,** Malignant granular cell tumor of the tongue, *Arch. Otolaryngol.,* 108, 603, 1982.
238. **Robertson, A. J., McIntosh, W., Lamont, P., and Guthrie, W.,** Malignant granular cell tumour (myoblastoma) of the vulva: report of a case and review of the literature, *Histopathology,* 5, 69, 1981.
238a. **Lattes, R.,** *Tumors of the Soft Tissues,* Fascicle 1/Revised, Second Series, *Atlas of Tumor Pathology,* Armed Forces Institute of Pathology, Washington, D.C., 1982.
239. **Glasunow, M.,** Über unreife, begrentzte und destruierend wachsende Rhabdomyoblastome, *Frankfurt Z.Pathol.,* 45, 328, 1933.

240. **Carnevale Ricci, F.,** Mioblastoma maligno della corda vocale, *Arch.Ital.O.R.L.*, 52, 436, 1940.
241. **Von Busanny-Caspari, W. and Hammar, C. H.,** Zur Malignität der sogenannten Myoblastenmyome, *Zentralbl.Allg.Pathol.*, 98, 401, 1958.
242. **Faleg, G.,** Due rare osservazioni di mioblastomiomi, benigno e maligno delle corde vocali, *Arch. De Vecchi Anat. Patol.*, 29, 847, 1959.
243. **Sobel, H. J., Marquet, E., Avrin, E., and Schwarz, R.,** Granular cell myoblastoma. An electron microscopic and cytochemical study illustrating the genesis of granules and aging of myoblastoma cells, *Am.J.Pathol.*, 65, 59, 1971.
244. **Usui, M., Ishii, S., Yamawaki, S., Sasaki, T., Minami, A., and Hizawa, K.,** Malignant granular cell tumor of the radial nerve. An autopsy observation with electron microscopic and tissue culture studies, *Cancer*, 39, 1547, 1977.
245. **Nakazato, Y., Ishizeki, J., Takahashi, K., and Yamaguchi, H.,** Immunohistochemical localization of S-100 protein in granular cell myoblastoma, *Cancer*, 49, 1624, 1982.
246. **Stefansson, K. and Wollmann, R. L.,** S-100 protein in granular cell tumors (granular cell myoblastomas), *Cancer*, 49, 1834, 1982.
247. **Al-Sarraf, M., Loud, A. V., and Vaitkevicius, V. K.,** Malignant granular cell tumor. Histochemical and electron microscopic study, *Arch. Pathol.*, 91, 550, 1971.
248. **Sobel, H. J., Schwarz, R., and Marquet, E.,** Light and electron microscope study of the origin of granular-cell myoblastoma, *J. Pathol.*, 109, 101, 1973.
249. **Shousha, S. and Lyssiotis, T.,** Granular cell myoblastoma: positive staining for carcinoembryonic antigen, *J. Clin. Pathol.*, 32, 219, 1979.

Chapter 2

MALIGNANT LYMPHOMAS AND RELATED CONDITIONS OF THE LARYNX

A. Ferlito

TABLE OF CONTENTS

I. NON-HODGKIN'S LYMPHOMAS

A. Introduction

Malignant lymphomas are neoplasms of the immune system and usually originate in the lymph nodes or from other lymphoid tissues. However, they may also arise in sites that normally contain no lymphoid tissue.

Freeman et al.[1] estimated that about one fourth of the malignant lymphomas collected by the End Results Group of Cancer Registries in the years 1950 to 1964 arose in extranodal sites, of which the larynx is one of the less common. They reported only 8 cases of laryngeal lymphomas on a series of 1467 Caucasian patients with nondisseminated lymphomas of extranodal origin.

Malignant lymphomas of the larynx correspond to those occurring elsewhere in the body. Sometimes the larynx is the primary site of the disease, and sometimes it alone is involved. The larynx may also be involved incidentally in the course of advanced and disseminated disease.

The lymphoid nodules contained in the lamina propria of the mucous membrane of the supraglottic region and the lymphoid tissue present in the ventricle of the larynx, referred to as the laryngeal tonsil,[1a] can explain the origin of these tumors in this organ.

In the presence of organ involvement by malignant non-Hodgkin's lymphomas, it is always mandatory to consider the lesion as potentially representing the first or most evident clinical finding of a disseminated malignant lymphoma. Before considering a laryngeal lymphoma as isolated, it is necessary to perform sequential staging procedures so as to determine the true extent of the disease. After histological examination of a primary lesion, adequate investigations consist of careful physical examination, bone marrow biopsy, chest X-ray, lymphangiogram, liver and kidney function tests, and other routine laboratory tests. Sometimes the investigations have limitations, as might be suggested by the subsequent occurrence of disseminated lymphomas. Therefore, several "isolated" or "localized" laryngeal lymphomas are not confined to that one area.

B. Terminology and Classification

The evolution of lymphoma terminology and classification during more than a century culminated in the Rappaport classification[2] that, with modifications, achieved broad application and became the standard classification for clinical therapeutic trials. In fact, in spite of recent and significant progress in the development of histochemical and immunologic methods for the identification of lympoid cells, morphology is still the most important tool for suggesting the behavior in non-Hodgkin's lymphoma.

At the present time several morphological classifications exist; each of these can separate the lymphomas into prognostic subgroups. The Lukes-Collins classification[3-5] is based on immunologic principles. Accurate application of this classification requires demonstrations that the tumor cells bear T-cell, B-cell, histiocytic, or no demonstrable markers. The Lennert[6] classification, also known as the Kiel classification, is based on cytologic features. Two main subgroups ("low" and "high" grades) with different prognosis are introduced. In the British classification,[7,8] like the Rappaport classification,[2] malignant lymphomas are subdivided mainly on the basis of the pattern of growth. Two grades (I and II) of malignancy are considered.

Other classifications are those of Dorfman[9-11] and of the WHO.[12] Nathwani[13] proposed a compromise classification of non-Hodgkin's lymphomas so as to reconcile the various classifications.

Recently, the National Cancer Institute (NCI) organized a large-scale international study to compare and evaluate the most prominent classification schemes for malignant non-

Hodgkin's lymphomas and attempted to formulate a unifying concept.[14] The best known classifications are compiled in Table 1.

The applicability of this current nomenclature is possible also in extranodal lymphomas. Table 2 shows the application of this concept in a series of non-Hodgkin's lymphomas of the larynx reported by Ferlito et al.[15]

C. Incidence

Laryngeal lymphomas are rare, and in our material the incidence is 0.23% of all laryngeal malignant neoplasms, excluding the plasmacytomas. In particular, primary involvement of the larynx is rare.[15-16a] A review of the world literature by De Santo and Weiland,[16] who reported 9 additional cases of their own treated at the Mayo Clinic from 1952 to 1968, revealed only 19 patients with laryngeal lymphoma, while Anderson et al.[17] found a total of 14 previously reported cases of isolated laryngeal lymphoma. Gregor[18] reported 5 instances of laryngeal lymphoma, of which 2 were localized, and found that 40 cases had been previously reported. The Japanese literature, during the decades 1960 to 1980,[19] recorded 24 cases of malignant lymphoma of the larynx.

Ferlito et al.[15] described the clinicopathologic features of six cases of non-Hodgkin's lymphoma observed through 1966 to 1979.

The larynx may be also involved by Lennert's lymphoma[20] and by mycosis fungoides in its terminal dissemination.[21-22a] Recently, I have observed a case of mycosis fungoides with involvement of the larynx and hypopharynx. Hood et al.[23] reported a case of the primary presentation of mycosis fungoides in the larynx. Widespread cutaneous lesions appeared 2 years after the original biopsy, which was initially interpreted as an undifferentiated small-cell malignant neoplasm. The patient died and the autopsy showed visceral involvement. Another case of mycosis fungoides involving the right half of the larynx has been described.[24]

D. Age and Sex

There is no sex predilection. The most affected are those between the ages of 50 to 70, but these tumors may also be seen in young individuals.

E. Site

Most lymphomas are located in the supraglottic region, in particular the epiglottis and aryepiglottic folds; the vocal cords may be involved.

F. Pathology

Gross pathology — The tumor appears as a more or less bulky mass, covered as a rule by an intact edematous mucosa.

Light microscopy (Figures 1 to 6) — The histological appearance of laryngeal lymphomas may be variable and it is quite similar to that described in involved lymph nodes and other organ lymphomas. However, a predominance of a diffuse pattern of growth, and a prevalence of the "lymphocytic" type of the Rappaport terminology have been noticed.

In most cases the lesion is composed of circumscribed masses of cytologically recognizable lymphoid elements that infiltrate the laryngeal structures, displaying a diffuse pattern of growth. Small, medium-sized, or large cleaved lymphoid cells may represent the predominant cell type or, less frequently, they comprise only a percentage of the proliferating cells, whereas the remaining ones are large non-cleaved follicular center cells and large cells of the immunoblastic type. The mitotic index is usually low or moderate. Necrosis is uncommon. Inflammatory elements such as neutrophils, plasma cells, and vessels are scanty or absent.

Particular clinicopathologic entities, mentioned in the incidence section, demonstrate in the larynx the same appearance that they may offer in other sites. In particular, a polymorphic

Table 1
MAJOR RECENTLY PROPOSED CLASSIFICATIONS OF NON-HODGKIN'S LYMPHOMAS AS MODIFIED BY RESPECTIVE AUTHORS

Rappaport classification

Nodular
- Lymphocytic, well differentiated
- Lymphocytic, poorly differentiated
- Mixed, lymphocytic and histiocytic
- Histiocytic

Diffuse
- Lymphocytic, well differentiated without plasmacytoid features
- Lymphocytic, well differentiated with plasmacytoid features
- Lymphocytic, poorly differentiated without plasmacytoid features
- Lymphocytic, poorly differentiated with plasmacytoid features
- Lymphoblastic, convoluted
- Lymphoblastic, nonconvoluted
- Mixed, lymphocytic and histiocytic
- Histiocytic without sclerosis
- Histiocytic with sclerosis
- Burkitt's tumor
- Undifferentiated

Malignant lymphoma, unclassified
Composite lymphoma

Lukes and Collins classification

Undefined cell type
T-cell type, small lymphocytic
T-cell type, Sezary-mycosis fungoides (cerebriform)
T-cell type, convoluted lymphocytic
T-cell type, immunoblastic sarcoma (T-cell)
B-cell type, small lymphocytic
B-cell type, plasmacytoid lymphocytic
Follicular center cell, small cleaved
Follicular center cell, large cleaved
Follicular center cell, small non-cleaved
Follicular center cell, large non-cleaved
Immunoblastic sarcoma (B-cell)
- Subtypes of follicular center cell lymphomas
  1. Follicular
  2. Follicular and diffuse
  3. Diffuse
  4. Sclerotic with follicles
  5. Sclerotic without follicles

Histiocytic
Malignant lymphoma, unclassified

Kiel classification

Low-grade malignancy
- Lymphocytic, chronic lymphocytic leukemia
- Lymphocytic, other
- Lymphoplasmacytoid
- Centrocytic
- Centroblastic-centrocytic, follicular, without sclerosis
- Centroblastic-centrocytic, follicular, with sclerosis
- Centroblastic-centrocytic, follicular and diffuse, without sclerosis
- Centroblastic-centrocytic, follicular and diffuse, with sclerosis
- Centroblastic-centrocytic, diffuse
- Low grade malignant lymphoma, unclassified

High-grade malignancy
- Centroblastic
- Lymphoblastic, Burkitt's type
- Lymphoblastic, convoluted cell type
- Lymphoblastic, other (unclassified)
- Immunoblastic
- High grade malignant lymphoma, unclassified

Malignant lymphoma, unclassified (Unable to specify "high grade" or "low grade")
Composite lymphoma

British National Lymphoma Investigation classification

Follicular lymphoma
- Follicle cells, predominantly small
- Follicle cells, mixed small and large
- Follicle cells, predominantly large

Diffuse lymphoma
- Lymphocytic, well differentiated (small round lymphocyte)
- Lymphocytic, intermediately differentiated (small follicle lymphocyte)
- Lymphocytic, poorly differentiated (lymphoblast)
  - (a) Non-Burkitt
  - (b) Burkitt's tumors
  - (c) Convoluted cell mediastinal lymphoma
- Lymphocytic/mixed small lymphoid and large cell (mixed follicle cells)
- Undifferentiated large cell (large lymphoid cell)
- Histiocytic cell (mononuclear phagocytic cell)
- Plasma cell (extramedullary plasma cell)
- Malignant lymphoma, unclassified
- Plasmacytoid differentiation
- Sclerosis, banded
- Sclerosis, fine

Working formulation

Low grade
- Malignant lymphoma
  - Small lymphocytic
    - Consistent with CLL
    - Plasmacytoid
- Malignant lymphoma, follicular

Table 1 (continued)
MAJOR RECENTLY PROPOSED CLASSIFICATIONS OF NON-HODGKIN'S LYMPHOMAS AS MODIFIED BY RESPECTIVE AUTHORS

    - Predominantly small cleaved cell
      - Diffuse areas
      - Sclerosis
  - Malignant lymphoma, follicular
    - Mixed, small cleaved and large cell
      - Diffuse areas
      - Sclerosis
- Intermediate grade
  - Malignant lymphoma, follicular
    - Predominantly large cell
      - Diffuse areas
      - Sclerosis
  - Malignant lymphoma, diffuse
    - Small cleaved cell
      - Sclerosis
  - Malignant lymphoma, diffuse
    - Mixed, small and large cell
      - Sclerosis
      - Epithelioid cell component
  - Malignant lymphoma, diffuse
    - Large cell
      - Cleaved cell
      - Noncleaved cell
      - Sclerosis
- High grade
  - Malignant lymphoma
    - Large cell, immunoblastic
      - Plasmacytoid
      - Clear cell
      - Polymorphous
      - Epithelioid cell component
  - Malignant lymphoma
    - Lymphoblastic
      - Convoluted cell
      - Nonconvoluted cell
  - Malignant lymphoma
    - Small noncleaved cell
      - Burkitt's follicular areas
  - Miscellaneous
    - Composite
    - Mycosis fungoides
    - Histiocytic
    - Extramedullary plasmacytoma
    - Unclassifiable
    - Other

lymphocytic infiltrate, mycosis cells with "cerebriform" nuclei, and mucosal Pautrier's microabscesses are distinguishing features of mycosis fungoides.

G. Diagnosis and Differential Diagnosis

Adequate biopsy is essential for diagnosis and has to be large enough to be representative of the whole neoplasm so as to assist in the identification of the pattern and the cytomorphological typing of the lesion.

Laryngeal malignant lymphomas, particularly of the "poorly differentiated lymphocytic type", must be differentiated from nonlymphomatous small-cell malignancies. In addition, some tumor-like or reactive conditions (pseudolymphomas) that, though rarely, can be encountered in the larynx,[24a,b] should be considered in histologically differential diagnosis (see Table 3).

The separation of a non-Hodgkin's lymphoma of the "lymphocyte type" from an "oat cell" carcinoma of the larynx may offer some serious difficulties.[25] Small cell carcinomas are usually composed of pleomorphic dark cells which are only moderately larger than mature lymphocytes. The detection of tumor areas consisting of spindle-shaped cells, as frequently displayed by these tumors, and the usually high mitotic index may be useful in their identification.

Lymphomatoid granulomatosis, a tumor-like lymphoreticular granulomatous disease, is another condition which may be very difficult to separate from malignant lymphomas arising in the larynx. The recognition of a polymorphous infiltrate containing atypical, especially plasmacytoid cells and varying numbers of cells in mitotic activity as well as the demonstration of vasculitis, destruction of vessels, and necrosis, are in favor of the diagnosis of lymphomatoid granulomatosis.[26]

Table 2
CLASSIFICATION OF SIX CASES OF LYMPHOID TUMORS OF LARYNX (ACCORDING TO VARIOUS CLASSIFICATIONS OF NON-HODGKIN'S MALIGNANT LYMPHOMAS)

Case no.	Pattern	Rappaport (1966)	Lukes and Collins (1977)	Henry et al. (1978)	Lennert and Mohri (1978)
1	Diffuse	PDLL	Small cleaved FCC	Lymphocytic intermediate differentiation (small follicle cell)	Centrocytic
2	Diffuse	H	Large noncleaved FCC	Undifferentiated large cell	Centroblastic (secondary)
3	Diffuse	H	Large noncleaved FCC	Undifferentiated large cell	Centroblastic (secondary)
4	Diffuse	PDLL	Small cleaved FCC	Lymphocytic intermediate differentiation (small follicle cell)	Centrocytic
5	Diffuse	Mixed	Large cleaved FCC	Lymphocytic intermediate differentiation (with undifferentiated large cell component)	Centrocytic (with large cell component)
6	Diffuse	PDLL	Small cleaved FCC	Lymphocytic intermediate differentiation (small follicle cell)	Centrocytic

PDLL = Poorly differentiated lymphocytic lymphoma; FCC = follicular center cell; H = "histiocytic".

From Ferlito, A. et al., *ORL*, 43, 61, 1981. With permission.

The differential diagnosis must also include Sjogren's syndrome involving the larynx,[27] and Wegener's granulomatosis that occasionally may extensively involve the larynx.[28-31]

The distinction of malignant lymphoma from a lymphoid reactive hyperplasia (or pseudolymphoma) is difficult.[32] Modern immunologic and cytochemical techniques are of diagnostic value for distinguishing between a benign hyperplastic or reactive extranodal lymphoid infiltration and an extranodal malignant lymphoma. Malignant lymphomas exhibit either k- or λ -light chain components in their surface immunoglobulins in accord with their immunological monoclonal nature, whereas pseudolymphomas, both the monomorphous and polymorphous types, are immunologically polyclonal.[33]

In general, the demonstration of monotypic immunoglobulin (single light chain type) by immunoperoxidase and immunofluorescence methods can help to resolve three common diagnostic problems:

1. The distinction between large-cell lymphomas and nonlymphoid neoplasms
2. The differentiation of neoplastic from reactive lymphoid infiltrates
3. The subclassification of malignant lymphomas according to their cell of origin

In addition to histochemistry and immunoperoxidase staining, electron microscopic studies may be helpful in most of the problems in differential diagnosis. According to Henry,[34] some of the advantages of the latter technique are

1. The confirmation of the diagnosis of lymphoma
2. The identification of the cell type involved in the neoplastic process
3. The identification of the degree of "differentiation" of the component cells

4. The demonstration of various inclusions, organelles, and cell-to-cell contact, which may prove useful as markers
5. The utilization of histochemical and immunoelectron microscopic techniques helpful in the identification of the different cell types

H. Behavior and Prognosis

Isolated (stage IE) non-Hodgkin's malignant lymphomas of the larynx can be successfully treated with radiation and locally cured.[16a] The basis of this effective treatment is, in addition to careful histopathologic diagnosis, an appropriate staging which may exclude dissemination of disease. Intensive investigations and long-term follow-up are indicated. Instead, the prognosis is poor in the presence of an advanced and disseminated disease.

II. HODGKIN'S DISEASE

No convincing example of primary isolated Hodgkin's disease in the larynx has been reported. The diagnosis of Hodgkin's disease in the larynx is based on the finding of distinctive Reed-Sternberg cells, as it would be in the lymph nodes. The correct diagnosis will result from careful identification of these cells in an appropriate context.[35]

Secondary laryngeal involvement in Hodgkin's disease is unusual, though several reports may be found.[36-39] Shilling et al.[38] reported three cases in which Hodgkin's disease had given no clinical evidence in the larynx, and in all three cases there was histologic involvement of the bone marrow of the laryngeal skeleton but no involvement of soft tissues and mucosa.

III. PLASMACYTOMA

A. Introduction

The neoplasms originating from plasma cells are considered and described as diseases originating both from the bone marrow (in the greatest majority of cases) and from extraskeletal sites (upper respiratory tract, GI tract, thyroid, lungs, lymph nodes). Their behavior may be benign or malignant, though the majority are malignant. Consequently, these diseases are labeled as osseous and extraosseous plasma cell tumors which may be benign or malignant, solitary or multiple, simultaneous or sequential, according to the clinicopathological characteristics.

B. Terminology and Classification

The terms adopted are numerous and among them we mention extramedullary plasmacytoma, plasmacytoma, plasma cell tumor, malignant plasmacytoma, extramedullary plasma cell tumor, secretory lymphoma, etc.

As a clear distinction between the proliferating diseases of the lymphocytic and plasmacytic lines appears to be no longer justified today, the neoplastic processes of plasma cells are included in several recent classifications of non-Hodgkin's lymphomas.

C. Incidence

Primary extraskeletal plasmacytomas are rare and many of those reported may represent a focus of extraskeletal dissemination from an occult multiple myeloma. More than 90% of the extramedullary plasmacytomas occur in the head and neck area,[40,41] and at least 75% of these develop in the upper respiratory tract.

A significant number of reports are available describing primary and secondary plasmacytomas involving the larynx. Pahor,[42] while reviewing the English literature on this subject, found 31 cases and added 1 personal case. Maniglia and Xue[43] reported 3 cases of laryngeal

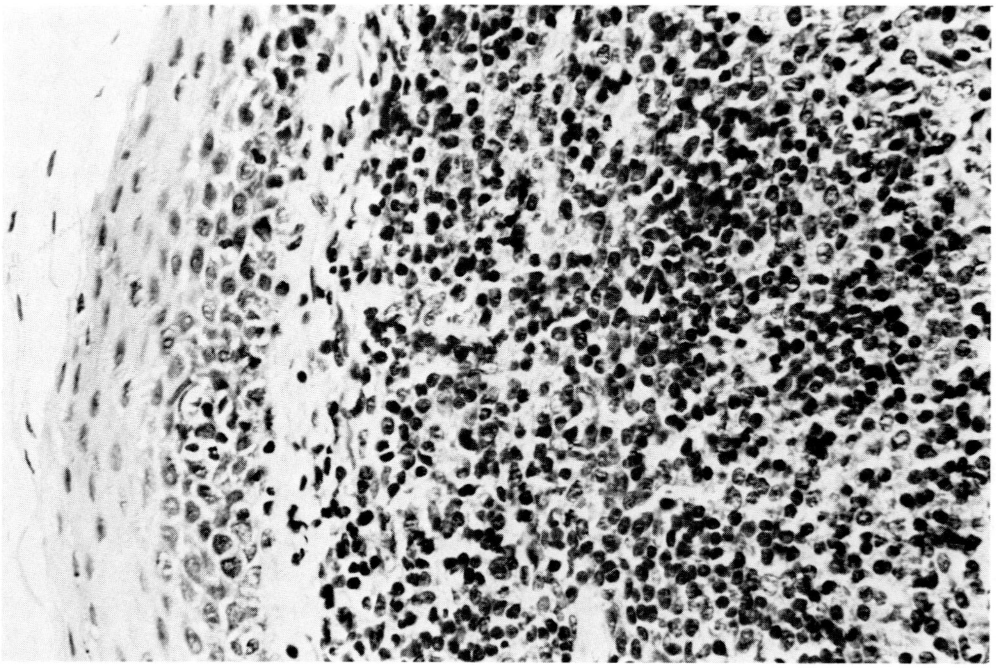

FIGURE 1. Non-Hodgkin's lymphoma. A subepithelial neoplastic infiltrate displaying a diffuse pattern of growth is characterized by small-sized lymphoid cells with hyperchromatic nuclei. (H.E.; Magnification × 100.)

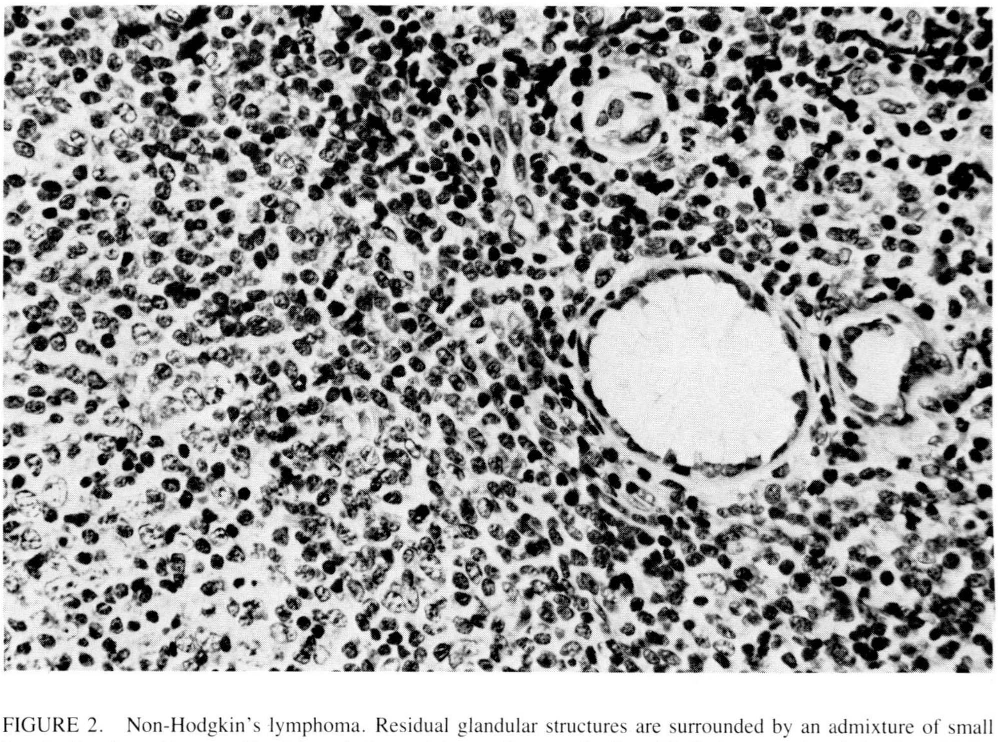

FIGURE 2. Non-Hodgkin's lymphoma. Residual glandular structures are surrounded by an admixture of small lymphoid cells and larger cells with vesicular nuclei, prominent nucleoli, and indistinct cytoplasmic borders. (H.E.; Magnification × 100.) (From Ferlito, A. et al., *ORL*, 43, 61, 1981. With permission.)

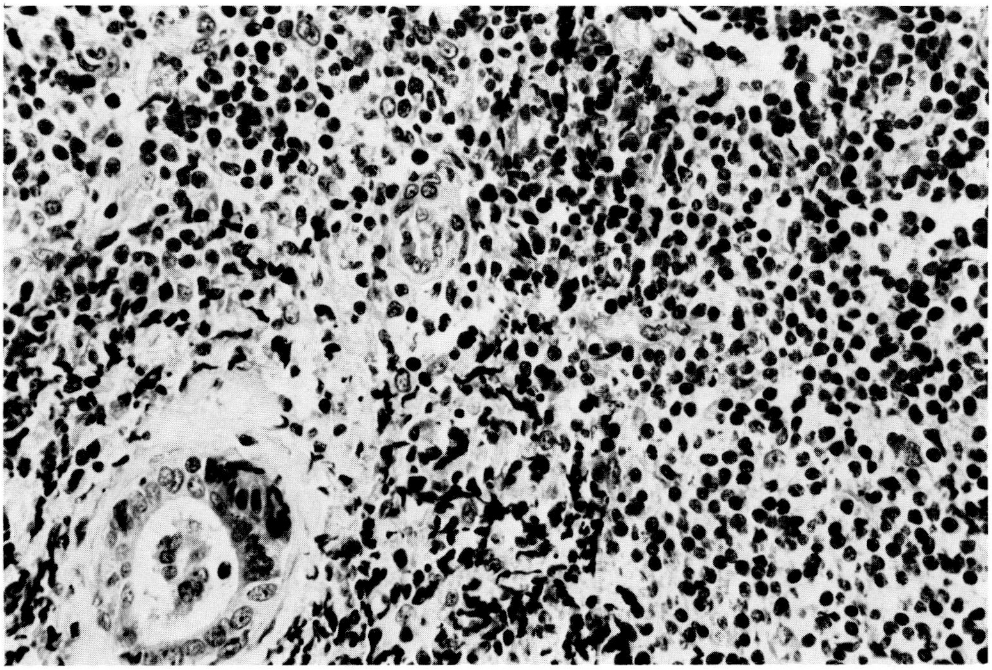

FIGURE 3. Non-Hodgkin's lymphoma. The laryngeal structures are replaced by a monotonous infiltrate consisting of small cells with hyperchromatic nuclei and scant cytoplasms. (H.E.; Magnification × 100.) (From Ferlito, A. et al., *ORL*, 43, 61, 1981. With permission.)

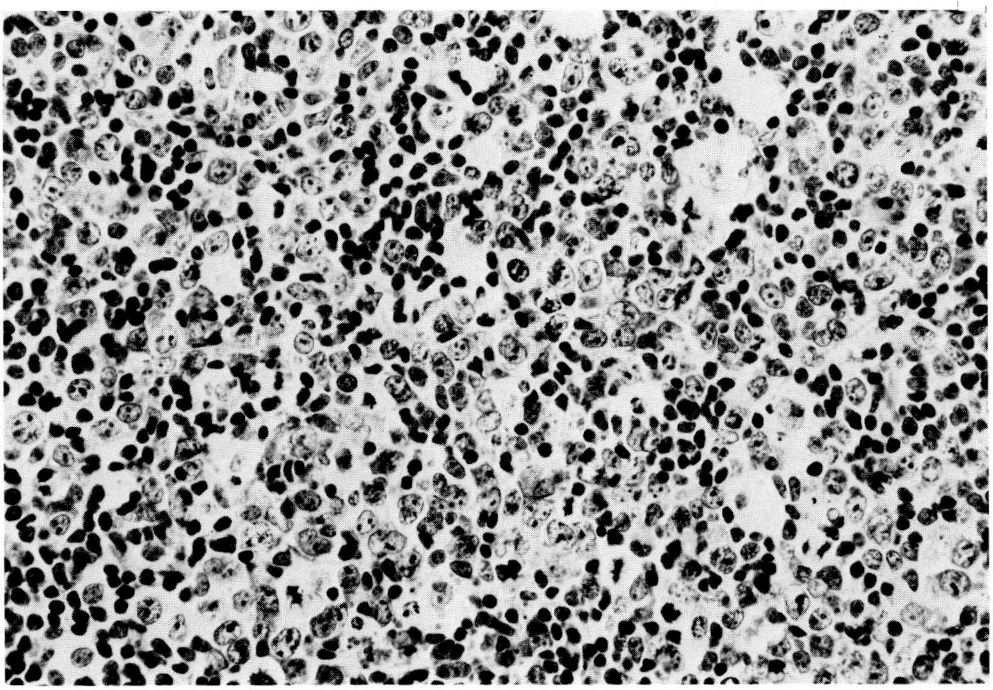

FIGURE 4. Non-Hodgkin's lymphoma. Medium-sized to large cells with round to ovoid nuclei and one to several nucleoli are numerous. (H.E.; Magnification × 100.) (From Ferlito, A. et al., *ORL*, 43, 61, 1981. With permission.)

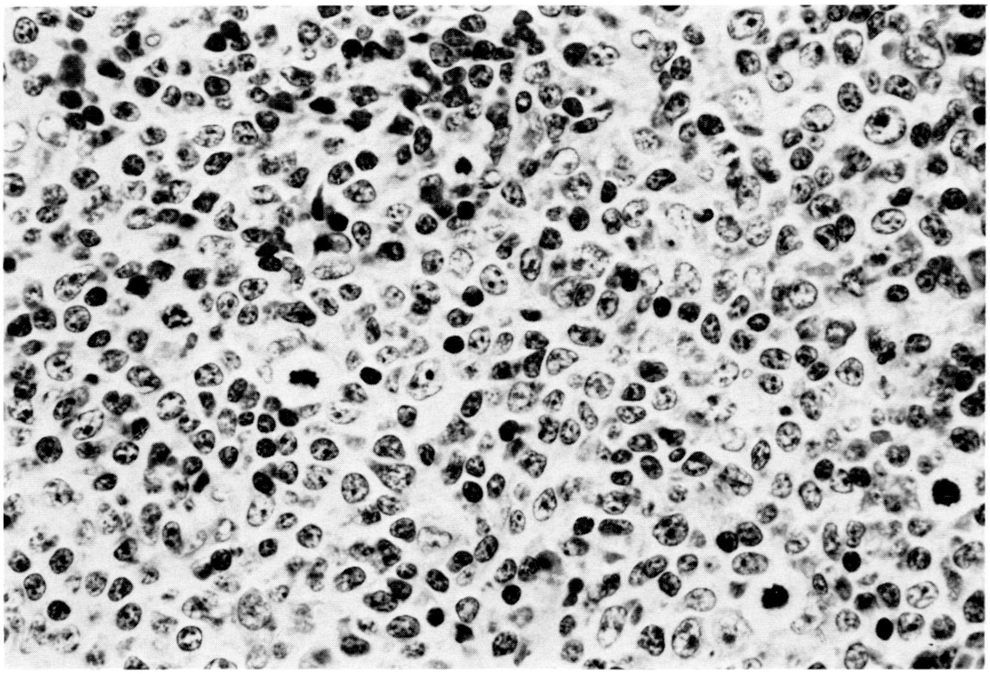

FIGURE 5. Non-Hodgkin's lymphoma. Some immunoblast-like cells are admixed with large and medium sized lymphoid cells. (H.E.; Magnification × 100.) (From Ferlito, A. et al., *ORL*, 43, 61, 1981. With permission.)

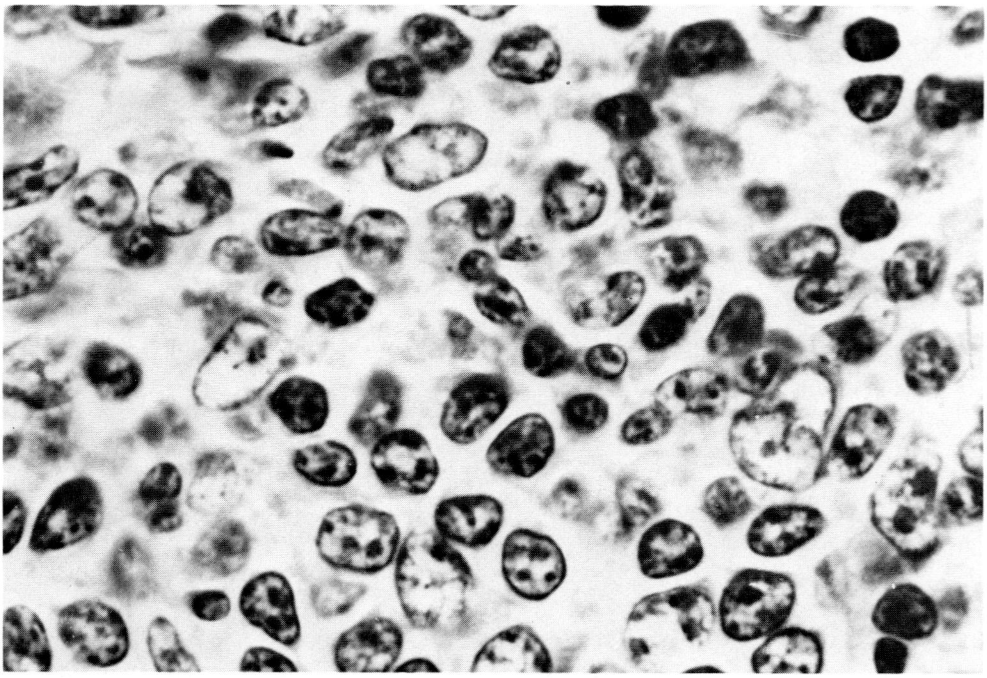

FIGURE 6. Non-Hodgkin's lymphoma. A high-power view of a neoplasm shows small angulated lymphocytes, larger cells with vesicular nuclei and some immunoblast-like cells. (H.E.; Magnification × 160.) (From Ferlito et al., *ORL*, 43, 61, 1981. With permission.)

Table 3
DIFFERENTIAL DIAGNOSTIC POSSIBILITIES OF LARYNGEAL LYMPHOMAS

Malignant conditions
Anaplastic carcinoma (oat-cell type)
Undifferentiated carcinoma (nasopharyngeal type)
Malignant melanoma
Chloroma
Plasmacytoma
Embryonal rhabdomyosarcoma
Non-neoplastic conditions
Lymphomatoid granulomatosis
Wegener's granulomatosis
Pseudolymphoma

plasmacytoma (2 cases associated with multiple myeloma and 1 considered to be solitary) and collected 79 other cases.

Actually, the cases reported in the world literature are about 100. The laryngeal localization, however, may be the sign of multiple myeloma, usually IgG or IgA and exceptionally, IgD.[44]

D. Age and Sex

The most affected age is between 40 and 60. The male to the female ratio is 2 to 3:1.

E. Site

The epiglottis and the ventricles are the most common sites, followed by the vocal cords and ventricular folds.[42]

F. Pathology

Gross pathology — The tumor may appear as a polypoid or pedunculated mass, with a smooth surface without ulceration of the mucosa. The lesion may be solitary or at times (though rarely) multiple, regardless of the fact that it may be associated or not with myeloma in other organs.

Light microscopy (Figures 7 to 11) — The tumor is composed of clusters of plasma cells, sometimes forming an alveolar arrangement, supported by a delicate stroma with numerous dilated capillaries. The tumor cells are round or oval in shape with eosinophilic cytoplasm, are hyperchromic, and are excentrically placed around nuclei displaying dense chromatin. Binucleated and multinucleated plasma cells may also be present, as well as Russell bodies. Not infrequently, an eosinophilic, amorphous, nonfibrillar substance resembling amyloid matter may be noted. Numerous giant cells of the foreign body type may be seen around these deposits.

G. Diagnosis and Differential Diagnosis

The diagnosis usually is not problematic. The neoplasm consists of pure populations of plasma cells of the Marschalkò type, which form compact sheets in a scanty connective tissue stroma. Amyloid deposits may be present.[45]

The plasmacytoma must be differentiated from anaplastic carcinoma, non-Hodgkin's lymphoma of the lymphoplasmacytic type, and plasma cell granuloma. The recognition of lymphocytes, plasmablasts, and immunoblasts represents the most important criterion in

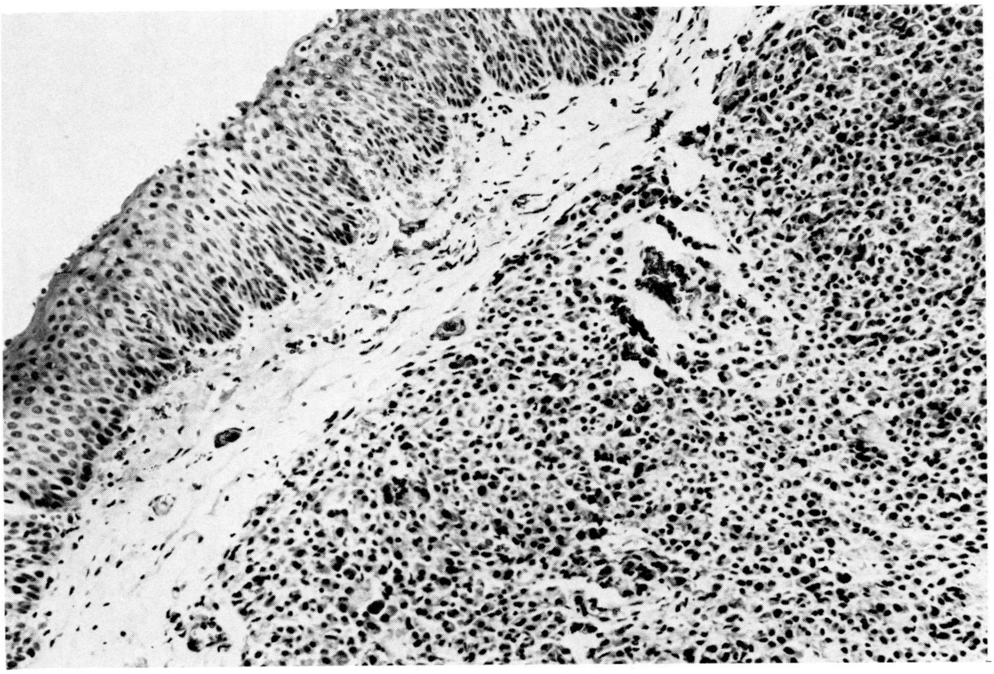

FIGURE 7. Plasmacytoma. A low-power view of a tumor shows a mucosal infiltration by polymorphous plasmacytic elements. (H.E.; Magnification × 40) (From Ferlito, A. et al., *J.Laryngol.Otol.*, 96, 759, 1982. With permission.)

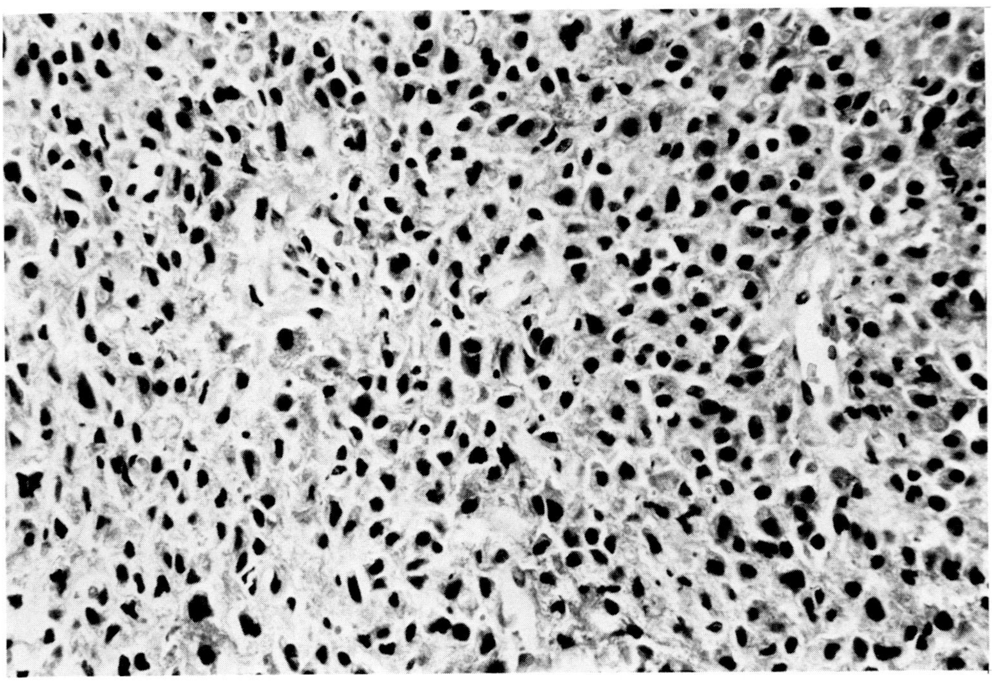

FIGURE 8. Plasmacytoma. Higher-power view showing mature and immature plasma cells. (H.E.; Magnification × 100.) (From Ferlito, A. et al., *J.Laryngol.Otol.*, 96, 579, 1982. With permission.)

preparations often reveal unrecognized lesions. The aryepiglottic folds, the epiglottis, the true and false vocal cords, and the subglottic regions are the most commonly affected sites.

Macroscopically, the lesion may be characterized by the presence of a nodular formation or edema of the affected regions. The mucosal lining is almost always intact, and becomes ulcerated only in advanced disease.

Microscopically, the laryngeal structures are infiltrated by leukemic cells, displaying different morphologic aspects according to the type of leukemia (myeloblastic, myelocytic, stem-cell, lymphocytic, or granulocytic leukemia). There is no particular type of leukemia which is more susceptible to produce lesions in the larynx.

In addition to true specific leukemic infiltrates, antileukemic treatment may cause extensive necrosis and ulcerations of the larynx.[50]

REFERENCES

1. **Freeman, C., Berg, J. W., and Cutler, S. J.,** Occurrence and prognosis of extranodal lymphomas, *Cancer,* 29, 252, 1972.

1a. **Eggston, A. A. and Wolff, O.,** *Histopathology of the Ear, Nose and Throat,* Williams & Wilkins, Baltimore, 1947.

2. **Rappaport, H.,** Tumors of the Hematopoietic System, in Atlas of Tumor Pathology, Section 3, Fascicle 8, Armed Forces Institute of Pathology, Washington, D.C., 1966.

3. **Lukes, R. J. and Collins, R. D.,** Immunologic characterization of human malignant lymphomas, *Cancer,* 34, 1488, 1974.

4. **Lukes, R. J. and Collins, R. D.,** New approaches to the classification of the lymphomata, *Br. J. Cancer,* 31(2), 1, 1975.

5. **Lukes, R. J. and Collins, R. D.,** Luke-Collins classification and its significance, *Cancer Treat. Rep.,* 61, 971, 1977.

6. **Lennert, K.,** *Malignant Lymphomas other than Hodgkin's Disease,* Springer-Verlag, N.Y., 1978.

7. **Bennett, M. H., Farrer-Brown, G., Henry, K., and Jelliffe, A. M.,** Classification of non-Hodgkin's lymphomas, *Lancet,* 2, 405, 1974.

8. **Henry, K., Bennett, M. H., and Farrer-Brown, G.,** Morphological classification of non-Hodgkin's lymphomas, *Recent Results Cancer Res.,* 64, 38, 1978.

9. **Dorfman, R. F.,** Classification of non-Hodgkin's lymphomas, *Lancet,* 1, 1295, 1974.

10. **Dorfman, R. F.,** Classifications of malignant lymphomas, *Am. J. Surg. Pathol.,* 1, 167, 1977.

11. **Dorfman, R. F.,** Pathology of the non-Hodgkin's lymphomas: new classifications, *Cancer Treat. Rep.,* 61, 945, 1977.

12. **Mathé, G., Rappaport, H., O'Conor, G. T., and Torloni, H.,** Histological and cytological typing of neoplastic disease of haematopoietic and lymphoid tissues, in International Histological Classification of Tumours, No. 14, World Health Organization, Geneva, 1976.

13. **Nathwani, B. N.,** A critical analysis of the classifications of non-Hodgkin's lymphomas, *Cancer,* 44, 347, 1979.

14. National Cancer Institute Sponsored Study of Classifications of Non-Hodgkin's Lymphomas, Summary and descriptions of a working formulation for clinical usage, *Cancer,* 49, 2112, 1982.

15. **Ferlito, A., Carbone, A., and Volpe, R.,** Diagnosis and assessment of non-Hodgkin's malignant lymphomas of the larynx, *ORL,* 43, 61, 1981.

16. **De Santo, L. W. and Weiland, L. H.,** Malignant lymphoma of the larynx, *Laryngoscope,* 80, 966, 1970.

16a. **Swerdlow, J. B., Merl, S. A., Davey, F. R., Gacek, R. R., and Gottlieb, A. J.,** Non Hodgkin's lymphoma limited to the larynx, *Cancer,* 53, 2546, 1984.

17. **Anderson, H. A., Maisel, R. H., and Cantrell, R. W.,** Isolated laryngeal lymphoma, *Laryngoscope,* 86, 1251, 1976.

18. **Gregor, R. T.,** Laryngeal malignant lymphoma. An entity? *J. Laryngol.Otol.,* 95, 81, 1981.

19. **Urabe, N.,** Malignant lymphomas of the larynx. A report of a case, *Otolaryngology,* 54, 119, 1982.

20. **Holinger, L. D., Soltes, S. F., Pellettiere, E. V., II, Delicata, D. S., and Murthy, A. K.,** The otolaryngologic manifestations of malignant lymphoma with a high content of epithelioid histiocytes (Lennert's lymphoma), *Am. J. Otolaryngol.,* 1, 229, 1980.

21. **Epstein, E. H., Jr., Levin, F. L., Croft, J. D., Jr., and Lutzner, M. A.,** Mycosis fungoides: survival, prognostic features, response to therapy, and autopsy findings, *Medicine,* 51, 61, 1972.

22. **Rappaport, H. and Thomas, L. B.,** Mycosis fungoides: the pathology of extracutaneous involvement, *Cancer,* 34, 1198, 1974.

22a. **Strahan, R. W. and Calcaterra, T. C.,** Otolaryngologic aspects of mycosis fungoides. A case report, *Laryngoscope,* 81, 1912, 1971.
23. **Hood, A. F., Mark, G. J., and Hunt, J. V.,** Laryngeal mycosis fungoides, *Cancer,* 43, 1527, 1979.
24. **Agarwal, M. K., Gupta, S., and Gupta, O. P.,** Mycosis fungoides of the larynx, *Asian Med. J.,* 25, 180, 1982.
24a. **Szmeja, Z., Obrebowski, A., and Burian, P.,** Ein Fall laryngealer Lokalisation eines sogenannten Castelman-Tumors, *HNO,* 32, 252, 1984.
24b. **Dindzans, L. J., Irvine, B. W. H., and Hayden, R. E.,** An unusual case of airway obstruction, *J.Otolaryngol.,* 13, 252, 1984.
25. **Ferlito, A.,** Histological classification of larynx and hypopharynx cancers and their clinical implications. Pathologic aspects of 2052 malignant neoplasms diagnosed at the ORL Department of Padua University from 1966 to 1976, *Acta Otolaryngol.,* Suppl. 342, 1, 1976.
26. **Saltzstein, S. L.,** Extranodal malignant lymphomas and pseudolymphomas, in *Pathology Annual,* Vol. 159, Appleton-Century-Crofts, N. Y., 1969.
27. **Barrs, D. M., McDonald, T. J., and Duffy, J.,** Sjogren's syndrome involving the larynx: report of a case, *J. Laryngol. Otol.,* 93, 933, 1979.
28. **Friedmann, I.,** The changing pattern of granulomas of the upper respiratory tract, *J. Laryngol.Otol.,* 85, 631, 1971.
29. **Howells, G. H. and Friedmann, I.,** Giant cell granuloma associated with lesions resembling polyarteritis nodosa, *J.Clin.Pathol.,* 3, 220, 1950.
30. **MacKinnon, D. M.,** Lethal midline granuloma of the face and larynx, *J.Laryngol.Otol.,* 84, 1193, 1970.
31. **Kurita, S. and Hirano, M.,** Wegener's granuloma localized in the larynx. Report of a case, *Auris, Nasus, Larynx (Tokyo),* Suppl. 10, 97, 1983.
32. **Ferlito, A., Doglioni, C., Bontempini, L., and Arrigoni, A.,** Metachronous coexistence of laryngeal pseudolymphoma and squamous cell carcinoma, An unreported case, *ORL,* 46, 202, 1984.
33. **Saraga, P., Hurlimann, J., and Ozzello, L.,** Lymphomas and pseudolymphomas of the alimentary tract. An immunohistochemical study with clinicopathologic correlations, *Hum. Pathol.,* 12, 713, 1981.
34. **Henry, K.,** Electron microscopy in the non-Hodgkin's lymphomata, *Br. J. Cancer,* 31(2), 73, 1975.
35. **Strum, S. B., Park, J. K., and Rappaport, H.,** Observations of cells resembling Sternberg-Reed cells in conditions other than Hodgkin's disease, *Cancer,* 26, 176, 1970.
36. **Lautz, H. A.,** Nasal and laryngeal involvement in abdominal Hodgkin's disease, *Arch. Otolaryngol.,* 67, 78, 1958.
37. **Ash, J. E., Beck, M. R., and Wilkes, J. D.,** Tumors of the Upper Respiratory Tract and Ear, in Atlas of Tumor Pathology, Section IV, Fascicles 12 and 13, Armed Forces Institute of Pathology, Washington, D.C.,1964.
38. **Shilling, B. B., Abell, M. R., and Work, W. P.,** Leukemic involvement of larynx, *Arch. Otolaryngol.,* 85, 658, 1967.
39. **Meyer-Breiting, E.,** Lymphogranulomatose des Kehlkopfes, *Laryngol. Rhinol. Otol.,* 54, 897, 1975.
40. **Batsakis, J. G., Friea, G. T., Goldman, R. T., and Karlsberg, R. C.,** Upper respiratory tract plasmacytoma, *Arch. Otolaryngol.,* 79, 613, 1964.
41. **Poole, A. G. and Marchetta, F. C.,** Extramedullary plasmacytoma of the head and neck, *Cancer,* 22, 14, 1968.
42. **Pahor, A.,** Plasmacytoma of the larynx, *J. Laryngol. Otol.,* 92, 223, 1978.
43. **Maniglia, A. J. and Xue, J. W.,** Plasmacytoma of the larynx, *Laryngoscope,* 93, 741, 1983.
44. **Ferlito, A., Carbone, A., Volpe, R., and Recher, G.,** Late occurrence of IgD myeloma in plasmacytoma of nasal cavity, cervical lymph node and larynx, *J.Laryngol.Otol.,* 96, 759, 1982.
45. **Michaels, L. and Hyams, V. J.,** Amyloid in localized deposits and plasmacytomas of the respiratory tract, *J. Pathol.,* 128, 29, 1979.
46. **Scott, F. E. T., Dupont, P. A., and Webb, J.,** Plasmacytoma of the stomach. Diagnosis with the aid of the immunoperoxidase technique, *Cancer,* 41, 675, 1978.
47. **Friedmann, I.and Osborn, D.A.,** The larynx, in *Systemic Pathology,* Vol. 1, 2nd ed., Symmers, W.St.C., Ed., Churchill Livingstone, Edinburgh, 1976.
48. **Ti, M., Villafuerte, R., Chase, P. H., and Dosik, H.,** Acute leukemia presenting as laryngeal obstruction, *Cancer,* 34, 427, 1974.
49. **Freeland, A. P., van Nostrand, A. W. P., and Jahn, A. F.,** Metastases to the larynx, *J. Otolaryngol.,* 8, 448, 1979.
50. **Ferlito, A. and Di Bonito, L.,** A propos d'une observation de laryngo-oesophagite ulcéro-nécrotique chez un malade atteint de leucose aiguë. Considérations étiopathogéniques, *Ann. Otolaryngol. Chir. Cervicofac.,* 91, 199, 1974.

Chapter 3

SECONDARY TUMORS OF THE LARYNX*

A. Ferlito

Secondary or metastatic tumors of the larynx are rare, in particular if laryngeal involvement in the course of systemic diseases is excluded, as in acute and chronic leukemia, Hodgkin's disease, lymphoma, and multiple myeloma, together with the involvement of the larynx by paralaryngeal or extrinsic laryngeal tumors. A few rare cases of thyroid tumors initially presenting as laryngeal problems have been reported,[1,2] but these are not to be considered as metastases.

A number of theories have been put forward to explain the rarity of secondary tumors to the larynx. In 1889, Paget[3] maintained that some tissues had a less favorable ground for neoplastic growth. In 1949, Coman et al,[4] by means of experimental studies on rabbits, excluded the hypothesis put forward by Paget and suggested as a more acceptable explanation that there were objective difficulties for neoplastic emboli to reach certain organs. This hypothesis was supported also by Loughead and Bushnell.[5] We agree with other investigators [6,7] that the rarity of the laryngeal metastases might be explained by considering the larynx as a terminal organ within the normal blood and lymph circulation.

It is widely accepted [8,9] that the number of reported cases of laryngeal metastases is lower than their actual frequency. Their true incidence might be obscured by other metastatic lesions and only a thorough autopsy examination of the larynx of patients who died of neoplastic disease would probably reveal a greater number of cases.

The first case of secondary cancer of the larynx was reported by Eppinger [10] in 1880 and concerned a malignant melanoma of the skin that had metastasized to the region above the left ventricular band. At the Mayo Clinic, from 1941 to 1971, only two cases of secondary cancers of the larynx have been seen.[7]

During the period from January 1966 through December 1983, only 4 cases of metastases in the larynx and hypopharynx from malignant melanoma have been observed at the ENT Department of Padua University in a series of 3012 primary and secondary malignant neoplasms of the larynx and hypopharynx recorded in the same period (0.13). The total number of metastatic spread to the larynx so far reported in the literature is 83.[6-8,10-64] The essential data are summarized in Table 1. It appears that there is a predilection for the male sex, with a male to female ratio of 2:1. It must be stressed that there is a different incidence in the two sexes of primary and secondary neoplasms of the larynx. The median age is 58 years, with a variability range between 24 to 83 years.

Malignant melanoma of the skin is the neoplasm most frequently metastasizing to the larynx (Figures 1 to 5). In fact, in 25 (30.1%) of the 83 cases, it was the primary neoplasm. Malignant melanoma forms 1.2% of all malignant neoplasms and is responsible for 0.74% of all deaths due to neoplasm.[9] Malignant melanoma may metastasize via the bloodstream and lymphatic channels to distant organs, including heart and skeletal muscle, which are only rarely affected by metastatic spread. A lower tendency to metastasize to the larynx characterizes the renal adenocarcinoma (or hypernephroma): 12 of the 83 reported cases with an incidence of 14.5%. This neoplasm may metastasize to all organs with a predilection, in decreasing order, for lungs, lymph nodes, liver, bones and adrenal glands. The incidence of secondaries from bronchial cancer was 10.8%, mammary cancer was 10.8%, and prostatic cancer was 6%. In Table 2 the 83 cases of metastases to the larynx are analyzed in relation

* This chapter is based on the paper by Ferlito, A. and Caruso, G., Secondary malignant melanoma of the larynx. Report of two cases and review of 79 laryngeal secondary cancers, *ORL*, 46, 117, 1984.

to the site of the primary neoplasm and oncotype. Only rarely are metastases to the larynx caused by mesenchymal tumors (5 cases). An exceptional instance is that of metastasis to the larynx from a neuroblastoma.[52]

From the data collected, the supraglottic region appears to be the most affected site. In fact, it is involved in 27 of 67 documented cases (40.3%). Another fairly frequent possibility is the simultaneous involvement of multiple laryngeal location, an occurrence seen in 23 cases (34.3%).

As to frequency, the subglottic region follows (12 cases out of 67, with a percentage of 17.9). Definitely less common is the occurrence of metastases to the glottic space (only 4 cases, with an incidence of 6%). In one case only was the metastasis located in the lateral wall of the hypopharynx. The more abundant vascularization, both hematic and lymphatic, of the supra- and subglottic region helps in understanding the different distribution. Furthermore, the epiglottis is the laryngeal cartilage offering less resistance to metastatic spread. The ossified cartilages are more easily invaded by metastatic tumors.[65] In contrast, the perichondrium [46] acts as a barrier against metastatic spread.

Symptoms of metastatic tumors of the larynx are not different from those of primary tumors and vary according to the site affected. Among the cases reported, some were asymptomatic, and the discovery of the laryngeal involvement was an autopsy finding.[8,32,37,46]

In other cases[29,39,41,57] however, the laryngeal location was the first symptom reported by the patient and led to the discovery of the primary neoplasm, which otherwise might have gone undetected. Beside hoarseness and dysphagia, hemoptysis is an important symptom of laryngeal metastasis from renal adenocarcinoma because of the abundant vascularization of the tumor.[41,60]

Neoplastic dissemination to the larynx occurs via the bloodstream, through lymphatic or the hemolymphatic circulation. Via the bloodstream, spread takes place through systemic circulation. This is the ‘‘vena cava’’ type of metastatic spread described by Walther:[25] inferior vena cava, right heart, lungs, left heart, aorta, external carotid artery, upper thyroid artery, upper laryngeal artery. The retrograde circulation through the vertebral venous plexus, which helps to explain some obscure cases of metastases also has considerable importance. In such cases, the pulmonary organ system is by-passed and the metastases to the head and neck develop without lung involvement (as described by Batson[66]) on the pattern of metastatic spread of prostatic adenocarcinoma. Anastomoses of vertebral veins and intercostal veins explain the metastases from breast cancer. Fisher and Fisher[67] have demonstrated that neoplastic emboli may, through the lymphatic system, by-pass all lymph node stations and enter the thoracic duct. In 1955, Zeidman [68] maintained that effluent lymphatic vessels connected the thoracic duct with the mediastinal, intercostal, and supraclavicular lymph nodes. The connections between supraclavicular and subglottic lymph vessels allow an understanding of the metastatic spread to the larynx through lymphatics.

Also, the metastases from neoplasm of the nasopharynx (one case) and from ovarian carcinoma (one case) may be explained by lymphatic dissemination. In the first instance, a retrograde flow from the internal jugular lymph node draining both nasopharynx and the supraglottic region may be suggested. Ovarian carcinoma may, in turn, spread to the larynx through the paraaortic, mediastinal, and paratracheal lymph nodes. The same pathway is suggested by Oku et al.[61] to explain laryngeal metastases from pancreatic carcinoma.

According to Freeland et al.,[8] even though dissemination through lymphatics follows a more orderly progression as compared with metastatic spread via the bloodstream, both modalities have the same possibilities of favoring tumor spread to the larynx. The mainly hematic or lymphohematic pathogenesis of laryngeal metastases is explained by their location, which is mainly submucosal.

At any rate, laryngeal involvement is bound to be more frequent in the terminal stages of a neoplastic disease, when other organs have been invaded, or diffuse carcinomatosis is present. However, an isolated metastatic deposit to the larynx can occur [7,45] and ought to be carefully evaluated. Treatment of a secondary lesion of the larynx is in fact justified when other organs have not yet been affected. In this case, partial or total laryngectomy may be performed, or radiotherapy or combination chemotherapy may be given.

Prognosis is almost generally unfavorable in the short term. There are unusual cases such as those reported by Chamberlain[44] and by Glanz and Kleinsasser[57] describing metastases from malignant melanoma of the skin and from embryonal carcinoma of testis, which at 6 years from the diagnosis of laryngeal involvement had remained free of recurrence to the larynx and of other metastases.

The histopathological differential diagnosis may be difficult. Metastases of a renal adenocarcinoma must be distinguished from the primary clear-cell carcinoma of the larynx.[69,70] Stains for glycogen and lipids are usually positive in the cells of renal adenocarcinoma, and histochemical stains with PAS, DPAS, Best's carmine, Oil Red and Sudan black may therefore assist in establishing the correct diagnosis.[71] Metastases from amelanotic malignant melanoma may be mistaken for anaplastic carcinoma. Finally, primary malignant melanoma of the larynx has to be distinguished from its secondary location in the same organ. The existence of primary laryngeal melanoma is well known.[72-80] It may develop from melanocytes present in the laryngeal mucosa.[81-84]

Though metastases to the larynx of malignant melanoma are rare, this possibility has to be borne in mind by the otolaryngologist in regard to patients with laryngeal symptoms. Shaheen[39] believes that even in the absence of a clinically detectable primary melanoma elsewhere, this can be the cause of metastatic melanoma in the larynx. The biological behavior of this neoplasm is in fact unpredictable as the lesion may metastasize at variable time intervals and also after the successful treatment of the primary neoplasm. Some melanomas may be self-eliminating. However, the clinical disappearance of the primary neoplasm does not prevent the production of distant metastases. It is then most probable that malignant melanomas of the larynx described as primary tumors are actually to be considered as secondary. It is important to demonstrate junctional activity for a diagnosis of primary malignant melanoma.[78]

In neoplastic patients and in particular in those "at risk" because of malignant melanoma of the skin or renal adenocarcinoma, it is important to perform routine indirect laryngoscopy. This is a simple investigation which, as Freeland et al.[8] have pointed out, should be part of the "metastatic" screening of all cancer patients, in particular if a curative treatment of the primary lesion is to be done.

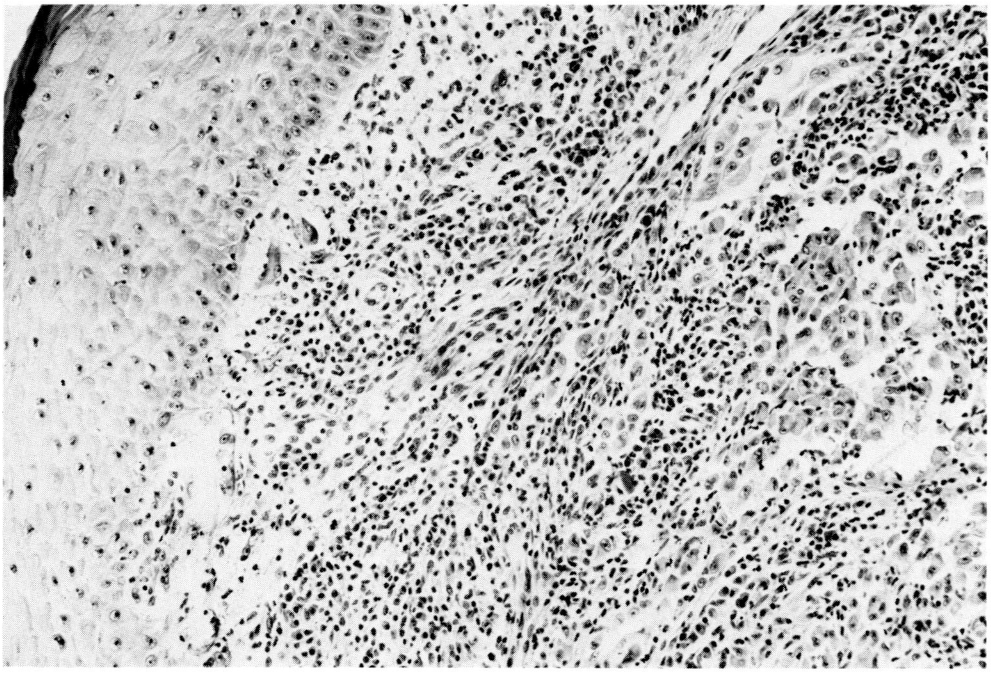

FIGURE 1. Larynx. Metastatic malignant melanoma from the skin of the cheek to larynx. Junctional nesting of the melanoma cells are not present. (H.E.; Magnification × 40.)

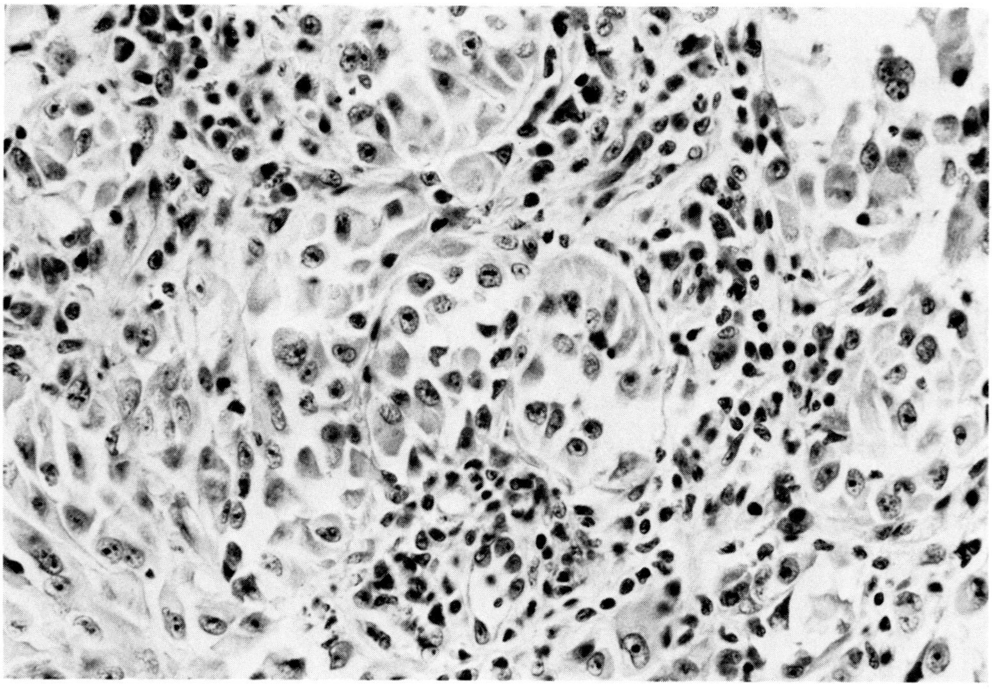

FIGURE 2. Larynx. Another area of the same tumor. Note the typical pattern of the neoplasm. (H.E.; Magnification × 100.)

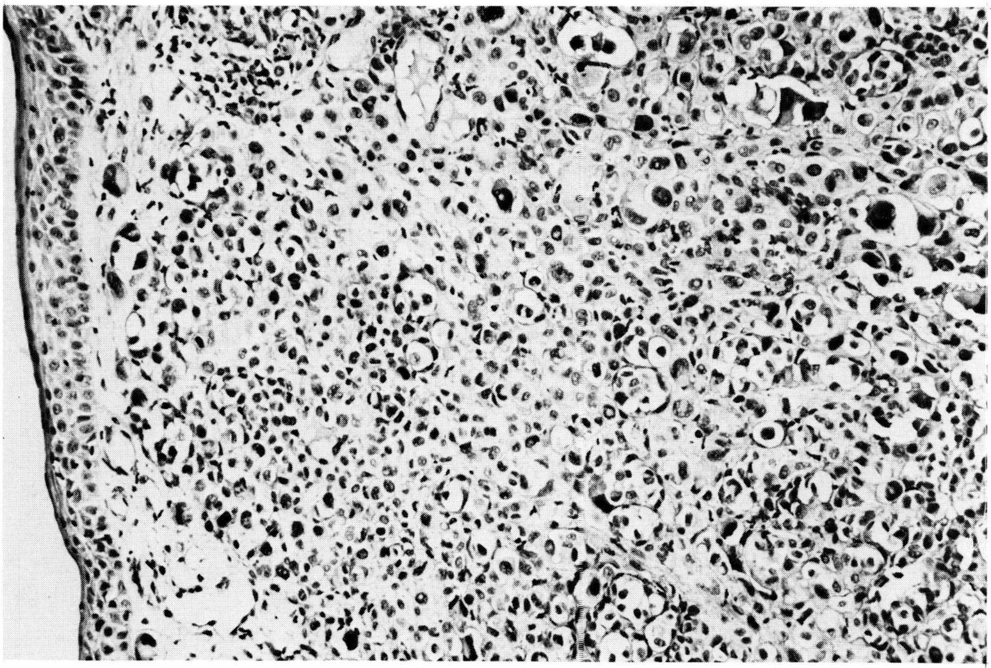

FIGURE 3. Larynx. Malignant melanoma of the medium third of the right leg to larynx. Junctional activity is absent. (H.E.; Magnification × 40.)

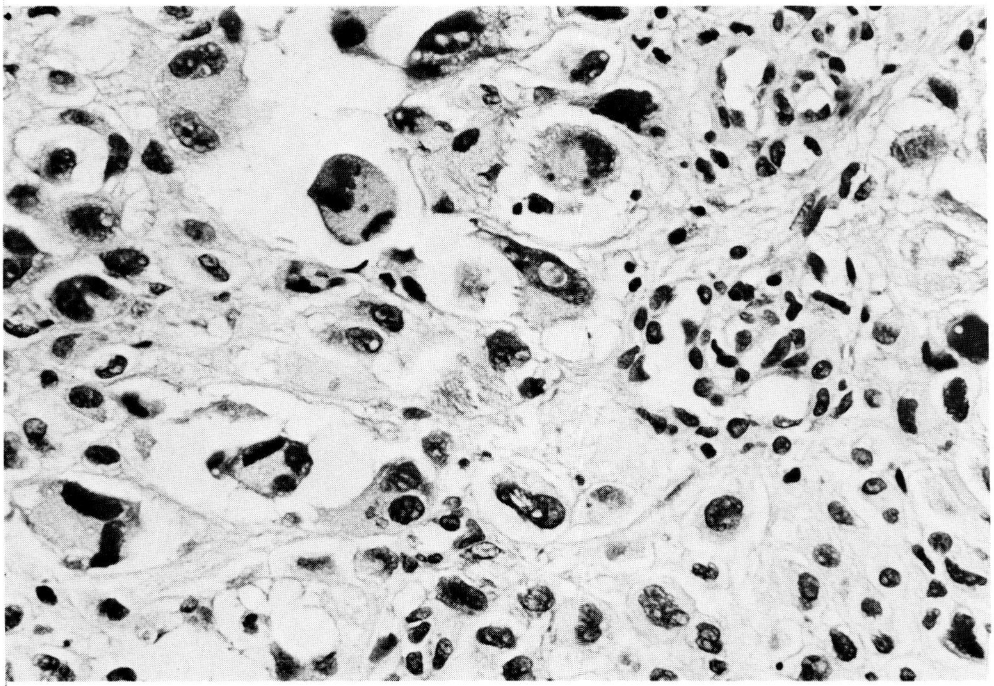

FIGURE 4. Larynx. Same case of Figure 3. Great cellular pleomorphism is present. Note the large and multinucleated giant cells. (H.E.; Magnification × 100.)

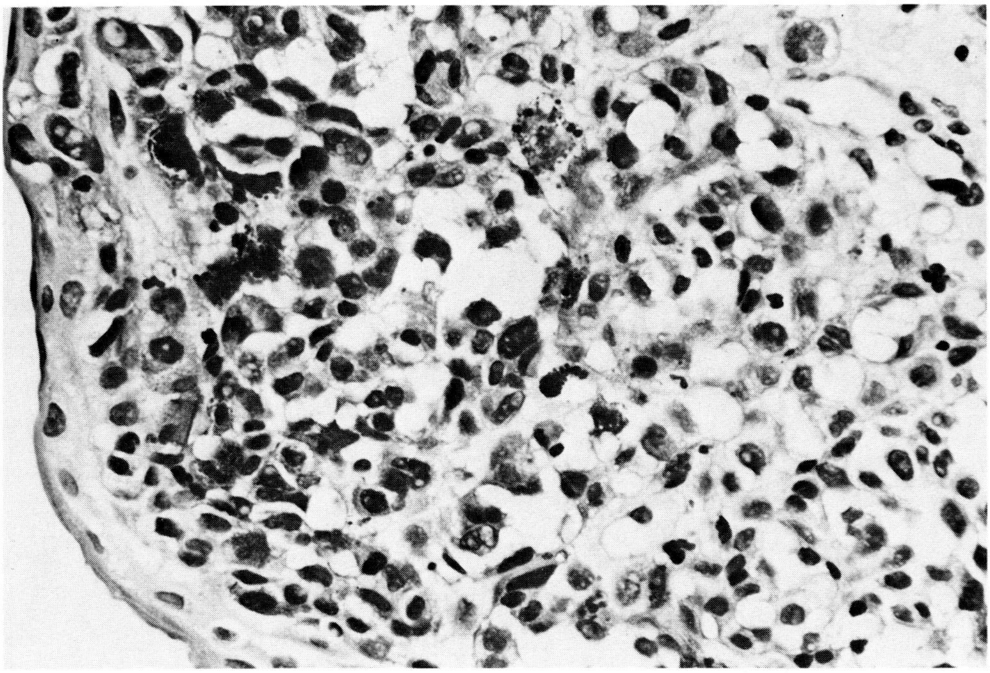

FIGURE 5. Larynx. Same case as Figure 3. Note the pigmented tumor melanocytes. (H.E.; Magnification × 100.)

Table 1
LARYNGEAL METASTASES

Age	Sex	Location of primary neoplasm	Histologic type	Location of laryngeal metastasis	Symptoms	Time interval between diagnosis of primary neoplasm and laryngeal symptoms	Treatment of laryngeal metastasis	Metastases to other organs	Follow-up	Remarks	Ref.
		Skin	Malignant melanoma	Above the left ventricular band							10
		Esophagus	Carcinoma	Vocal cords							11
		Bone		Ventricular band							12
52	M	Skin	Malignant melanoma	Subglottic region				Scalp and oropharynx			13
49	M	Skin	Malignant melanoma	Epiglottis, true and false vocal cords							
50	M	Skin	Malignant melanoma	Epiglottis			Excision at indirect laryngoscopy				
78	M	Skin	Malignant melanoma	Right aryepiglottic fold			Excision				
48	M	Skin	Malignant melanoma	Right hemilarynx			Excision				
		Kidney	Adenocarcinoma							Author failed to specify the exact site of the secondary laryngeal tumor	14
		Breast									
		Prostate									16
		Stomach									17

Table 1 (continued)
LARYNGEAL METASTASES

Age	Sex	Location of primary neoplasm	Histologic type	Location of laryngeal metastasis	Symptoms	Time interval between diagnosis of primary neoplasm and laryngeal symptoms	Treatment of laryngeal metastasis	Metastases to other organs	Follow-up	Remarks	Ref.
		Kidney	Adenocarcinoma	Right ventricle invading the ventricular band							
54	M	Stomach	Adenocarcinoma	Subglottic region			Total laryngectomy	Thyroid			
52	M	Kidney	Adenocarcinoma	Subglottic region below right vocal cord	Hoarseness			Thyroid, liver, pancreas, adrenals, regional lymph nodes, lungs		Autopsy disclosed the primary tumor	18
63	M	Skin	Malignant melanoma	Subglottic region		6 months		Lungs			19
52	M	Lung	Carcinoma		Dyspnea		Radiotherapy				
63	M	Mediastinum	Sarcoma	Subglottic region				Lungs			21
		Breast									22
63	M	Kidney	Adenocarcinoma	Epiglottis	Dysphagia	6 years	Radiotherapy and excision			1 year and 6 months after removal of laryngeal neoplasm, there were no other metastases	23
67	M	Kidney	Adenocarcinoma	Posterior wall of the larynx	Hoarseness						24
74	M	Kidney	Adenocarcinoma	Left arytenoid	Hoarseness, dysphagia						

49	F	Lung	Adenocarcinoma	Right Arytenoid			Hemilaryngectomy, radiotherapy	Thyroid			25
39	M	Adrenal	Sympathicoblastoma	Epiglottis, left aryepiglottic fold	Hoarseness, dysphagia			Kidney, lumbosacral muscles, cauda equina, cervical, hilar and lumbo-sacral lymph nodes	Died 11 months after laryngeal symptoms	Primary neoplasm diagnosed at autopsy	26
64	M	Kidney	Sarcoma	Subglottic region							27
63	F	Skin	Malignant melanoma	Right vocal cord	Hoarseness, mild dyspnea	1 year	Removal of right true and false vocal cords through laryngofissure, radiotherapy, total laryngectomy, and removal of the upper end of the esophagus after 1 year 5 months	Skin, cervical esophagus		In the interval between excision of primary tumor and hospital admission for laryngeal symptoms, 63 metastatic lesions (malignant melanoma) occured in the subcutaneous tissues	
68	M	Skin	Malignant melanoma	Left true vocal cord	Hoarseness		Removal at direct laryngoscopy	Right supraclavicular and axillary lymph nodes, occipital bone	Alive, without laryngeal recurrences at 3 months 10 days from removal of laryngeal lesion	Primary lesion was discovered after laryngeal metastasis	29
		Retroperitoneum	Sarcoma								30
46	F	Skin	Malignant melanoma	Left arytenoid	Dysphagia	2 years	Radiotherapy roentgen irradiation of the hypophysis	Liver, left lung 6 and 7 months respectively, after laryngeal diagnosis	Died about 9 months after laryngeal diagnosis	Autopsy not performed	31
72	M	Lung	Anaplastic carcinoma	Cricoid and thyroid cartilages				Peribronchial lymph nodes, bones, liver, diaphragm	Died 7 months after onset of symptoms	Author also reports 3 cases of laryngeal metastases from mul-	32

Table 1 (continued)
LARYNGEAL METASTASES

Age	Sex	Location of primary neoplasm	Histologic type	Location of laryngeal metastasis	Symptoms	Time interval between diagnosis of primary neoplasm and laryngeal symptoms	Treatment of laryngeal metastasis	Metastases to other organs	Follow-up	Remarks	Ref.
49	M	Lung	Anaplastic carcinoma	Cricoid and thyroid cartilages				Vertebral bodies, lungs, liver, stomach, brain	Died 5 months after diagnosis of primary neoplasm	tiple myeloma (1 case) and from chronic myelogenous leukemia (2 cases)	
70	M	Prostate	Adenocarcinoma	Cricoid and thyroid cartilages				Bones, liver, adrenals, lungs	Died 4 years after diagnosis of primary neoplasm	Laryngeal involvement was disclosed only by histologic examination following 100 consecutive autopsies of patients who died of neoplastic disease. In all cases bony metaplasia of laryngeal cartilages was present	
42	F	Breast	Anaplastic carcinoma	Cricoid and thyroid cartilages				Lymph nodes, bones, liver, kidney	Died 2 years, 2 months after radical mastectomy		
60	F	Breast	Anaplastic carcinoma	Cricoid and thyroid cartilages				Bones, lymph nodes, liver, brain	Died 1 year 6 months after radical mastectomy		

72	M	Skin	Malignant melanoma	Epiglottis			Total laryngectomy				33
49	M	Kidney	Adenocarcinoma	Anterior commissure	Hoarseness, sensation of a lump in the throat	5 months	Excision at indirect laryngoscopy		Alive, without recurrence at 6 months from removal of laryngeal lesion	Right nephrectomy was made	34
66	F	Breast	Carcinoma	Right vocal cord, right laryngeal ventricle, right pyriform sinus, cricoid and thyroid cartilages	Hoarseness	3 years 2 months	Radiotherapy (5685 R)	Bones (pelvis and probably spine	No evidence of laryngeal recurrence after nearly 3 years	Favorable response to radiotherapy	35
83	M	Prostate	Adenocarcinoma	Left arytenoid	Pain in the throat radiated to the left ear	Simultaneous				Few months before admission, the patient had symptoms of urinary obstruction	6
74	M	Prostate	Adenocarcinoma	Thyroid cartilage	Hoarseness, mass in the midanterior cervical region	Simultaneous					
		Lung	Carcinoma								36
72	F	Gallbladder	Carcinoma	Thyroid, cricoid, and arythenoid cartilages	Laryngeal pain			Left subclavicular lymph nodes, liver, rectum, periadrenal fat, bones, brain, spleen	Died 3 months after onset of laryngeal symptoms	Autopsy disclosed primary tumor Laryngeal cartilages were wholly ossified in all cases	
73	F	Breast	Carcinoma	Thyroid, cricoid, and arytenoid cartilages				Mediastinum, lungs, adrenals, kidneys, liver, bones	Died nearly 4 years after radical mastectomy		
38	M	Lung	Anaplastic carcinoma	Thyroid and cricoid cartilages	Laryngeal pain nearly 9 months			Pericardium, mediastinum	Died 10 months after diagnosis of primary tumor		

Table 1 (continued)
LARYNGEAL METASTASES

Age	Sex	Location of primary neoplasm	Histologic type	Location of laryngeal metastasis	Symptoms	Time interval between diagnosis of primary neoplasm and laryngeal symptoms	Treatment of laryngeal metastasis	Metastases to other organs	Follow-up	Remarks	Ref.
64	M	Lung	Epidermoid carcinoma	Thyroid, cricoid, and arytenoid cartilages	Laryngeal pain			Peribronchial and peritracheal lymph nodes, bones, liver	Died 2 years from diagnosis of primary tumor		
38	M	Skin	Malignant melanoma	Epiglottis, aryepiglottic fold, hypopharynx				Skin, lungs, liver, spleen, testis, heart, adrenals	Died 1 year after removal of primary tumor	Laryngeal location was disclosed at autopsy	
24	M	Testis	Seminoma	Right false vocal cord	Hoarseness	13 months	Excision at indirect laryngoscopy	Skin	Died 1 year 10 months from left orchiectomy		38
65	M	Eye	Amelanotic malignant melanoma	Left arytenoid, left false vocal cord	Hoarseness		Removal at direct laryngoscopy, lateral neck dissection, radiotherapy to larynx and neck (3000 R)	Lymph nodes, skin, mediastinum, heart, pancreas	Died 5 years 9 months after diagnosis of the laryngeal metastasis	Laryngeal symptoms occurred 3 years prior to discovery of primary neoplasm; no liver metastases; no evidence of laryngeal lesion at autopsy	39
70	F	Skin	Malignant melanoma	Right true and false vocal cords	Hoarseness, dyspnea	Nearly 8 years	Radiotherapy (750 R, 6MeV)	Skin	Died 3 months after laryngeal diagnosis		40
60	F	Kidney	Adenocarcinoma	Left aryepiglottic fold	Melena, hemoptisis, vomiting of blood		Removal at direct laryngoscopy	Adrenals	Alive without signs of other metastases 2 years 9 months from nephrectomy	Laryngeal involvement seen before diagnosis of primary tumor; 18 years earlier patient underwent radical mastectomy	41

										for solid Ca. of right breast	
38	F	Breast	Ductal carcinoma	Right false vocal cord	Hoarseness, dyspnea, dysphagia	4 months	Removal at direct laryngoscopy, radiotherapy	Axillary lymph nodes, lungs			42
59	M	Skin	Amelanotic malignant melanoma	Epiglottis, left false vocal cord	Dry cough, dyspnea, hoarseness	Some years	Total laryngectomy, radical neck dissection, radiotherapy	Skin (dorsum and left ear)lymph nodes	Died 1 year after surgery (probably of disseminated disease)		43
55	M	Skin	Malignant melanoma	Right arytenoid, right true and false vocal cords	Hoarseness laryngeal dyspnea	14 years	Radiotherapy (6000 rad)	Axillary lymph nodes, skin	At 6 years no laryngeal recurrence or evidence of distant metastases		44
61	F	Kidney	Adenocarcinoma	Subglottic region	Sore throat, hoarseness, choking spasms	1 year	Removal at direct laryngoscopy		Alive at 5 months from laryngeal recurrence and at 2 years from renal surgery	Laryngeal recurrence 4 months later (right ventricular band); this case represents an example of isolated solitary metastatic spread	45
81	F	Breast	Ductal carcinoma	Cricoid, thyroid, arytenoid cartilages				Left axillary lymph nodes, lungs, pleura, liver, perihepatic lymph nodes, spleen, bones, adrenals	Died 20 hours after admission	Laryngeal infiltration stopped abruptly at the perichondrium without invading the surrounding soft tissues; patient was asymptomatic	46
60	M	Lung	Oat cell carcinoma	Right true and false vocal cords	Hoarseness dry cough	Simultaneous	Radiotherapy		Died 6 months after laryngeal diagnosis		
		Skin	Malignant melanoma								
		Jaw	**Sarcoma**								49
		Kidney	**Adenocarcinoma**								50
75	**M**	**Colon**	**Adenocarcinoma**	Subglottic region	Hoarseness,	2 years 1 month	Radiotherapy		At 6 months	Clinical examina-	7

Table 1 (continued)
LARYNGEAL METASTASES

Age	Sex	Location of primary neoplasm	Histologic type	Location of laryngeal metastasis	Symptoms	Time interval between diagnosis of primary neoplasm and laryngeal symptoms	Treatment of laryngeal metastasis	Metastases to other organs	Follow-up	Remarks	Ref.
					stridor		(6000 rad)		from radiotherapy no residual disease or laryngeal recurrence	tion and laboratory tests did not reveal other metastases	
79	M	Kidney	Adenocarcinoma	Right aryepiglottic fold	Intermittent dysphagia, hoarseness, choking sensations	17 years	Removal at direct laryngoscopy		Died 6 months after laryngeal diagnosis from cardiac decompensation		51
51	F	Nose	Esthesioneuroblastoma	Subglottic region	Laryngeal dyspnea	13 years	Radiotherapy	Cervical lymph nodes, ribs		Very favorable response to radiotherapy	52
		Breast	Carcinoma							Authors reported only one case of laryngeal secondary tumor observed in the last 30 years in the collection of the Institute Gustave-Roussy	53
		Colon	Adenocarcinoma								54
		Colon	Adenocarcinoma								
55	M	Lung	Epidermoid carcinoma	Subglottic region	Dyspnea, hemoptisis	3 years 4 months	Radiotherapy (6000 rad)		Died about 1 year after laryngeal diagnosis; no evidence of laryngeal recurrence		55
36	F	Skin	Malignant melanoma	Left aryepiglottic fold	Hoarseness, sensation of a lump in the throat	10 months	Radiotherapy				56

35	M	Testis	Embryonal carcinoma	Epiglottis	Dysphagia	4 years	Removal at direct laryngoscopy radiotherapy (3500 R)		At 6 years absence of local recurrence and metastases		57
40	M	Skin	Malignant melanoma	Left false vocal cord	Hoarseness	5 years	Immunotherapy	Lymph nodes	Died 4 months after laryngeal diagnosis	Autopsy not performed	
68	M	Prostate	Adenocarcinoma	Epiglottis	Hoarseness		Removal at direct laryngoscopy radiotherapy	Liver, hypophysis, soft tissues	Died 9 months after laryngeal diagnosis of complication following surgery for perforated gastric ulcer	First symptoms due to secondary laryngeal location; No sign of laryngeal lesion at autopsy	
58	F	Uterus (cervix)	Carcinoma	Right arytenoid, cricoid region, laryngeal ventricle, pyriform sinus, cervical esophagus	Dyspnea, dysphagia	5 years 4 months	Total laryngectomy	Cervical lymph nodes, lungs (from uterine Ca. or follicular Ca. of the thyroid?)	Died 5 months after surgery	Patient underwent arytenoidopexy and hemicordectomy for bilateral recurrent palsy; lesion was associated with follicular Ca. of the thyroid; autopsy not performed	
57	M	Trachea	Oat cell carcinoma	Subglottic region	Dyspnea, dysphagia	2 years 2 months	Radiotherapy (4000 rad) chemotherapy	Liver, esophagus, lymph nodes, pancreas, brain	Died 3 months after laryngeal diagnosis		58
		Skin	Malignant melanoma	Aryepiglottic fold						Authors observed only one case of laryngeal metastasis from 1957 to 1973	59
43	F	Skin	Malignant melanoma	Left aryepiglottic fold, epiglottis, subglottic region				Widespread systemic dissemination (skin, lungs, brain)		Authors report also 1 case of infiltration of the larynx by acute myeloblastic leukemia	8
54	F	Ovary	Cystadenocarcinoma	Subglottic region				Lungs, liver, lymph nodes			
57	M	Nasopharynx	Carcinoma	Supraglottic region, pyriform sinus				Cervical lymph nodes, liver, bones, lungs			

Table 1 (continued)
LARYNGEAL METASTASES

Age	Sex	Location of primary neoplasm	Histologic type	Location of laryngeal metastasis	Symptoms	Time interval between diagnosis of primary neoplasm and laryngeal symptoms	Treatment of laryngeal metastasis	Metastases to other organs	Follow-up	Remarks	Ref.
55	F	Kidney	Adenocarcinoma	Epiglottis	Hemoptisis	5 months		Brain, lungs		Brain metastasis allowed detection of the primary neoplasm	60
70	M	Pancreas	Pleomorphic carcinoma	Epiglottis	Cough, sore throat, bloody sputum		Supraglottic laryngectomy, left suprahyoid and right radical neck dissection	Lymph nodes, carcinomatous peritonitis	Died 1 month after admission	Primary neoplasm was found only at autopsy	61
		Scalp-face	Angiosarcoma								62
		Skin	Malignant melanoma							There was secondary tumor even on base of the tongue	63
75	F	Skin	Malignant melanoma	Epiglottis, pharyngeal wall, left false vocal cord	Hoarseness	2 years, 8 months	Radiotherapy (6000 R)		Alive. No dysphagia or dyspnea are present	No other metastases found	64
60	M	Skin	Malignant melanoma	Epiglottis, right false vocal cord	Symptomless	10 months		Lymph nodes of the groin, skin, lungs, bones	Died 3 months after laryngeal diagnosis	Hemoptisis due to lung metastasis. Autopsy not performed.	
54	F	Skin	Malignant melanoma	Hypopharynx	Symptomless	13 years		Widespread systemic dissemination	Died 4 months after hypopharyngeal diagnosis		
52	M	Skin	Malignant melanoma	Interarytenoid region	Dysphagia	14 years	Excision	Submandibular lymph node	Alive at 1 year, 3 months from removal of laryngeal lesion		

Table 2
ANALYSIS OF 83 CASES OF LARYNGEAL METASTASES WITH REGARD TO PRIMARY TUMOR

Site of primary tumor	Histologic type		Cases	Incidence %
Skin	Malignant melanoma		25	30.1
Eye	Malignant melanoma		1	1.2
Kidney	Adenocarcinoma (hypernephroma)		12	14.5
	Sarcoma		1	1.2
Lung	Carcinoma NOS	2		
	Anaplastic carcinoma	3		
	Epidermoid carcinoma	2	9	10.8
	Adenocarcinoma	1		
	Oat cell carcinoma	1		
Breast	Carcinoma NOS	3		10.8
	Anaplastic carcinoma	2	9	
	Ductal carcinoma	2		
	?	2		
Prostate	Adenocarcinoma	4	5	6.0
	?	1		
Colon	Adenocarcinoma		3	3.6
Stomach	Adenocarcinoma	1	2	2.4
	?	1		
Testis	Seminoma	1	2	2.4
	Embryonal carcinoma	1		
Nose	Esthesioneuroblastoma		1	1.2
Nasopharynx	Carcinoma NOS		1	1.2
Trachea	Oat cell carcinoma		1	1.2
Esophagus	Carcinoma NOS		1	1.2
Gallbladder	Carcinoma NOS		1	1.2
Pancreas	Pleomorphic carcinoma		1	1.2
Uterine cervix	Carcinoma NOS		1	1.2
Ovary	Cystadenocarcinoma		1	1.2
Adrenal gland	Sympathicoblastoma		1	1.2
Scalp-face	Angiosarcoma		1	1.2
Jaw	Sarcoma		1	1.2
Mediastinum	Sarcoma		1	1.2
Retroperitoneum	Sarcoma		1	1.2
Bone	?		1	1.2

REFERENCES

1. **Thinakkal, R., Cabel, G., and Borkenhagen, R.,** Medullary carcinoma of the thyroid as a laryngeal problem, *Laryngoscope,* 89, 283, 1979.
2. **Sweeney, E. C., McDonnell, L., and O'Brien, C.,** Medullary carcinoma of the thyroid presenting as tumours of the pharynx and larynx, *Histopathology,* 5, 263, 1981.
3. **Paget, S.,** 1889, Quoted by **Mazzarella, L. A., Pina, L. H., and Wolff, D.,** Asymptomatic metastasis to the larynx, *Laryngoscope,* 76, 1547, 1966.
4. **Coman, D. F., Eisenberg, R. B., and McCutcheon, M.,** Factors affecting the distribution of tumor metastasis. Experiments with V_2 carcinoma of rabbits, *Cancer Res.,* 9, 649, 1949.

5. **Loughead, J.R. and Bushnell, J.**, Metastasis of malignant tumors to the larynx, *Laryngoscope*, 64, 50, 1954.
6. **Quinn, F. B., Jr. and McCabe, B. F.**, Laryngeal metastases from malignant tumors in distant organs, *Ann. Otol. Rhinol. Laryngol.*, 66, 139, 1957.
7. **Whicker, J.H., Carder, G. A., and Devine, K. D.**, Metastasis to the larynx. Report of a case and review of the literature, *Arch. Otolaryngol.*, 96, 182, 1972.
8. **Freeland, A. P., van Nostrand, A. W. P., and Jahn, A. F.**, Metastases to the larynx, *J. Otolaryngol.*, 8, 448, 1979.
9. **Batsakis, J. G.**, *Tumors of the Head and Neck, Clinical and Pathological Considerations*, 2nd ed., Williams & Wilkins, Baltimore, 1979.
10. **Eppinger, H.**, 1880, Quoted by **Ellis, M. and Winston, P.**, Secondary carcinoma of the larynx, *J. Laryngol. Otol.*, 71, 16, 1957.
11. **Landgraf**, 1888, Quoted by **Ellis, M. and Winston, P.**, Secondary carcinoma of the larynx, *J. Laryngol.Otol.*, 71, 16, 1957.
12. **Chapuis**, 1896, Quoted by **Ellis, M. and Winston, P.**, Secondary carcinoma of the larynx, *J. Laryngol.Otol.*, 71, 16, 1957.
13. **Massei, F.**, 1900, Quoted by **Bolognesi, C. and Nucci, C.**, Metastasi laringea da neoplasia della mammella, *Otorinolaringol. Ital.*, 32, 280, 1963.
14. **Neumann, H.**, 1905, Quoted by **Ellis, M. and Winston, P.**, Secondary carcinoma of the larynx, *J. Laryngol. Otol.*, 71, 16, 1957.
15. **Schmorl, G.**, 1908, Quoted by **Auriol, M., Chomette, G., and Abelanet, R.**, Métastases larygées des tumeurs malignes (à propos de quelques observations), *Gaz. Méd. Fr.*, 66, 233, 1959.
16. **Menzel, K.,M.**, 1912, Quoted by **Ellis, M. and Winston, P.**, Secondary carcinoma of the larynx, *J. Layngol. Otol.*, 71, 16, 1957.
17. **Hofer, G.**, 1922, Quoted by **Bolognesi, C. and Nucci, C.**, Metastasi laringea da neoplasia della mammella, *Otorinolaringol. Ital.*, 32, 280, 1963.
18. **Turner, A. L.**, Metastatic, malignant tumor of the larynx secondary to the adenocarcinoma of the right kidney, *J. Laryngol. Otol.*, 39, 181, 1924.
19. **Motloch, E.**, 1927, Quoted by **Bolognesi, C. and Nucci, C.**, Metastasi laringea da neoplasia della mammella, *Otorinolaringol. Ital.*, 32, 180, 1963.
20. **Hajek, M.**, 1928, Quoted by **Bolognesi, C. and Nucci, C.**, Metastasi laringea da neoplasia della mammella, *Otorinolaringol. Ital.*, 32, 280, 1963.
21. **Caboche, H. and Paisseau**, 1930, Quoted by **Bolognesi, C. and Nucci, C.**, Metastasi laringea da neoplasia della mammella, *Otorinolaringol. Ital.*, 32, 280, 1963.
22. **Mullin, M. V. and Langston, F. V.**, 1930, Quoted by **Auriol, M., Chomette, G., and Abelanet, R.**, Métastases larygées des tumeurs malignes, (à propos de quelques observations), *Gaz. Méd. Fr.*, 66, 233, 1959.
23. **Oppikofer, E.**, 1932, Quoted by **Bolognesi, C. and Nucci, C.**, Metastasi laringea da neoplasia della mammella, *Otorinolaringol. Ital.*, 32, 280, 1963.
24. **Maxwell, J. H.**, 1942, Quoted by **Bolognesi, C. and Nucci, C.**, Metastasi laringea da neoplasia della mammella, *Otorinolaringol. Ital.*, 32, 280, 1963.
25. **Walther, H. E.**, 1948, Quoted by **Bolognesi, C. and Nucci, C.**, Metastasi laringea da neoplasia della mammella, *Otorinolaringol. Ital.*, 32, 280, 1963.
26. **Fabbi, F.**, Metastasi laringea di simpatico-blastoma primitivo della surrenale destra. Sindrome della coda equina da metastasi midollare, *Otorinolaringol. Ital.*, 17, 75, 1948.
27. **Rebattu, J., Martin, H., and Takizawa,** 1950, Quoted by **Bolognesi, C. and Nucci, C.**, Metastasi laringea da neoplasia della mammella, *Otoringolarinol. Ital.*, 32, 280, 1963.
28. **Fisher, G. E. and Odess, J. S.**, Metastatic malignant melanoma of the larynx, *Arch. Otolaryngol.*, 54, 639, 1951.
29. **Loughead, J. R.**, Malignant melanoma of the larynx, *Ann. Otol. Rhinol. Laryngol.*, 61, 154, 1952.
30. **Willis, R. A.**, *The Spread of Tumors in the Human Body*, Butterworth, London, 1952.
31. **Faaborg-Andersen, K.**, Melanoma malignum laryngis, *Acta Otolaryngol.*, 43, 529, 1953.
32. **Ehrlich, A.**, Tumor involving the laryngeal cartilages, *Arch. Otolaryngol.*, 59, 178, 1954.
33. **Juan, P.**, 1956, Quoted by **Franzoni, M.**, I melanomi della laringe, *Boll. Mal. Orecchio Gola Naso*, 82, 113, 1964.
34. **Tamura, H. and Nakamoto, M.**, Ein Fall von Grawitz-Tumor mit Metastase im Kehlkopf, *Monatsschr. Ohrenheilkd.*, 90, 354, 1956.
35. **Ellis, M. and Winston, P.**, Secondary carcinoma of the larynx, *J. Laryngol. Otol.*, 71, 16, 1957.
36. **Freire, F., Camara, J., and Paiva, L.**, 1958, Quoted by **Glantz, H. and Kleinsasser, O.**, Metastasen im Kehlkopf, *HNO*, 26, 163, 1978.
37. **Auriol, M., Chomette, G., and Abelanet, R.**, Métastases laryngées des tumeurs malignes (à propos de quelques observations), *Gaz. Méd. Fr.*, 66, 233, 1959.

38. **Bolognesi, C. and Caliceti, G.,** Seminoma metastatico della laringe, *Otorinolaringol. Ital.*, 29, 15, 1960.
39. **Shaheen, O. H.,** A case of metastatic amelanotic melanoma of the larynx, *J. Laryngol. Otol.*, 74, 182, 1960.
40. **Bauer, J. and Fuchs, G.,** Lokalisation und Therapie der Melanome im Ohren-Nasen-Hals-Bereich, *Krebsarzt*, 16, 411, 1961.
41. **Bergstedt, M. and Herberts, G.,** Hypernephrometastasis in the larynx. Radical extirpation before diagnosis of primary tumour, *Acta Otolaryngol.*, 54, 95, 1962.
42. **Bolognesi, C. and Nucci, C.,** Metastasi laringea da neoplasia della mammella, *Otorinolaringol.Ital.*, 32, 280, 1963.
43. **Franzoni, M.,** I melanomi metastatici della laringe, *Boll.Mal.Orecchio.Gola.Naso.*, 82, 113, 1964.
44. **Chamberlain, D.,** Malignant melanoma, metastatic to the larynx, *Arch.Otolaryngol.*, 83, 231, 1966.
45. **Fields, J. A.,** Renal carcinoma metastasis to the larynx, *Laryngoscope*, 76, 99, 1966.
46. **Mazzarella, L. A., Pina., L.H., and Wolff, D.,** Asymptomatic metastasis to the larynx, *Laryngoscope*, 76, 1547, 1966.
47. **Bolla, A., Cabassa, N., and Scolari, R.,** Metastasi solitaria al laringe da microcitoma polmonare, *Arch.Ital.,Otol.*, 79, 74, 1968.
48. **Kubo, R., and Ono, M.,** 1968, Quoted by **Glanz, H. and Kleinsasser, O.,** Metastasen im Kehlkopf, *HNO*, 26, 163, 1978.
49. **Bardach, J. and Korzon, T.,** 1969, Quoted by **Stankiewicz, C. and Mostowski, L.,** Przerzut raka jasnokomorkowego nerki do krtani, *Otolaryngol.Pol.*, 32, 543, 1979.
50. **Palacios, E. J., Hanchey, C. C., and White, H. J.,** 1970, Quoted by **Glanz, H. and Kleinsasser, O.,** Metastasen im Kehlkopf, *HNO*, 26, 163, 1978.
51. **Miyamoto, R. and Helmus, C.,** Hypernephroma metastatic to the head and neck, *Laryngoscope*, 83, 898, 1973.
52. **Rachel, T. and Reinfuss, M.,** 1974, Quoted by **Stankiewicz, C. and Mostowski, L.,** Przerzut raka jasnokomorkowego nerki do krtani, *Otolaryngol.Pol.*, 32, 543, 1979.
53. **Eschwege, F., Cachin, Y., and Micheau, C.,** Treatment of adenocarcinoma of the larynx, *Can.J.Otolaryngol.*, 4, 291, 1975.
54. **Levine, H. L. and Applebaum, E. L.,** 1976, Quoted by **Glanz, H. and Kleinsasser, O.,** Metastasen im Kehlkopf, *HNO*, 26, 163, 1978.
55. **Zuchowska-Vogelgesang, B., Sokolowski, S. and Skolyszewski, J.,** 1976, Quoted by Glanz, H. and Kleinsasser, O., Metastasen im Kehlkopf,*HNO*, 26, 163, 1978.
56. **Tolstov, U. P. and Saburov, P. A.,** Metastatic melanoma of the larynx (translation), *Vestn.Otorinolaringol.*, 2, 99, 1977.
57. **Glanz, H. and Kleinsasser, O.,** Metastasen im Kehlkopf, *HNO*, 26, 163, 1978.
58. **Kyriakos, M., Berlin, B. P., and DeSchryver-Kecskemeti, K.,** Oat cell carcinoma of the larynx, *Arch.Otolaryngol.*, 104, 168, 1978.
59. **Snow, G. B., Esch, E. P. van der, and Slooten, E. A. van,** Mucosal melanomas of the head and neck, *Head Neck Surg.*, 1, 24, 1978.
60. **Stankiewicz, C. and Mostowski, L.,** Przerzut raka jasnokomorkowego nerki do krtani, *Otolaryngol.Pol.*, 32, 543, 1979.
61. **Oku, T., Hasegawa, M., Watanabe, I., Nasu, M., and Aoki, N.,** Pancreatic cancer with metastasis to the larynx, *J.Laryngol.Otol.*, 94, 1205, 1980.
62. **Maddox, J. C., and Evans, H. L.,** Angiosarcoma of skin and soft tissue: a study of forty-four cases, *Cancer*, 48, 1907, 1981.
63. **Batsakis, J. G., Regezi, J. A., Solomon, A. R., and Rice, D. H.,** The pathology of head and neck tumors. Mucosal melanomas, part 13, *Head Neck Surg.*, 5, 404, 1982.
64. **Ferlito, A. and Caruso, G.,** Secondary malignant melanoma of the larynx. Report of 2 cases and review of 79 laryngeal secondary cancers, *ORL*, 46, 117, 1984.
65. **Carter, R. L. and Tanner, N. S. B.,** Local invasion of laryngeal cancer. The importance of focal (metaplastic) ossification within laryngeal cartilage, *Clin.Otolaryngol.*, 4, 283, 1979.
66. **Batson, O. V.,** The function of the vertebral veins and their role in the spread of metastases, *Ann.Surg.*, 112, 138, 1940.
67. **Fisher, B. and Fisher, E. R.,** Significance of the interrelationship of lymph and blood vascular systems in tumor cell dissemination, *Prog.Clin.Cancer*, 4, 84, 1970.
68. **Zeidman, I.,** Experimental studies on the spread of cancer in the lymphatic system. III. Tumor emboli in the thoracic duct. The pathogenesis of Virchow's node, *Cancer Res.*, 15, 719, 1955.
69. **Ferlito, A.,** Histological classification of larynx and hypopharynx cancers and their clinical implications. Pathologic aspects of 2,052 malignant neoplasms diagnosed at the ORL Department of Padua University from 1966 to 1976, *Acta Otolaryngol.*, Suppl. 342, 1, 1976.
70. **Pesavento, G., Ferlito, A., and Recher, G.,** Primary clear cell carcinoma of the larynx, *J.Clin.Pathol.*, 33, 1160, 1980.

71. **Ferlito, A., Recher, G., and Polidoro, F.,** Nasal metastasis from primary cancer of the kidney, *J.Laryngol.Otol.,* 93, 1115, 1979.
72. **Havens, F. Z. and Parkhill, E. M.,** Tumors of the larynx other than squamous cell epithelioma, *Arch.Otolaryngol.,* 34, 1113, 1941.
73. **Curtiss, C. and Kosinski, A. A.,** Primary melanoma of the larynx. Report of a case and review of the literature, *Cancer,* 8, 961, 1955.
74. **Fenning, F. R.,** Malignant melanoma of the larynx, *Ann.Otol.Rhinol.Laryngol.,* 64, 1281, 1955.
75. **Cremonesi, G.,** Su un eccezionale reperto di sarcoma melanotico primitivo della laringe, *Minerva Otorinolaringol.,* 6, 333, 1956.
76. **Welsh, L. W. and Welsh, J. J.,** Malignant melanoma of the larynx, *Laryngoscope,* 71, 185, 1961.
77. **Pentazopoulos, P. E.,** Primary malignant melanoma of the larynx, *Laryngoscope,* 74, 95, 1964.
78. **Frable, W. J. and Frable, M. A. S.,** The larynx and trachea, in *Principles and Practice of Surgical Pathology,* Silverberg, S. G., Ed. John Wiley & Sons, N. Y., 1983.
79. **Moore, E. S. and Martin H.,** Melanoma of the upper respiratory tract and oral cavity, *Cancer,* 8, 1167, 1955.
80. **Lorentz, E.,** Das maligne Melanom des Kehlkopfes, *HNO,* 27, 275, 1979.
81. **Goldman, J. L., Lawson, W., Zak, F. G. and Roffman, J. D.,** The presence of melanocytes in the human larynx, *Laryngoscope,* 82, 824, 1972.
82. **Busuttil, A.,** Dendritic pigmented cells within human laryngeal mucosa, *Arch.Otolaryngol.,* 102, 43, 1976.
83. **DiGregorio, C. and DeGaetani, C. F.,** Melanosis of the larynx: a case report, *Appl.Pathol.,* 1, 10, 1983.
84. **Pesce, C. and Toncini, C.,** Melanin pigmentation of the larynx, *Acta Otolaryngol.,* 96, 189, 1983.

Chapter 4

SPREAD OF CANCER OF THE LARYNX

A. Ferlito

TABLE OF CONTENTS

I. INTRODUCTION

Laryngeal cancer may spread by direct infiltration, by the lymphatic, and by the hematogenous route. Tumor dissemination may be affected by various factors, such as the site of the primary neoplasm, the oncotype, the degree of cellular differentiation, the presence or absence of some barriers to its spread, as well as by some biological factors (largely related to tumor-host relationship). All these factors may act independently or synergically in cancer patients.

Now it may be pointed out that neoplastic infiltration is generally linked with the histologic type of the neoplasm. In fact, there are tumors such as small cell carcinoma which display a higher infiltrative power than squamous cell carcinoma, and others, such as verrucous squamous cell carcinoma, featuring "pushing" margins and a poor infiltrative ability, or adenoid cystic carcinoma, with a definite tendency to spread along neural and perineural pathways.

II. DIRECT INFILTRATION

Spread of laryngeal cancer is in three dimensions and the tumor may infiltrate the anatomical boundaries of the organ at various places.[1] The pattern of direct infiltration by laryngeal cancer is largely determined by anatomical and mechanical features.[2,3] The principal structures forming a barrier to tumor spread are the hyoepiglottic ligament, the conus elasticus, and the cartilages with their perichondrium (Figures 1 to 3).[4-6] The importance of the hyoepiglottic ligament as a barrier should not be overestimated. The membranous partition between the paraglottic space and the preepiglottic space does offer some resistance to tumor invasion (Figures 4 to 9) in the early stages of laryngeal cancer.[7] Less resistant to tumor invasion are the thyroepiglottic ligament and the cricothyroid membrane. Glandular structures may facilitate tumor spread.[8,9] Muscle fibers are easily dissociated by neoplastic infiltration.

The tumor may extend directly into the adjacent normal structures, and it may infiltrate the glossoepiglottic valleculae, the hypopharynx, the thyroid (Figure 10) and the trachea.[10] Occasionally, the neoplasm may invade the prelaryngeal muscles, subcutaneous tissues, and the overlying skin.

The behavior of laryngeal cancer varies, depending on the site of origin. Within the larynx, the extension in the mucosa and submucosa is common.[11]

Cancer of the vocal cord originating on the free margin of the anterior half spreads initially on the surface along the length of the cord. The anterior commissure and occasionally also the contralateral cord may be invaded. More rarely, the tumor grows posteriorly, involving the vocal process or anterior face of the arytenoid. Still more posteriorly, glottic cancer may involve the posterior commissure and the mucosa overlying the posterior plate of the cricoid cartilage.[12] The neoplasm may also invade both the laryngeal ventricle and the subglottic region.[3,10,13] An extension of the tumor into the subglottic region was found by Shaw[14] in 62 of his 306 cases with glottic cancer. In the advanced stage, cancer of the vocal cord invades the intrinsic muscles and the thyroid cartilage. Vertical extension of glottic tumors into the sub- or supraglottic regions occurs more often than horizontal extension to the opposite hemilarynx.[13,15] Cancer of the anterior commissure spreads in all directions, involving both vocal cords, the ventricle, the ventricular fold, the base of the epiglottis, and the subglottic region. Not uncommonly, cancer of the anterior commissure invades the lower margin of the thyroid ala and extends outside the laryngeal framework through the cricothyroid membrane. Infiltration of the Delphian lymph node is possible.

Supraglottic cancers have been divided into various subgroups, on the basis of the site apparently involved, as cancer of the laryngeal surface of the epiglottis, of the ventricular fold, of the ventricle, of the aryepiglottic fold, and of the arytenoid.

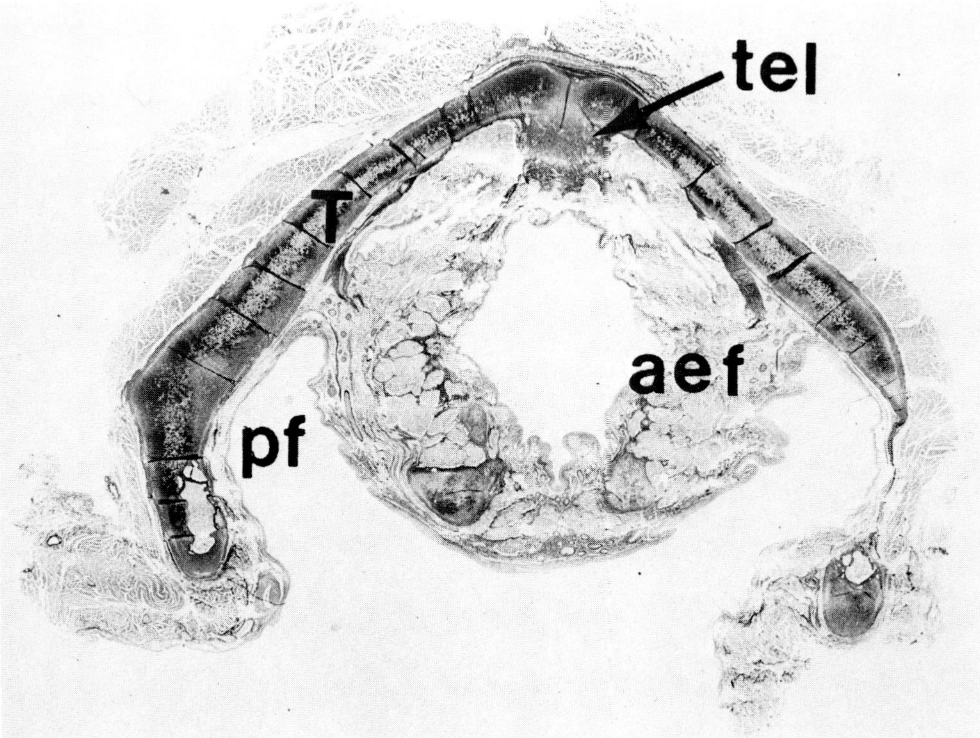

FIGURE 1. Horizontal sections of normal larynx at supraglottic level. (Victoria blue-van Gieson stain; Magnification × 3.)(A) Section through thyroepiglottic ligament; (B) section through lower epiglottis; (C) section through midepiglottis. *Right:* relative sites of these three levels. (T indicates thyroid cartilage; tel, thyroepiglottic ligament; aef, aryepiglottic fold; pf, piriform fossa; s, saccule; thm, thyrohyoid membrane; pes, preepiglottic space; m, membrane partition between preepiglottic and paraglottic spaces; hel, hyoepiglottic ligament; E; epiglottic cartilage; H, hyoid bone) (By courtesy of Prof. K. H. Lam.)

Supraglottic cancers have also been divided into suprahyoid laryngeal cancers (posterior surface of suprahyoid epiglottis, aryepiglottic fold, and arytenoid) and infrahyoid laryngeal cancers (infrahyoid epiglottis, ventricular fold, and ventricle). The tumors belonging to the second group are more common than those of the first group, and have been called cancers of the vestibulum. They have a clear tendency to spreading towards the preepiglottic space (Figure 7) because of the early destruction of the thyroepiglottic ligament either by direct passage through the orifices of the epiglottic cartilage or by direct destruction of the cartilage itself.[1,3,10,13] Suprahyoid laryngeal cancers tend to invade tongue base and pyriform sinus rather than the preepiglottic space.

Tumors of the supraglottic region may infiltrate the glottic plane and the subglottis, though clinically the neoplasm may appear to be restricted to the supraglottic region.[3,10,13,16-20] When a supraglottic tumor invades the paraglottic space (instead of the preepiglottic space), inferior invasion to the glottis can easily occur.[7] This occurs because the paraglottic space extends into the glottis along the medial surface of the thyroid cartilage (Figure 2).

Cancer of the ventricle is rare and may extend superiorly, inferiorly, and laterally, but Michaels and Hassmann[21] described 11 cases of ventriculosaccular cancer in which the malignant process was confined to the ventricle.

Subglottic cancer may not be detected at an early stage because of the absence of the symptoms. It extends to the whole subglottis and in the advanced stage presents as a circumferential growth,[10,22] but it may also extend upwards to the vocal cords and downwards

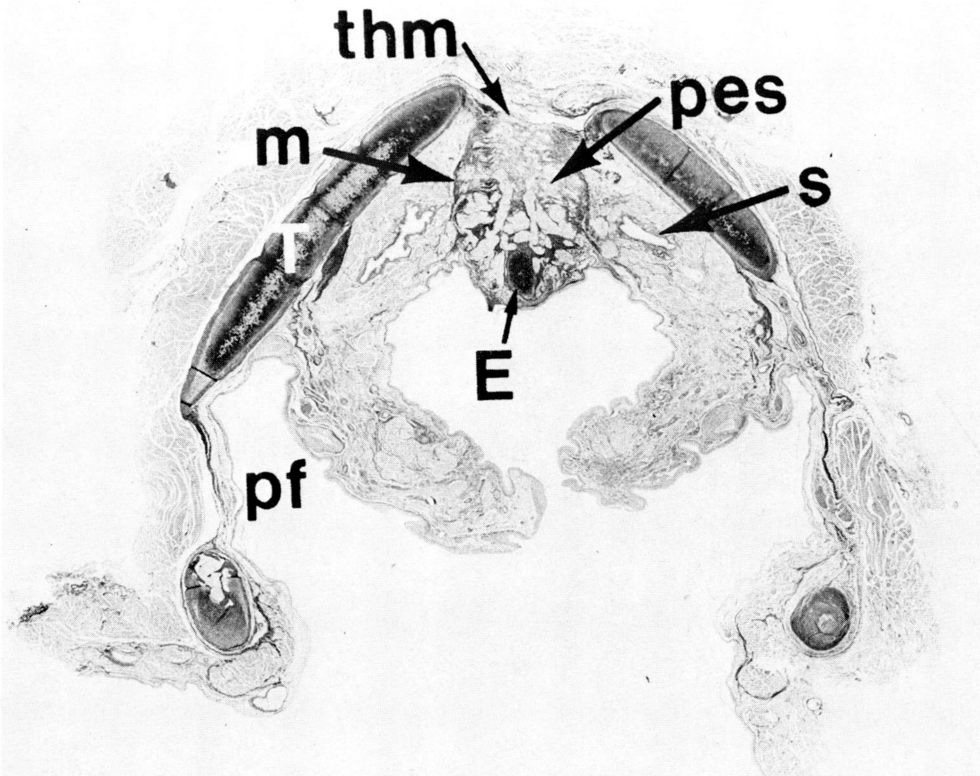

FIGURE 1B

to the trachea. When the tumor grows anteriorly, it may perforate the cricothyroid membrane and invade the thyroid gland,[23] anterior soft tissues, and later, the skin. If the tumor affects the posterior wall of the subglottis it may also infiltrate the cervical esophagus.[23] These tumors may resemble those of the trachea.[3]

Invasion of the laryngeal framework is a common feature of the transglottic cancers.[24-30] This term, originally adopted by McGavran et al.,[31] was used to describe "cancers that cross the ventricle of Morgagni, thus involving two or three of the preceding sites (i.e., glottis, infraglottic, supraglottic)". Transglottic tumors have a prominent tendency to spread outside the larynx.[1]

Laryngeal malignant tumors display some tendency to direct perineural and vascular invasion.[13,31,32] Perineural invasion is frequent and often spreads along the branches of the recurrent laryngeal nerve into the thyroarytenoid muscle, near the lower end of the thyroid ala. The longitudinal arrangement of the nerve trunks and the tendency of cancer to invade nerve sheaths enables its spread from one region to another.

Direct diffuse permeation of the submucosal lymphatics is well known in laryngeal and hypopharyngeal cancer with frequent lymph node involvement. Direct infiltration may affect adjacent lymph nodes, particularly the prelaryngeal lymph nodes (or Delphian nodes).

Direct invasion can occur into the laryngeal cartilages (Figures 11 and 12) and into the metaplastic bone of ossified laryngeal cartilages.[25,28,30] Nonossified cartilage is resistant to osteoclastic erosion and direct destruction by tumor cells may remain undetected. In ossified laryngeal cartilages the tumor cells stimulate the osteoclasts to destroy the bone in front of the tumor margin.[33] Nonossified cartilages appear to be more resistant to tumor invasion than ossified cartilages.[30,30a]

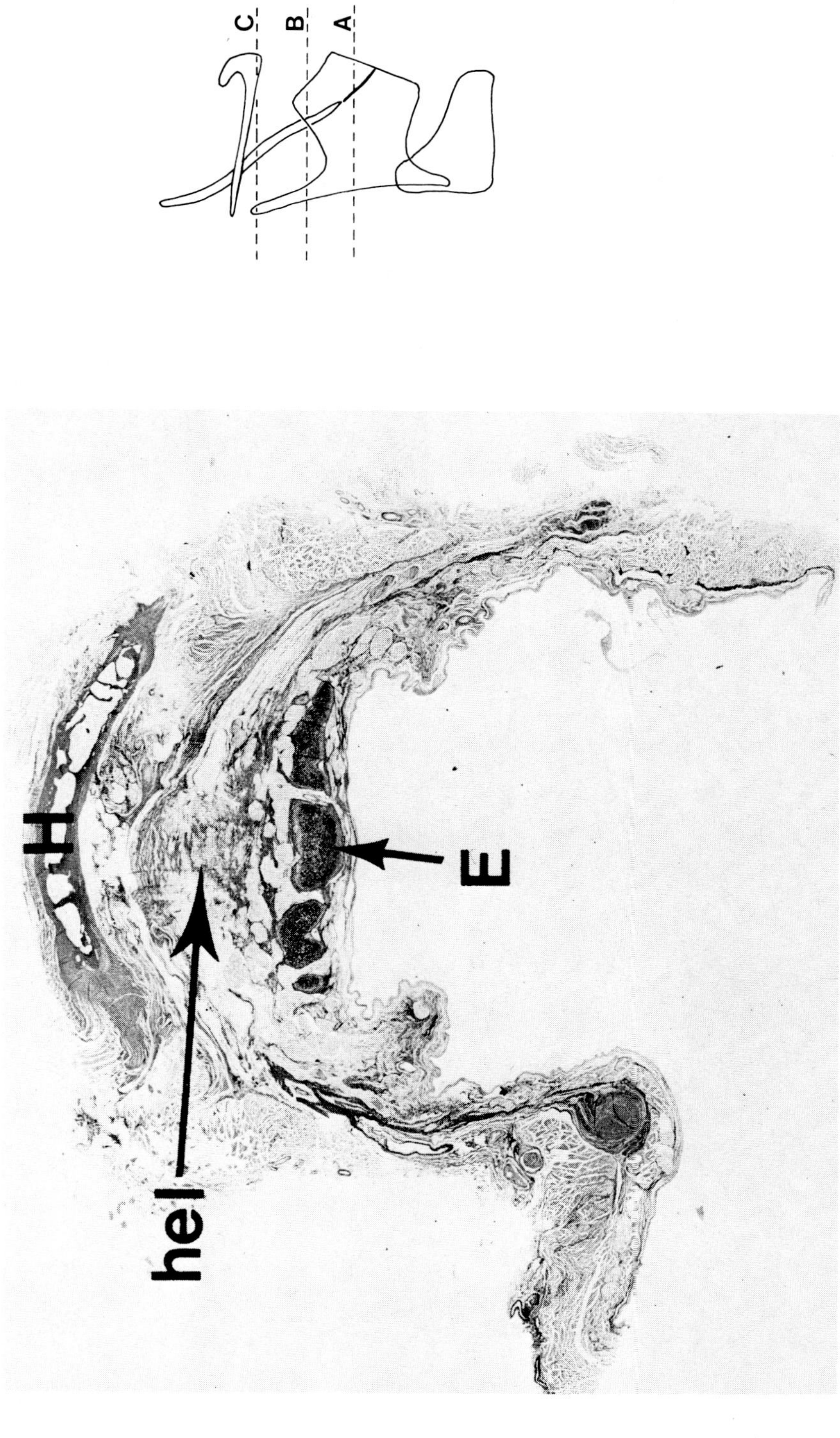

FIGURE 1C

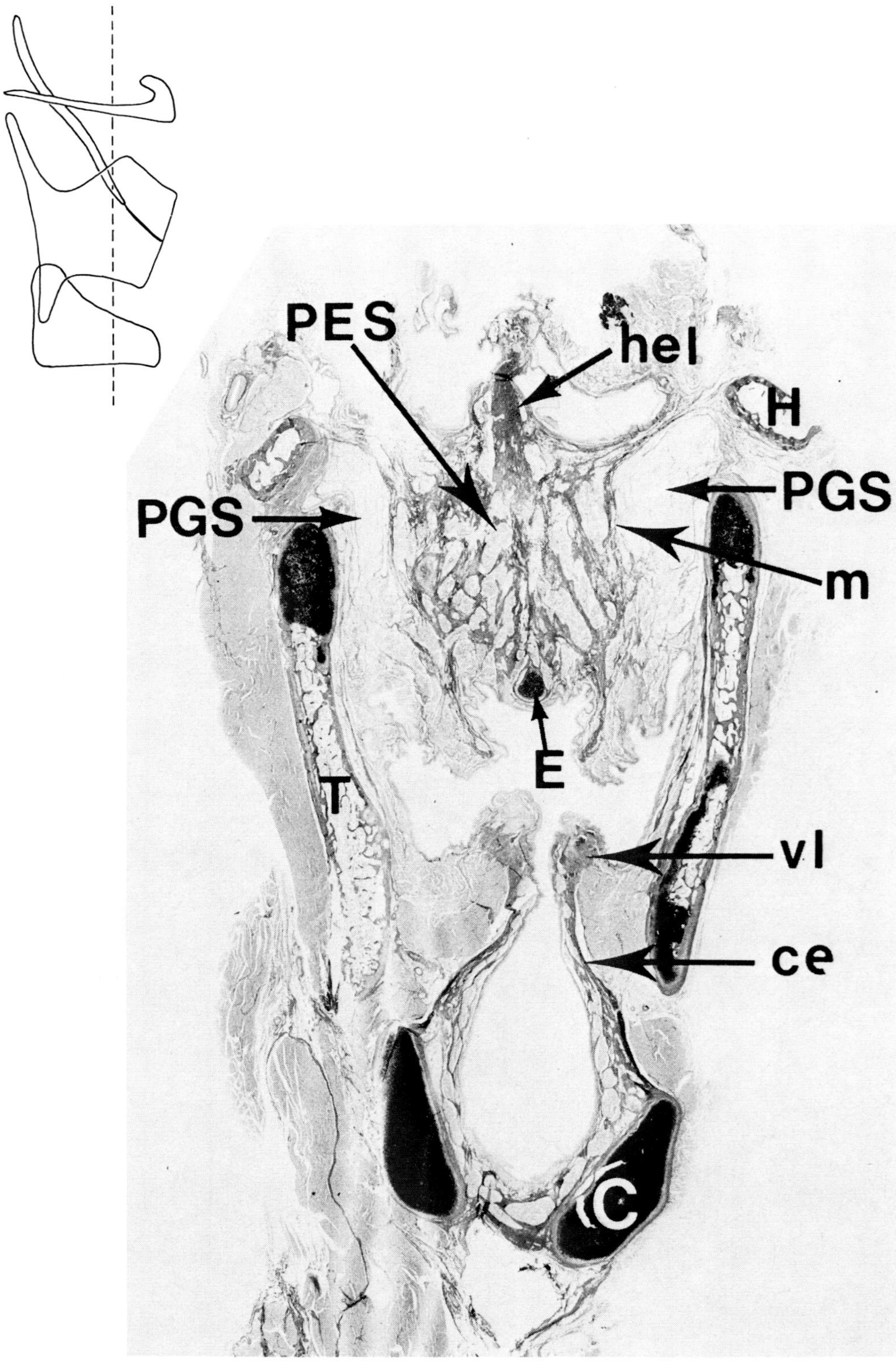

FIGURE 2. Coronal section of normal larynx through preepiglottic space. (Victoria blue-van Gieson stain; Magnification × 2.5.) T indicates thyroid cartilage; hel, hyoepiglottic ligament; vl, vocal ligament; ce, conus elasticus; PES, preepiglottic space; PGS, paraglottic space; m, membranous partition between PES and PGS; H, hyoid bone; E, epiglottic cartilage; C, cricoid cartilage. *Above:* level of section. (By courtesy of Prof. K. H. Lam.)

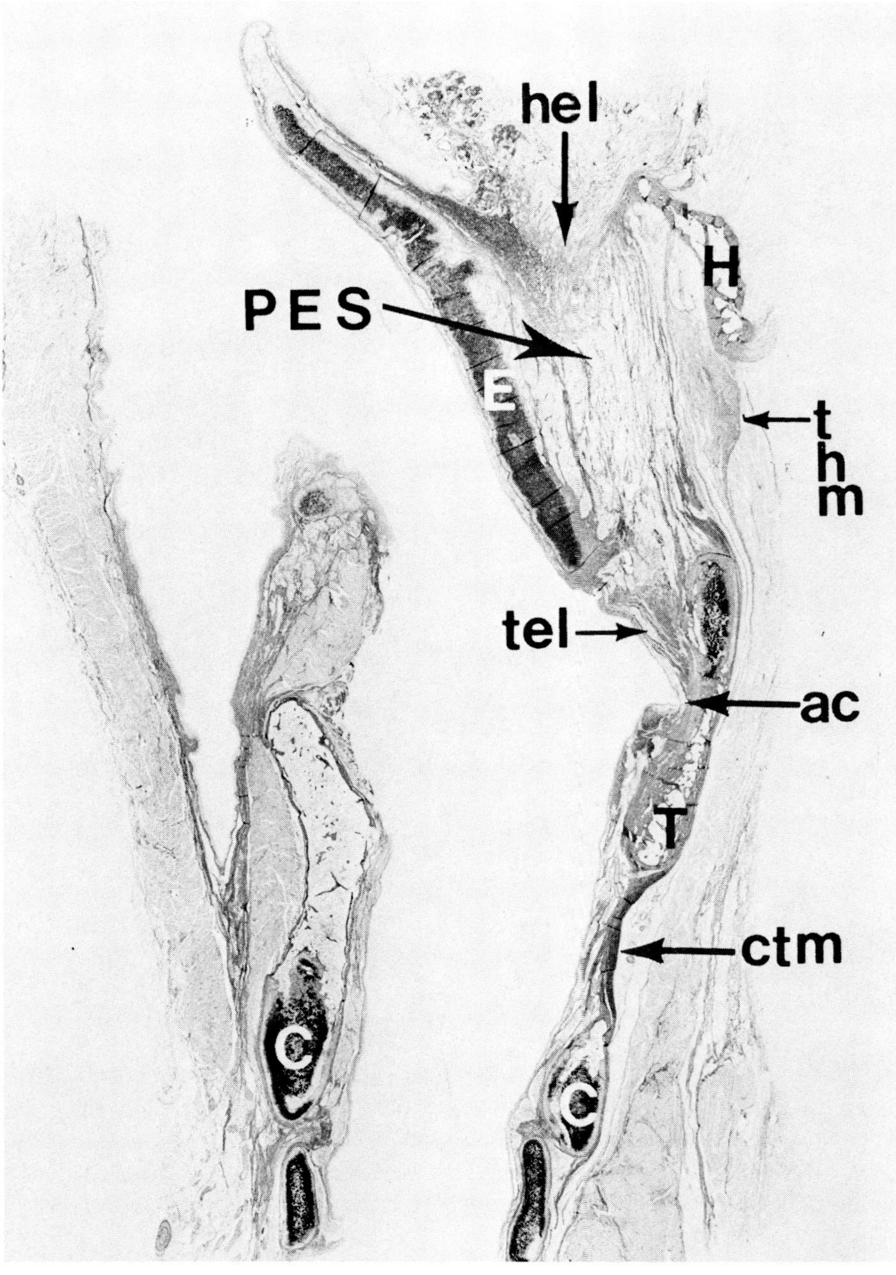

FIGURE 3. Sagittal section of normal larynx. (Victoria blue-van Gieson stain; Magnification × 2.5.) T indicates thyroid cartilage; hel, hyoepiglottic ligament; thm, thyrohyoid membrane; tel, thyroepiglottic ligament; ac, anterior commissure; ctm, cricothyroid membrane; PES, preepiglottic space; H, hyoid bone; E, epiglottic cartilage; C, cricoid cartilage. (By courtesy of Prof. K. H. Lam.)

III. LYMPHOGENOUS SPREAD

There are two major metastatic pathways: the lymphatic and the hematogenous route. The process whereby tumor cells penetrate the endothelial barrier of the lymphatic vessels is still unknown. Mechanical pressure by mobile neoplastic cells and the local release of substances may cause endothelial retraction or minute lesions on or near the junctional complexes.[34]

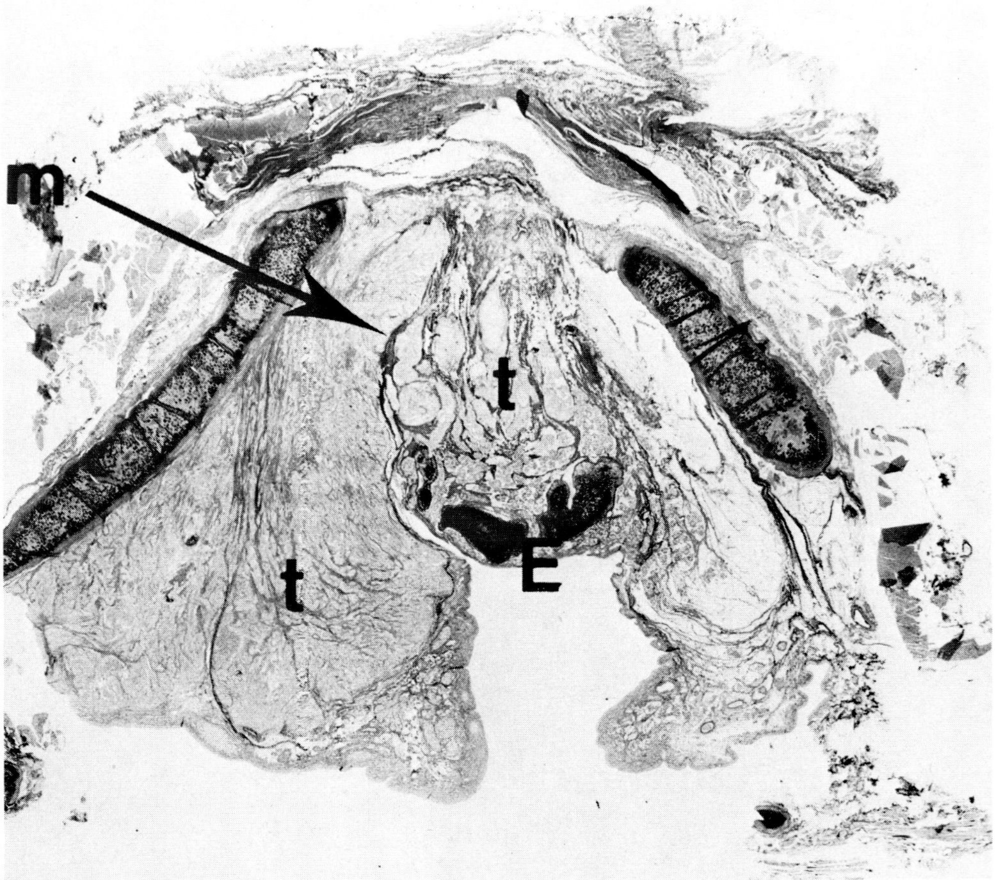

FIGURE 4. Horizontal section of larynx showing tumor(t) lying in both the left paraglottic and the preepiglottic spaces. The membranous portion(m) between these two spaces is preserved. E indicates epiglottis. (Victoria blue-van Gieson stain; Magnification × 3.) (By courtesy of Prof. K. H. Lam.)

The neoplastic cells — singly or in small emboli — are carried in afferent lymphatics and become trapped in the nodal sinus system where nodal deposits may develop. The necessary local conditions for their development have remained obscure.[34]

The development of cervical lymph node metastases is the most valid prognostic sign for predicting the evolution of a laryngeal neoplasm and is taken into account in determining the clinical stage of the tumor.

The spread to the lymphatic vessels is mainly by embolization, appearing first in the subcapsular sinus and subsequently spreading to the whole parenchyma of the node.

Nodal deposits may be confined by an intact capsule, but the lesion may penetrate the capsule of the node and invade the surrounding fat and the adjacent tissues.

Metastases are usually ipsilateral, often bilateral, and exceptionally, contralateral. Metastatic spread to the cervical lymph nodes occurs in 25 to 60 % of supraglottic tumors.[20,31,35-55] Subglottic cancers metastasize to the paratracheal lymph nodes in 50% of the cases, even though the affected lymph nodes may be clinically obscured.[10,22] Cancer of the vocal cord seldom causes lymph node secondaries because of the paucity of lymphatic vessels.

The localization of the cervical lymph node metastases is closely linked with the site of the primary lesion. Tumors of the supraglottic region metastasize primarily to subdigastric and upper jugular nodes, followed closely by the midjugular nodes. The posterior cervical

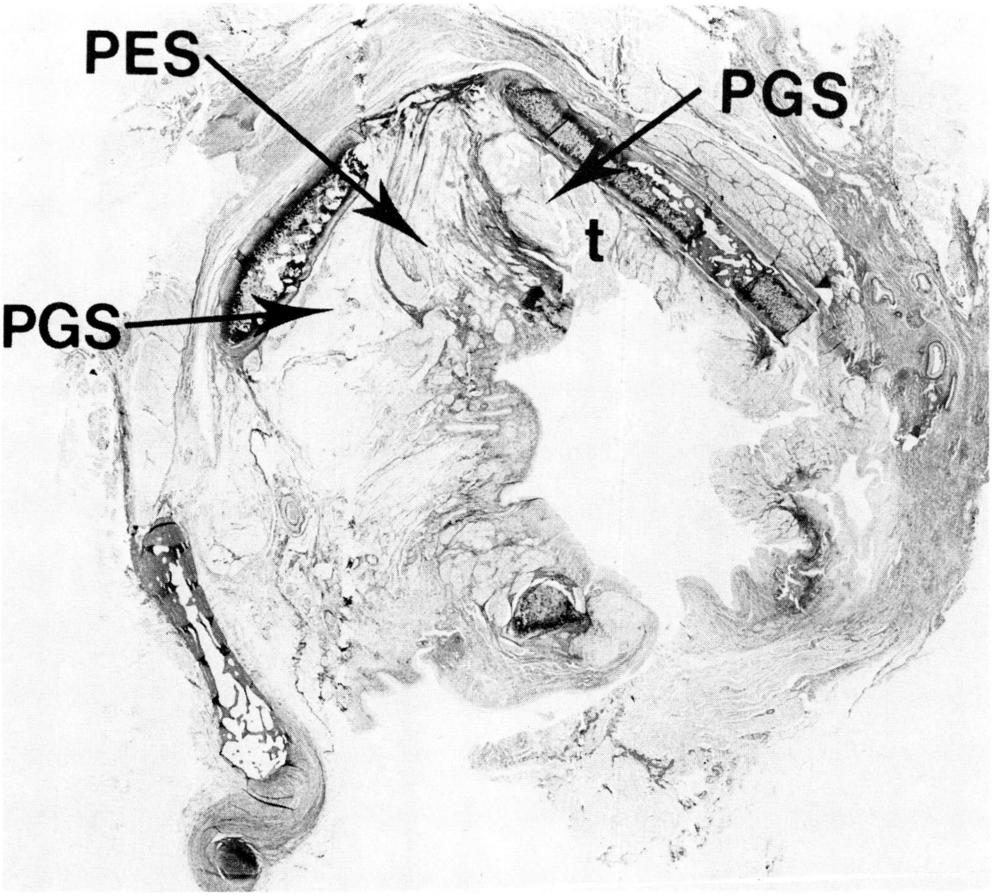

FIGURE 5. Horizontal section of larynx bearing a transglottic carcinoma showing tumor(t) in the right paraglottic space (PGS) pushing forward between the thyroid cartilage and the membranous partition between the spaces. The preepiglottic space (PES) remains clear of tumor. (Victoria blue-van Gieson stain; Magnification × 3.) (By courtesy of Prof. K. H. Lam.)

nodes are seldom involved, and the nodes of the submandibular triangle and submental areas are rarely affected.[56-59] Retrograde lymph flow may produce anomalous secondary deposits.

Subglottic tumors metastasize at an early stage and frequently to the lower deep cervical jugular chain, to the prelaryngeal node or nodes (Delphian node or nodes),[23] to the paratracheal nodes, to the lymph nodes of the recurrent nerve chain, and to the supraclavicular nodes. One or more lymph nodes — the prelaryngeal or Delphian node or nodes — will usually be found above the thyroid isthmus anterior to the lower portion of the thyroid cartilage.

Very rarely, squamous cell carcinoma[60] and small cell carcinoma[61] metastasize to the axillary lymph nodes, along the lymphatic pathways between the supraclavicular and the axillary nodes.

Neoplasms with a tendency to lymph node metastases are the squamous cell carcinoma,[62,63] spindle cell squamous carcinoma,[63-69] undifferentiated carcinoma,[64] anaplastic carcinoma with a lymphoid component (or lymphoepithelioma),[70-73] adenosquamous carcinoma,[74,75] clear cell carcinoma,[64,76] giant cell carcinoma,[77] small cell carcinoma,[61,78] carcinoid tumor,[79-84] and mucoepidermoid carcinoma.[85,86]

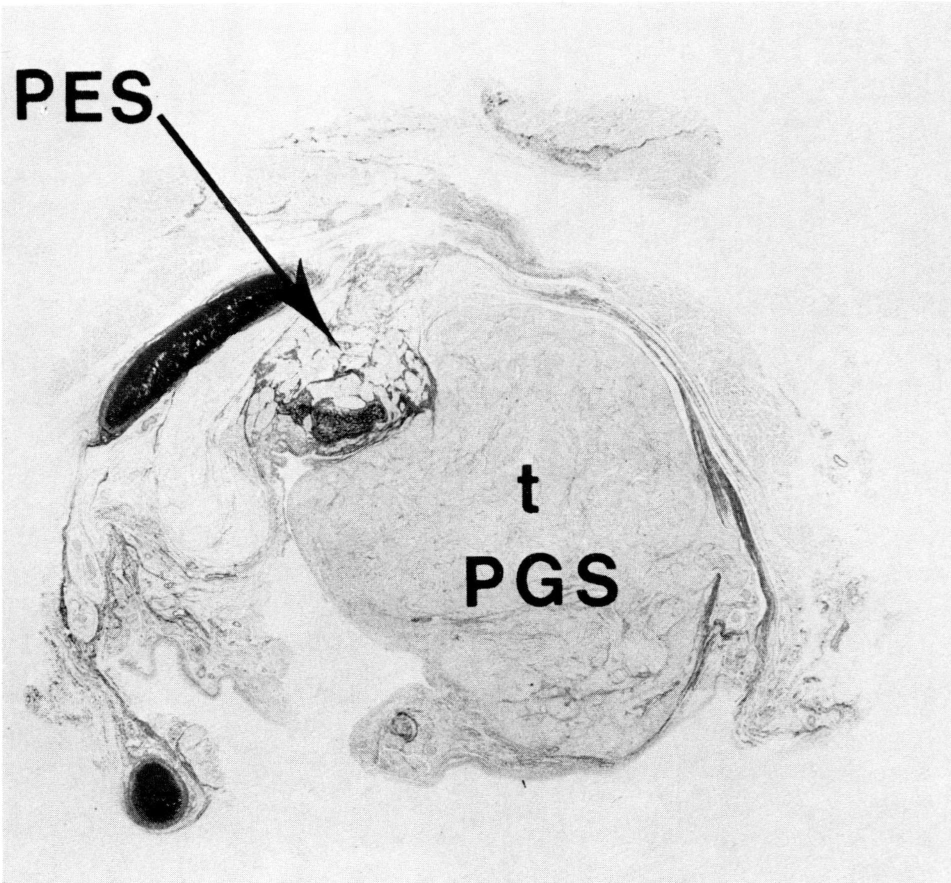

FIGURE 6. Horizontal section of larynx bearing a supraglottic carcinoma showing tumor(t) localized within the paraglottic space (PGS). The preepiglottic space (PES) is not invaded. (Victoria blue-van Gieson stain; Magnification × 3.) (By courtesy of Prof. K. H. Lam.)

Acinic cell carcinoma of the larynx may occasionally metastasize to the cervical lymph nodes,[87] although in some of the cases reported there were no metastases present.[88-90]

Verrucous squamous cell carcinoma does not metastasize to the lymph nodes.[91-95] However, Fisher[96] has noted 5 cases presenting lymph node metastases (out of 31) of verrucous squamous cell carcinoma of the larynx. The relatively high incidence of lymph node metastases might well be due to the fact that the author has classified some well-differentiated squamous cell carcinomas as verrucous cancer, too. From the series by Kraus and Perez-Mesa[97] of 105 verrucous squamous cell carcinomas, only 4 patients treated by irradiation developed lymph node secondaries, probably as a result of the changed biological character of the neoplasm.

Adenoid cystic carcinoma of the larynx does not metastasize to the cervical lymph nodes, but may infiltrate them by contiguity. Ferlito and Caruso,[98] who reviewed the literature on this subject, have found no well-documented case of laryngeal adenoid cystic carcinoma with lymph node metastases, even in those cases in which metastases to distant sites (lung, bone, brain) were present.

Primary malignant melanoma[99-101] and malignant paraganglioma[102,109a] of the larynx may spread to cervical lymph nodes.

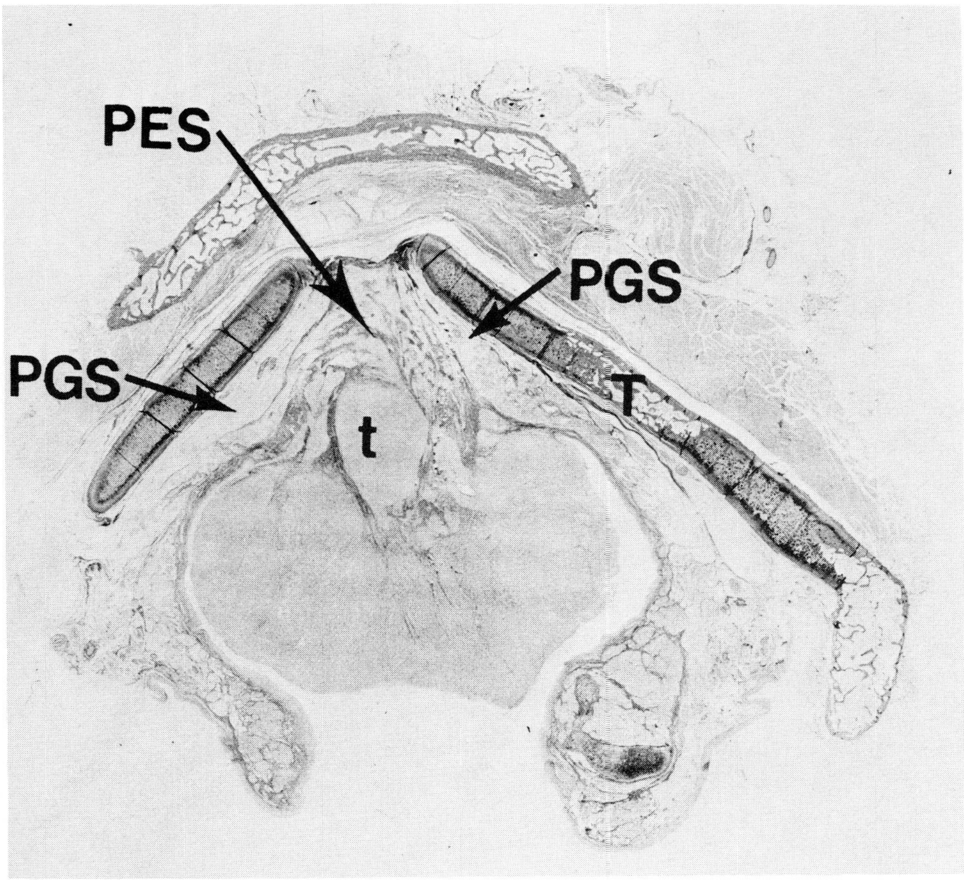

FIGURE 7. Horizontal section of larynx bearing an epiglottic tumor showing tumor(t) invading the preepiglottic space (PES). The paraglottic space (PGS) remains clear. T indicates thyroid cartilage. (Victoria blue-van Gieson stain; Magnification × 3.) (By courtesy of Prof. K. H. Lam.)

The rare liposarcoma of the larynx[110-118a] and the hemangiopericytoma[119-125] form no lymph node metastases. Also, in laryngeal angiosarcomas[126-129] and laryngo-hypopharyngeal synovial sarcomas,[130-143b] notwithstanding the presence of widespread metastases to distant organs, no involvement of the cervical lymph nodes has ever been seen.

Laryngeal lesions of Kaposi's sarcoma have usually been associated with classical skin changes, and lymph node involvement has been reported[144] in connection with this kind of tumor.

Malignant fibrous histiocytoma of the larynx (Figure 13) rarely metastasizes to the cervical lymph nodes, even when dissemination to distant organs (Figure 14) has occurred.[145-146]

Fibrosarcoma rarely metastasizes to the cervical lymph nodes.[147] It occasionally involves the regional lymph nodes by direct extension.

Chondrosarcoma of the larynx too (Figure 15), with the exception of some cases,[148-152a] does not spread to the cervical lymph nodes, also in the presence of pulmonary metastases (Figure 16). A few cases of well-documented laryngeal osteosarcoma have been described in the literature[147,153-156a] and regional metastases have been reported.[153,154]

Laryngeal leiomyosarcoma and rhabdomyosarcoma display a tendency to metastasize to cervical lymph nodes.[157] Lymphatic spread is uncommon in laryngeal malignant schwannoma,[158] but has occurred.[147]

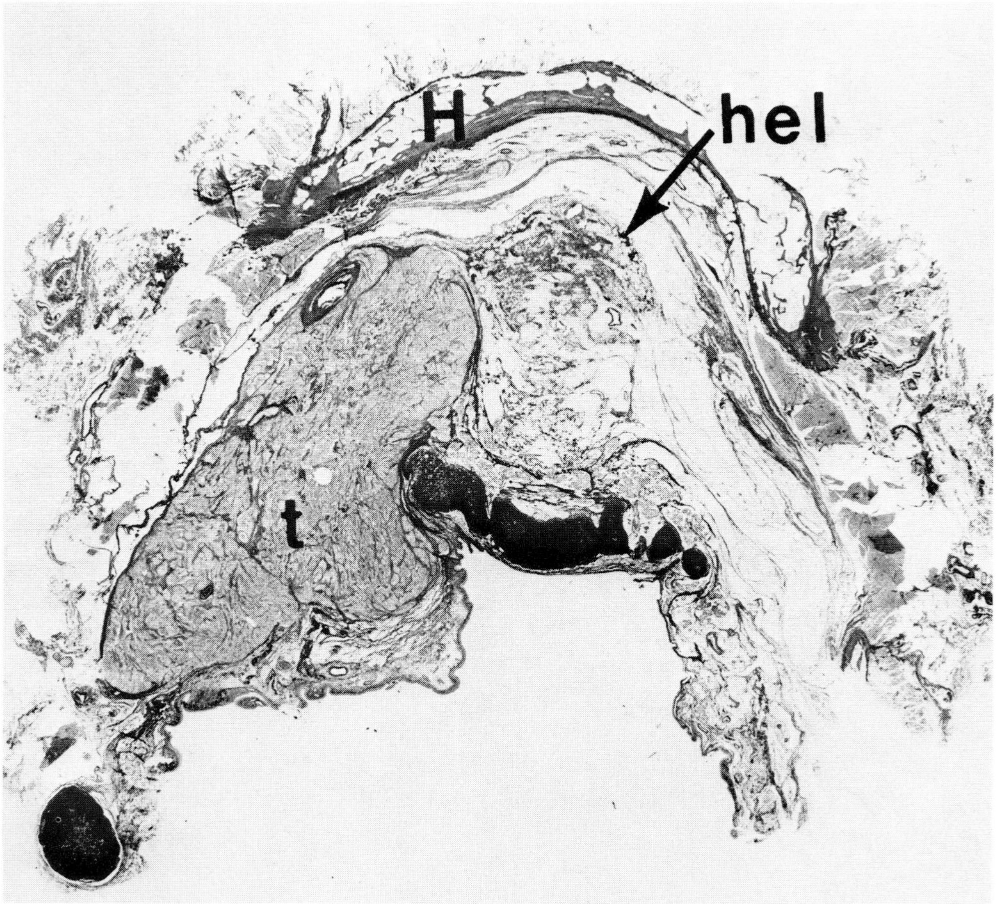

A

FIGURE 8. Horizontal sections of larynx; same specimen as Figure 4 but at a more cranial level. Tumor (t) is confined to the left side of the larynx as it spreads upward within the left paraglottic space. (Victoria blue-van Gieson stain; Magnification × 3.) (A) Section across middle of epiglottis (H indicates hyoid bone; hel, hyoepiglottic ligament). (B) section across hyoid bone. (By courtesy of Prof. K. H. Lam.)

Cervical lymph node metastases by malignant granular cell myoblastoma of the larynx have been reported.[159]

IV. HEMATOGENOUS SPREAD

Blood-borne metastases are uncommon, but in advanced stages of laryngeal cancer, widespread dissemination to various viscera may occur.[160-164] In the study by Ormerod and Shaw,[160] the incidence of proven distant metastases was 16%. Harrer and Lewis [165] noted that 16 of 18 patients with laryngeal cancer presented diffuse metastases at autopsy, 4 of which were squamous cell carcinomas with gross and microscopic evidence of cardiac and pericardiac metastases. One of these patients bore signs and symptoms of myocardial infarction.

Other cases of cardiac metastases from laryngeal cancer have been observed.[166-170] O'Brien et al.[162] reported 18 cases with distant spread out of 29 patients with laryngeal cancer. Abramson et al.[161] studied 650 patients with cancer of the larynx (75 of which were autopsied) and found that 34% had developed distant metastatic spread. It is interesting to note that at

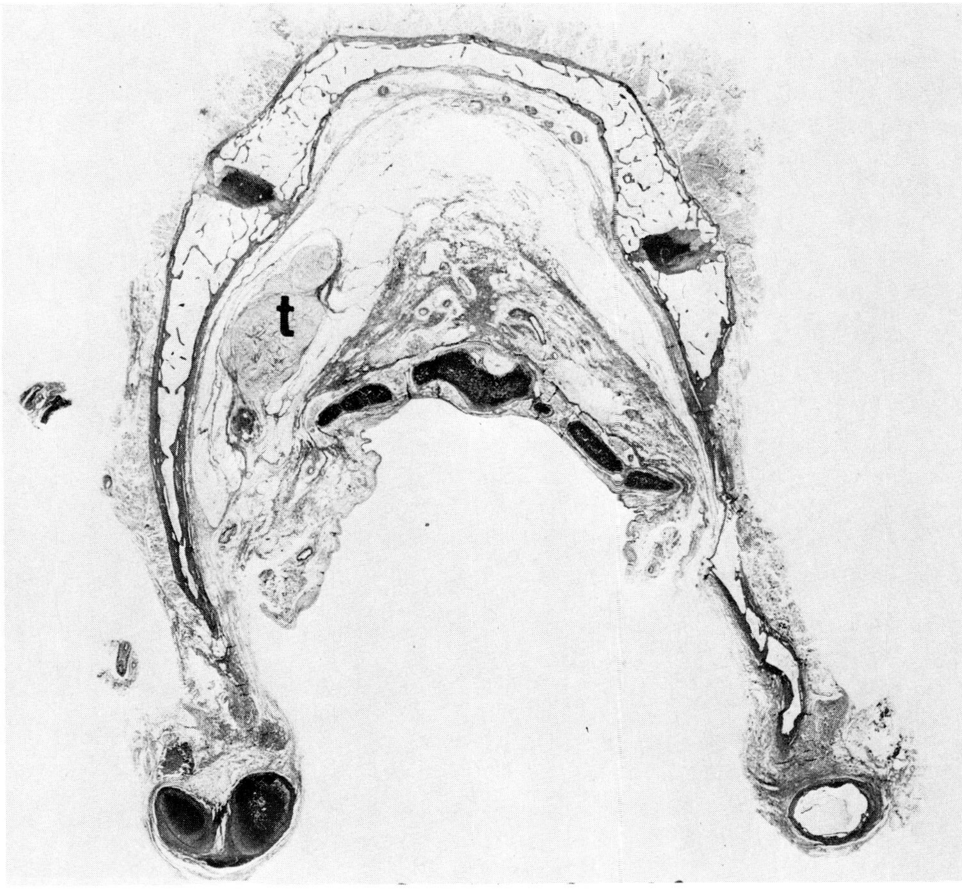

FIGURE 8B

autopsy, 80% of these patients displaying wide dissemination of the tumors had local neck involvement.

The sites which appear to be most affected by metastastic spread of squamous cell carcinoma and spindle cell squamous carcinoma are lungs and mediastinum, but also liver, skeletal system, brain, kidney, heart, and skin may be involved (Figures 17 to 23). Gnepp et al.[61] found in 43 cases of primary small cell carcinoma of the larynx that the most common sites of metastatic spread, excluding cervical lymph nodes, were liver (13 cases), lungs (11 cases), and bone (10 cases) (see Figures 24 and 25). Laryngeal metastasis to the temporal bone causing facial paralysis has also been reported.[171]

In most cases, metastases appear within the first few years; however there are tumors which may metastasize even after decades, such as the adenoid cystic carcinoma.

Finally, it must be remembered that occasionally, primary malignant neoplasms of the lung have been mistaken for metastases from a laryngeal cancer.[172]

The distinction between lymphatic and hematogenous spread is an artificial one since dissemination of most tumors occur by both routes.[173] There is some convincing experimental evidence that the two systems are linked since tumor cells injected into the bloodstream can be recovered in thoracic duct lymph.[174,175]

Communications between the lymphatic and venous systems are present in the neck region. The collecting lymphatic trunks from the head and neck terminate in the confluence of the subclavian and internal jugular vein, on the right side in the lymphatic duct and on the left side in the thoracic duct.[176] Since the lymph nodes are well supplied with blood vessels, and since they are usually situated in close proximity to large veins, metastases in lymph nodes may grow into veins and shed emboli into the venous stream. Lymph node involvement thus threatens bloodstream dissemination.[176] Also, the in vivo data have directly documented the intimate relationship that exists between the vascular and lymphatic systems in the spread of cancer:[174]

SPREAD OF CANCER OF THE LARYNX

Direct infiltration	Internal laryngeal structures	Mucosa Submucosa Laryngeal muscles Laryngeal cartilages Cricothyroid membrane Thyrohyoid membrane Lymph vessels Blood vessels Nerve sheaths
	External laryngeal structures	Prelaryngeal muscles Subcutaneous tissues Skin Prelaryngeal lymph nodes Paratracheal lymph nodes Preepiglottic space
	Adjacent organs	Tongue base Hypopharynx and cervical esophagus Thyroid gland Trachea
Lymphogenous spread	Cervical lymph nodes (particularly the jugular chain) Distant lymph nodes (exceptionally)	
↕ through thoracic duct and lymphaticovenous communications		
Hematogenous spread	Several organs (lungs, liver, bone, brain, cutis)	

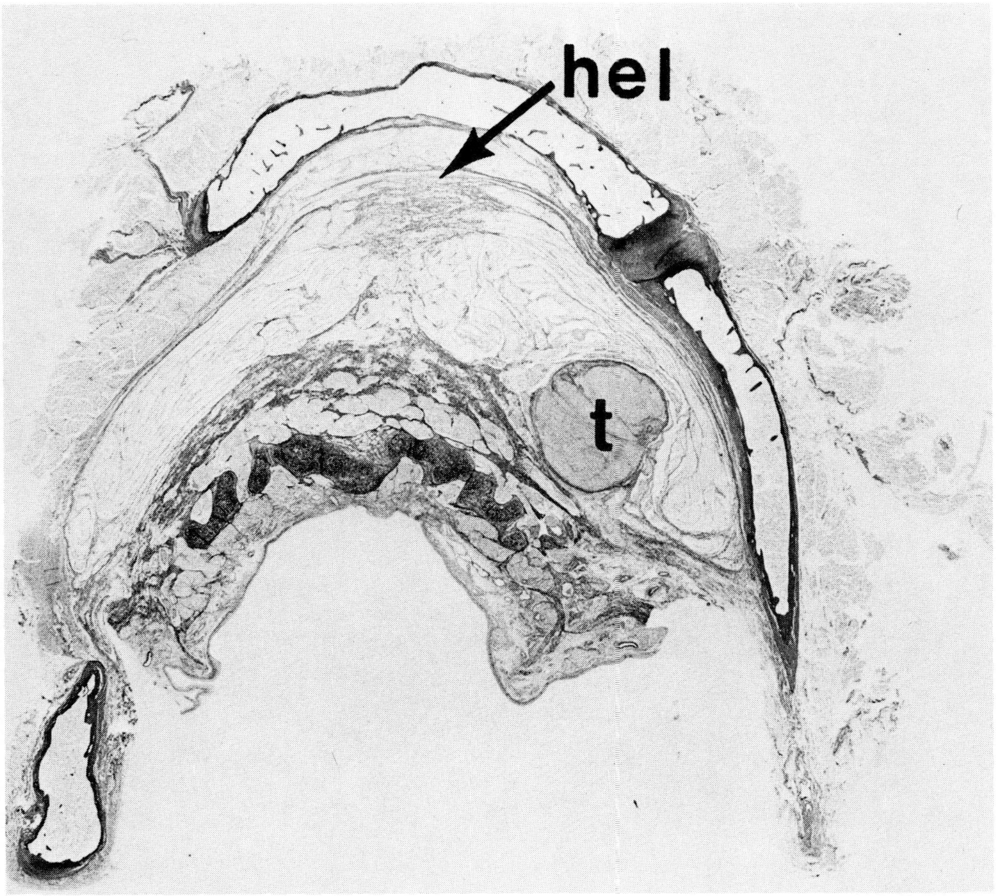

FIGURE 9. Horizontal section of larynx; same specimen as Figure 6 but at a more cranial level. Notice that the tumor(t) stays on the right side as it ascends in the paraglottic space; hel indicates hyoepiglottic ligament. (Victoria blue-van Gieson stain; Magnification × 3.) (By courtesy of Prof. K. H. Lam.)

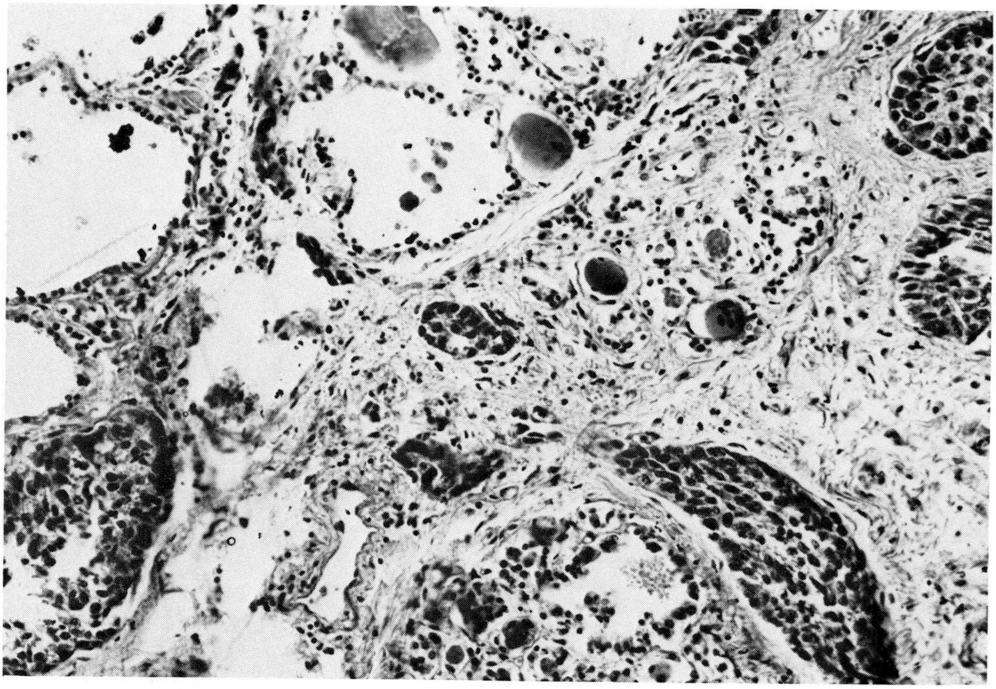

FIGURE 10. Direct invasion of the thyroid gland by poorly differentiated squamous cell carcinoma. (H.E.; magnification × 40.)

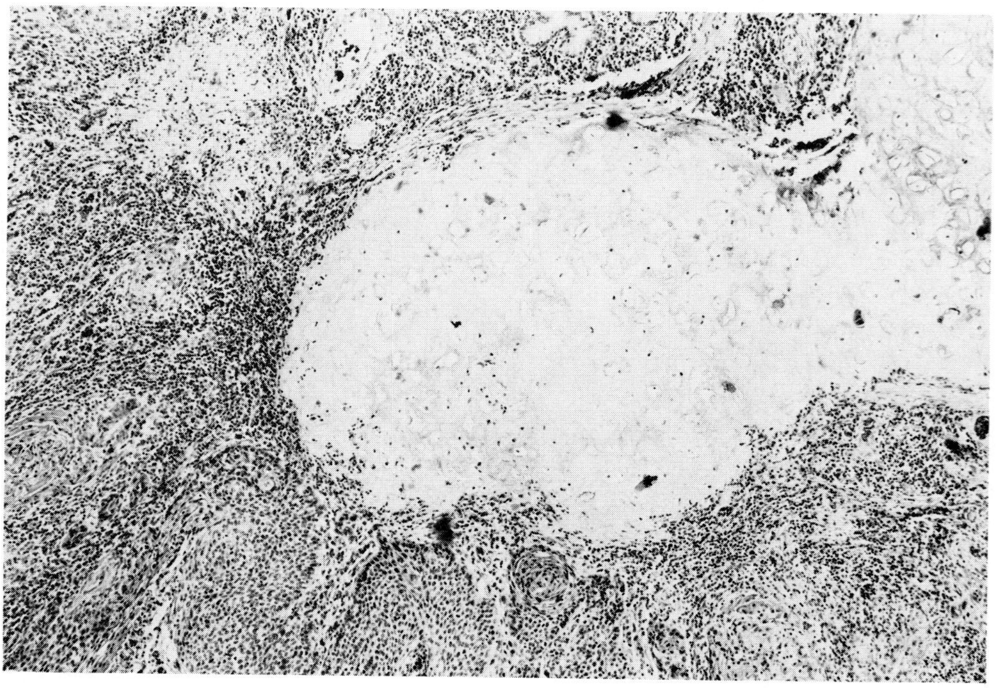

FIGURE 11. Direct invasion of the elastic cartilage of the epiglottis by squamous cell carcinoma. (H.E.; magnification × 16.)

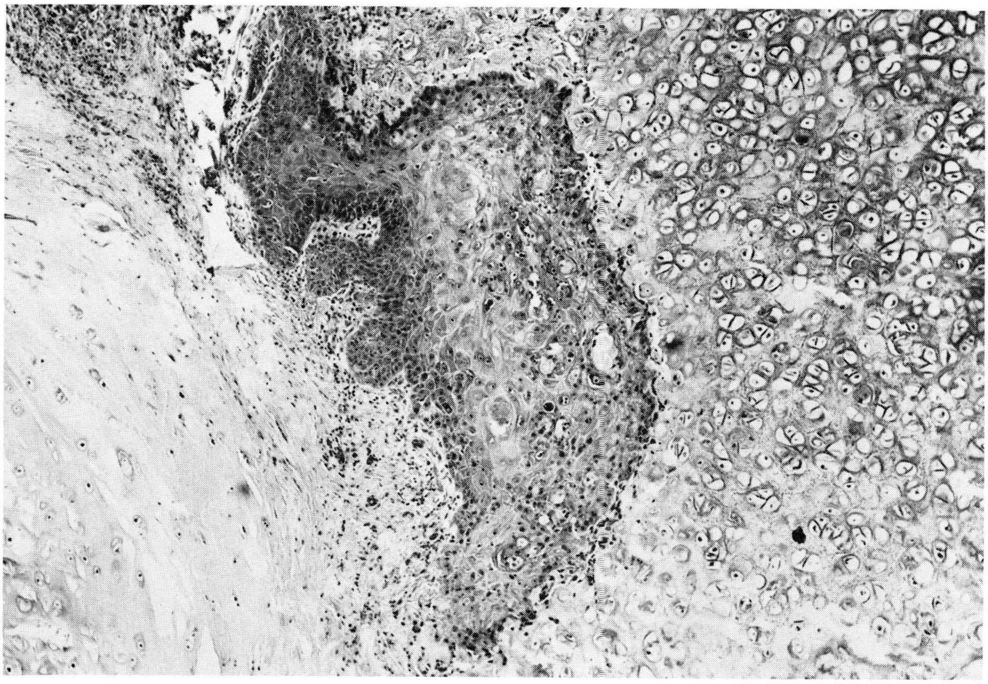

FIGURE 12. Direct invasion of the arytenoid cartilage by squamous cell carcinoma. (H.E.; magnification × 40.)

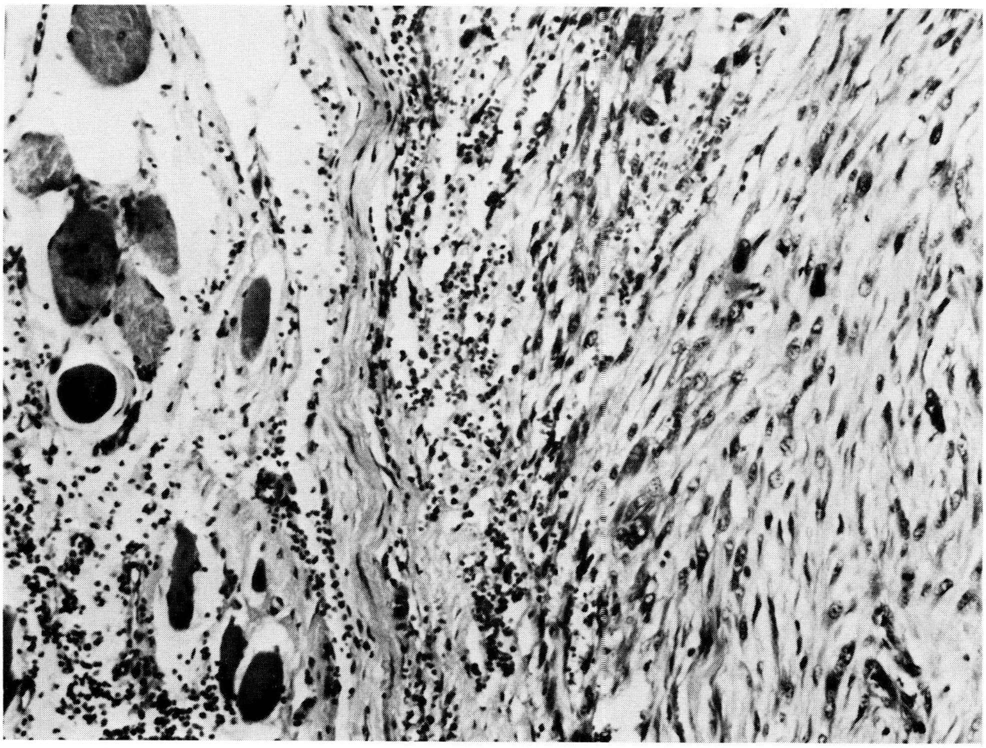

FIGURE 13. Malignant fibrous histiocytoma. Cellular area of the tumor mainly composed of spindle cells. (H.E.; magnification × 40.)

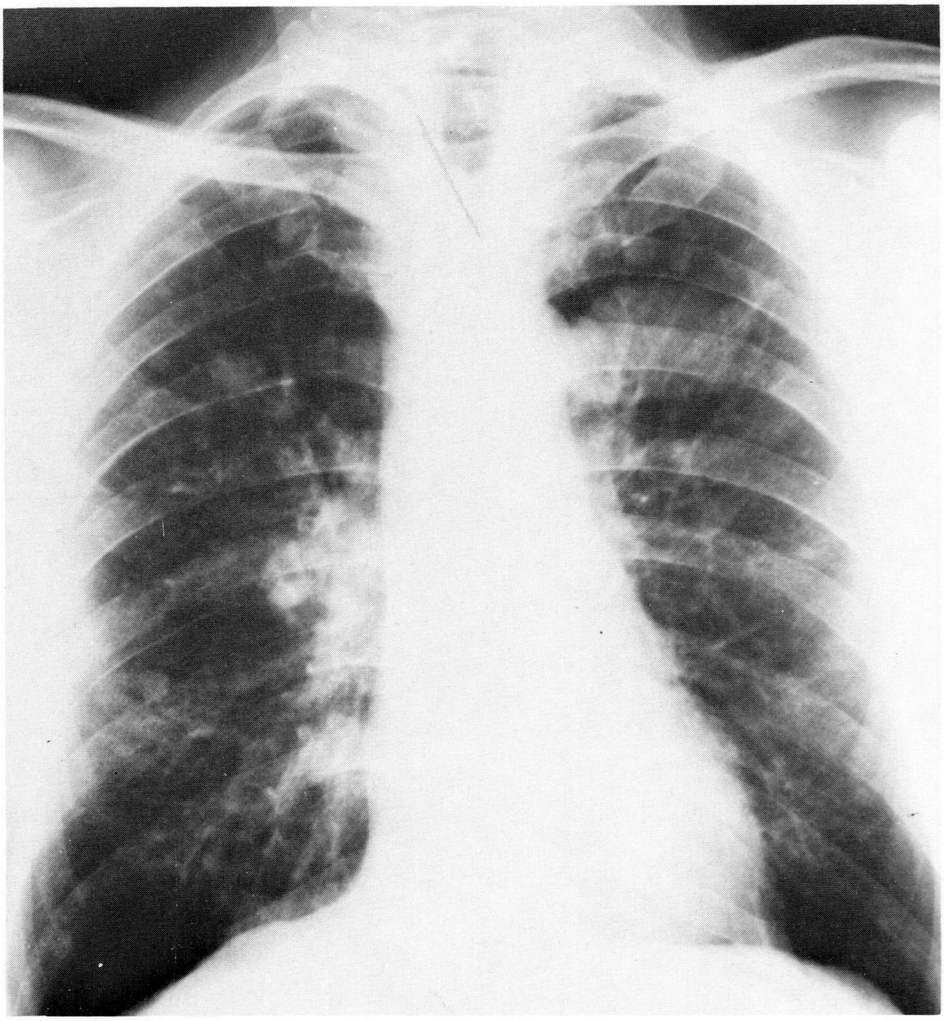

FIGURE 14. Chest roentgenogram demonstrates multiple lung metastases from malignant fibrous histiocytoma. This pulmonary pattern was present in the terminal stage of the disease. (From Ferlito, A., *Cancer*, 42, 611, 1978. With permission.)

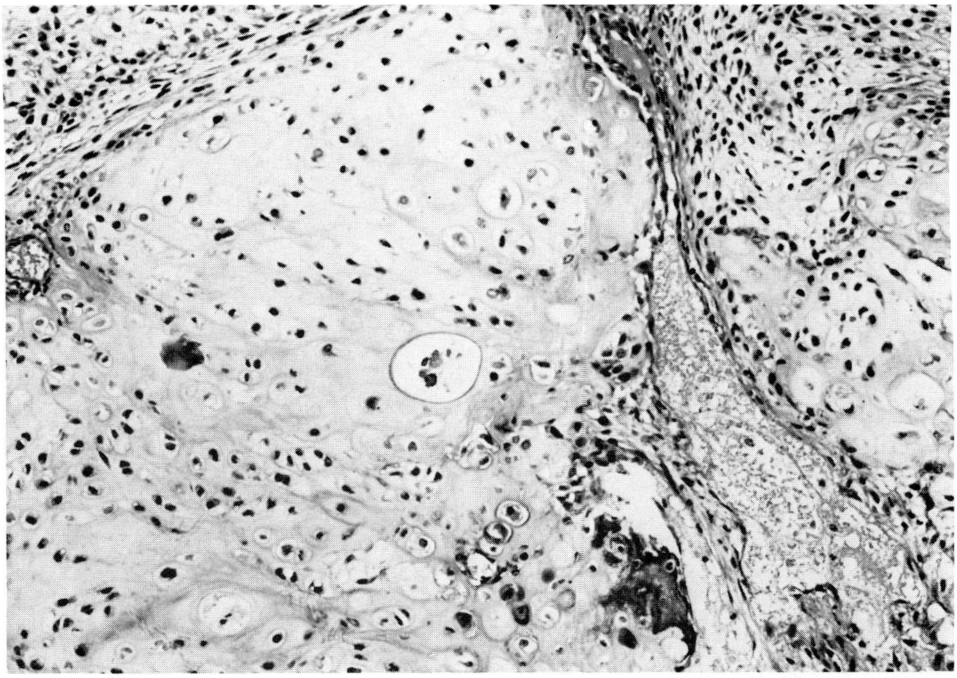

FIGURE 15. Chondrosarcoma (grade II). Several binucleated cells are present. (H.E.; magnification × 40.)

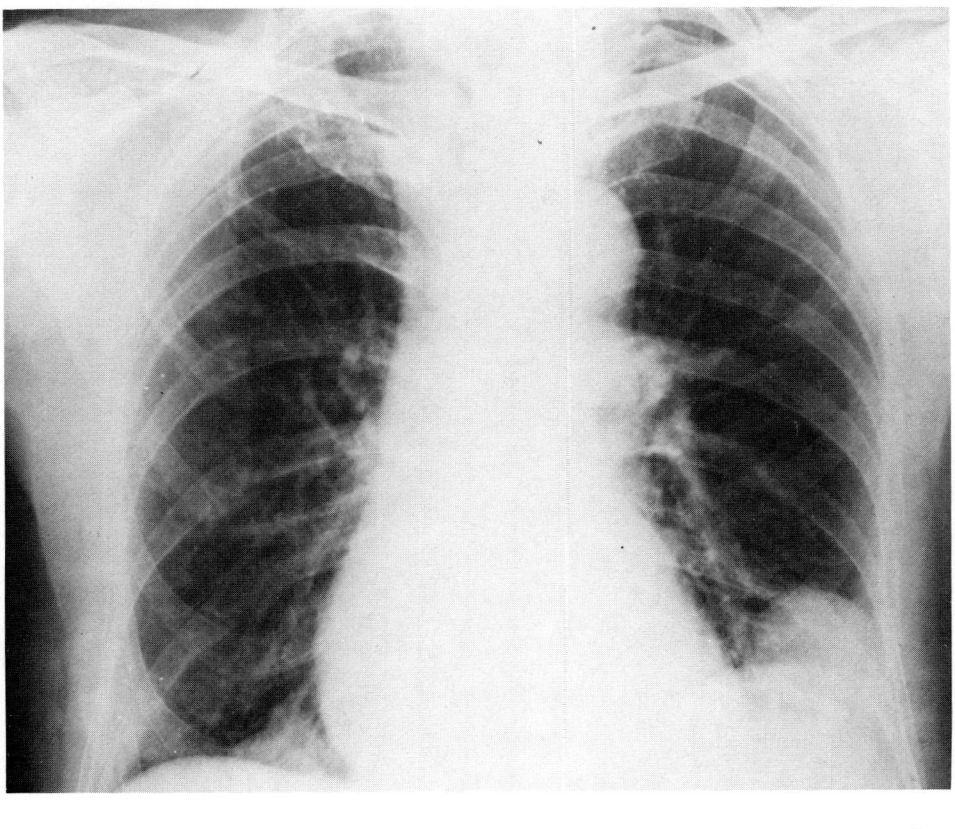

FIGURE 16. Chest roentgenogram showing bilateral pulmonary metastases from chondrosarcoma. (From Ferlito, A. et al., *Am. J. Otolaryngol.*, 5, 350, 1984. With permission.)

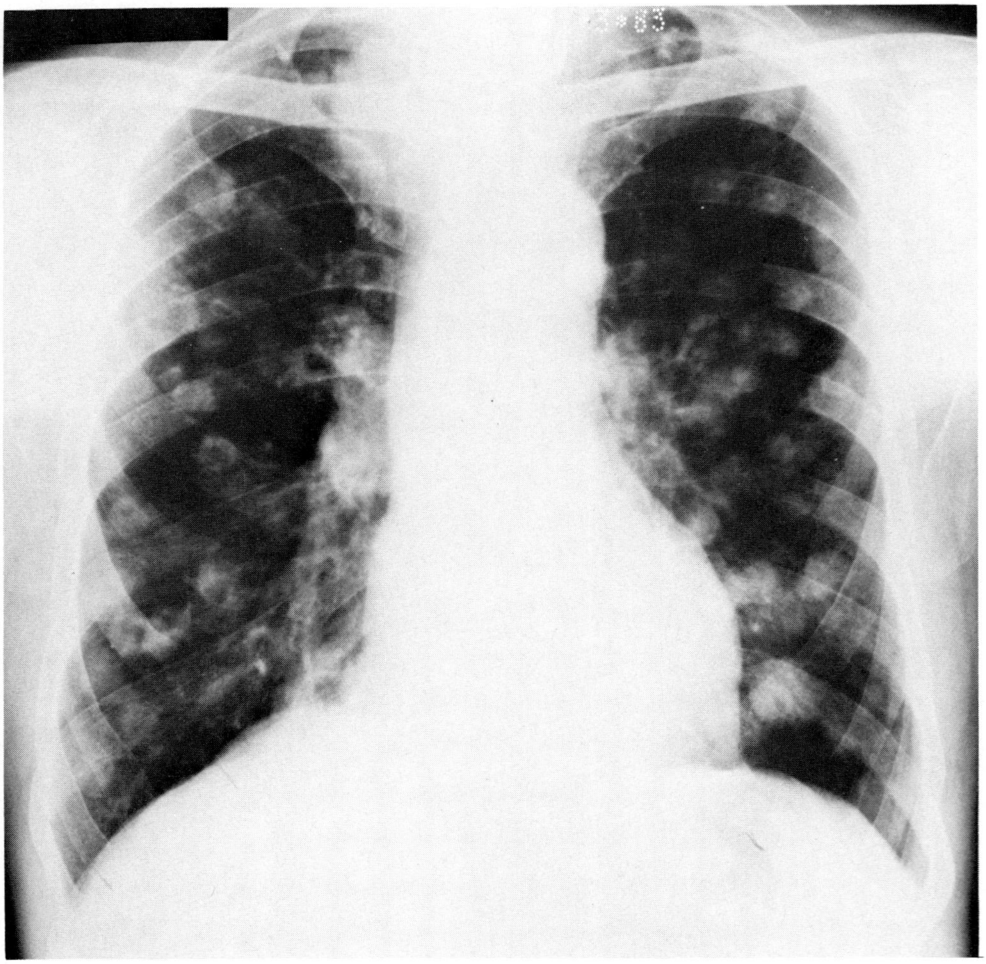

FIGURE 17. Chest roentgenogram showing multiple lung metastases from poorly differentiated squamous cell carcinoma.

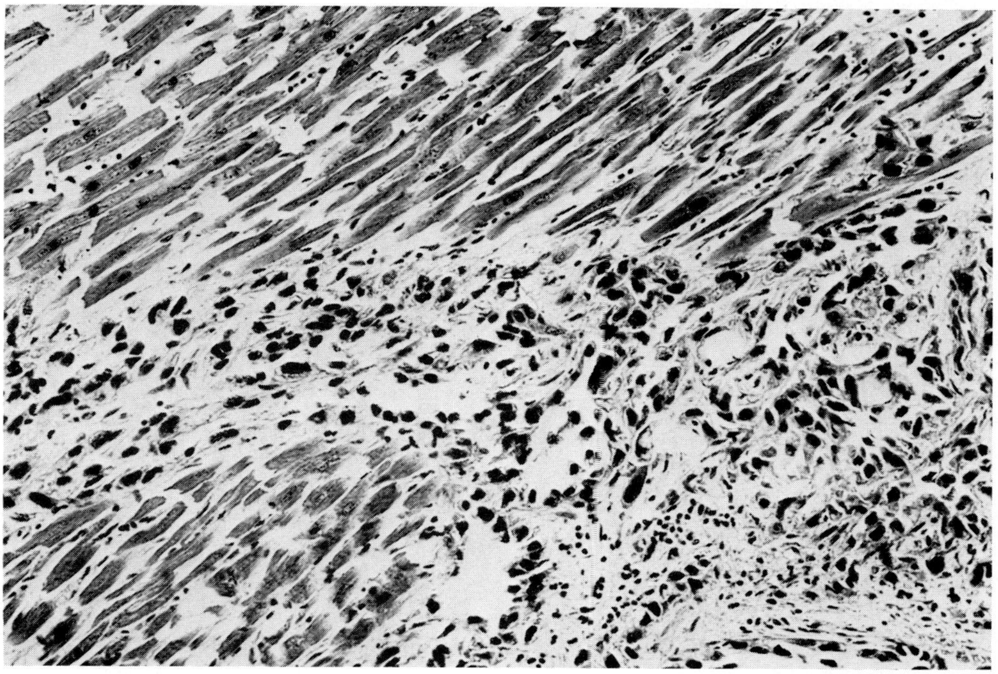

FIGURE 18. Cardiac metastasis from poorly differentiated squamous cell carcinoma. (H.E.; magnification × 40.)

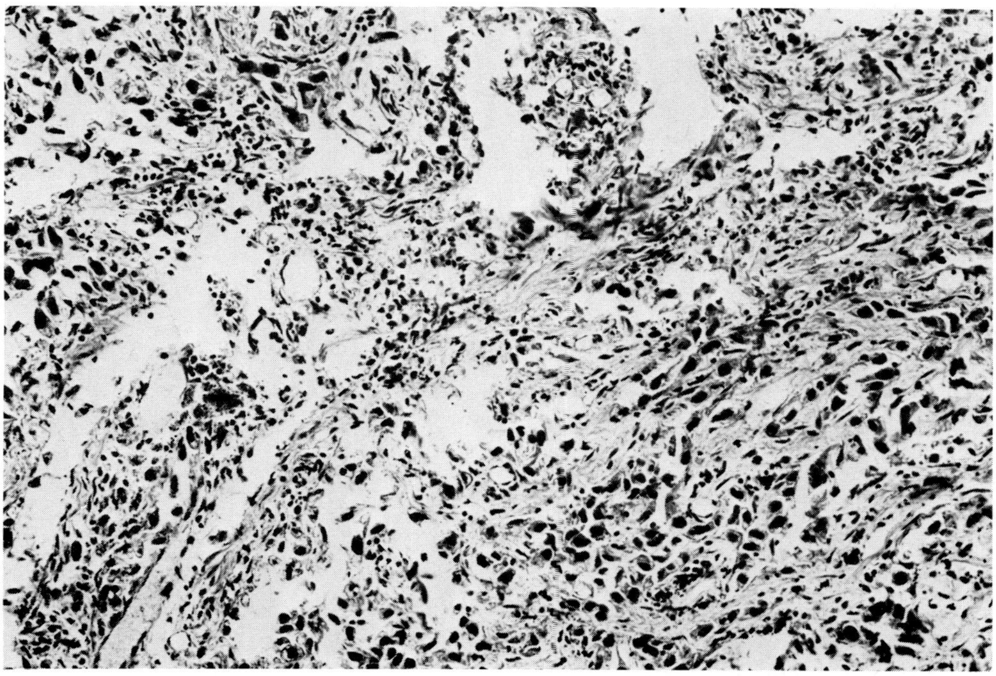

FIGURE 19. Lung metastasis from poorly differentiated squamous cell carcinoma. (H.E.; magnification × 16.)

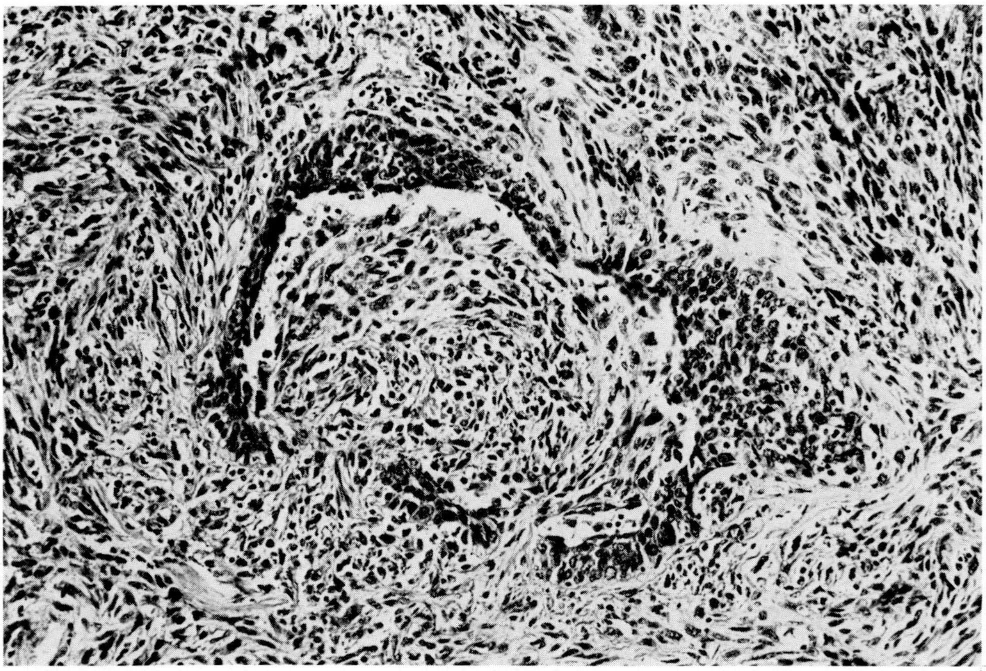

FIGURE 20. Spindle cell squamous carcinoma. Small nest of poorly differentiated squamous carcinoma in sarcoma-like tissue. (H.E.; magnification × 40.)

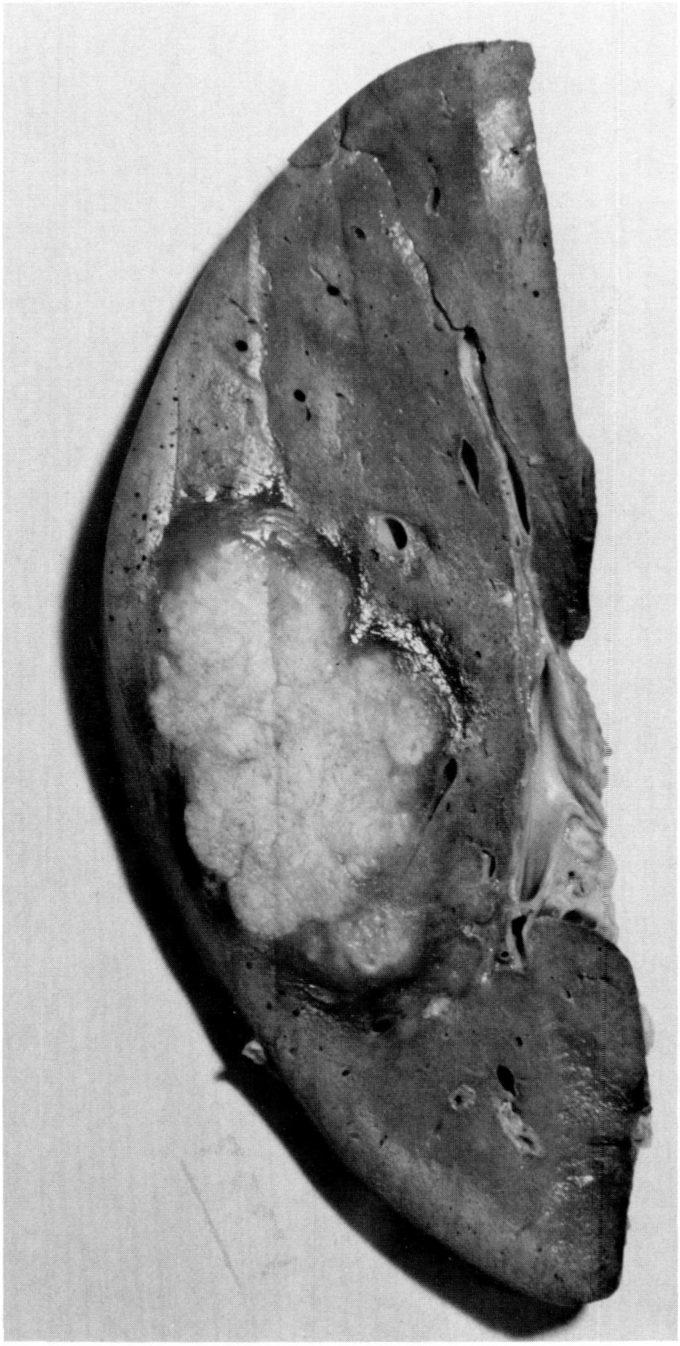

FIGURE 21. Secondary deposit in the liver of spindle cell squamous carcinoma.

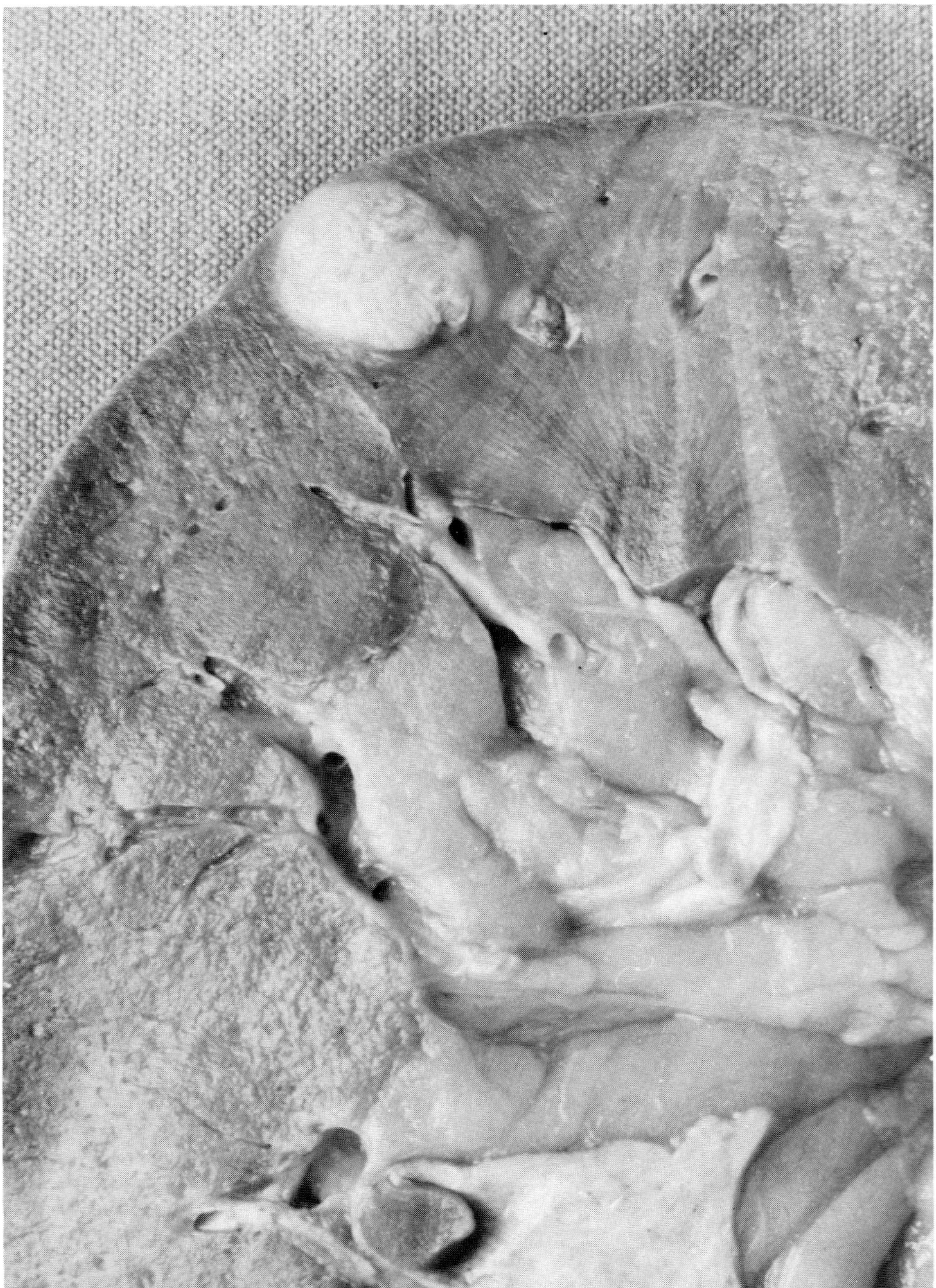

FIGURE 22. Isolated blood-borne deposit in the kidney of spindle cell squamous carcinoma.

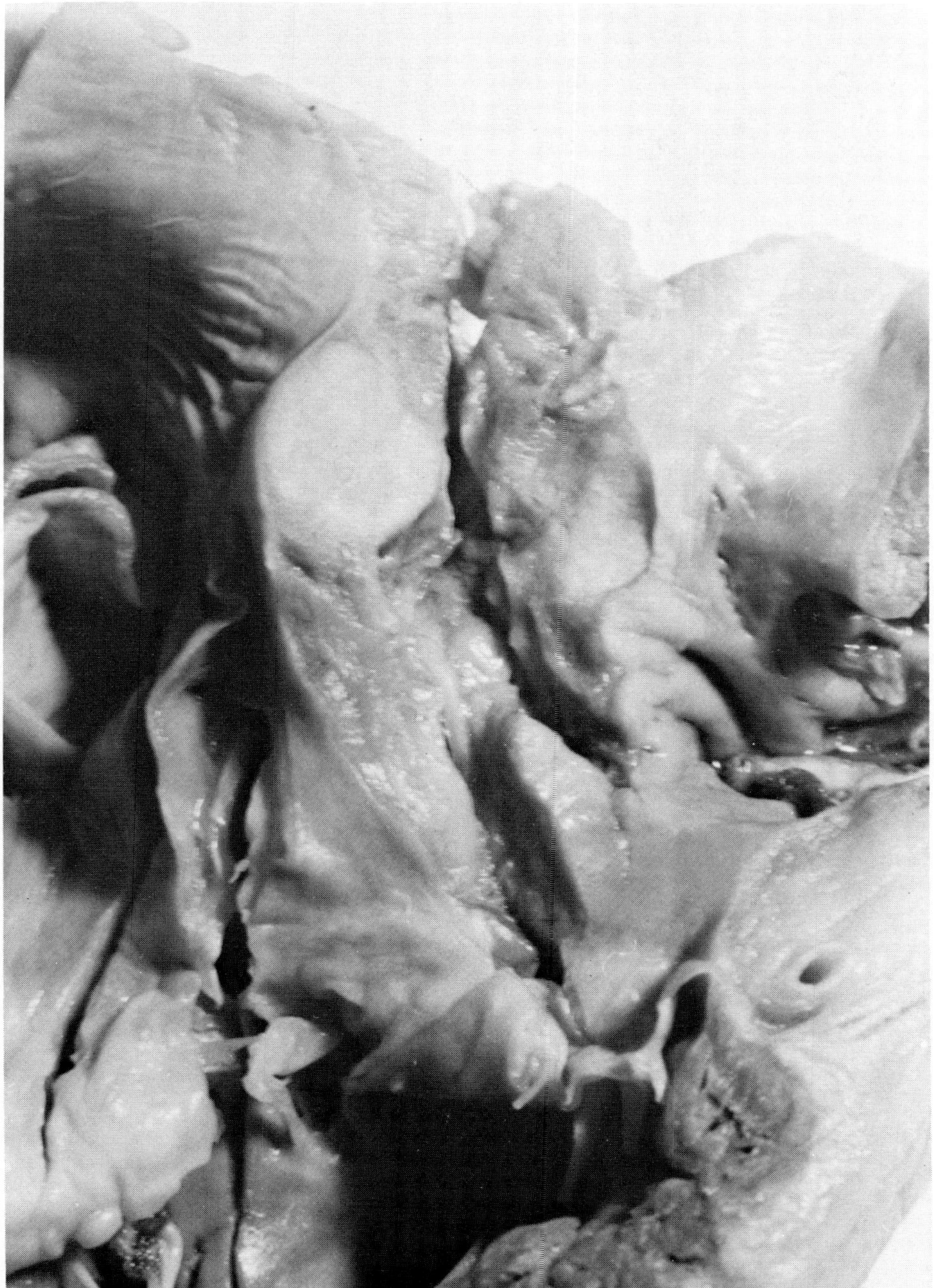

FIGURE 23. Cardiac metastasis from spindle cell squamous carcinoma.

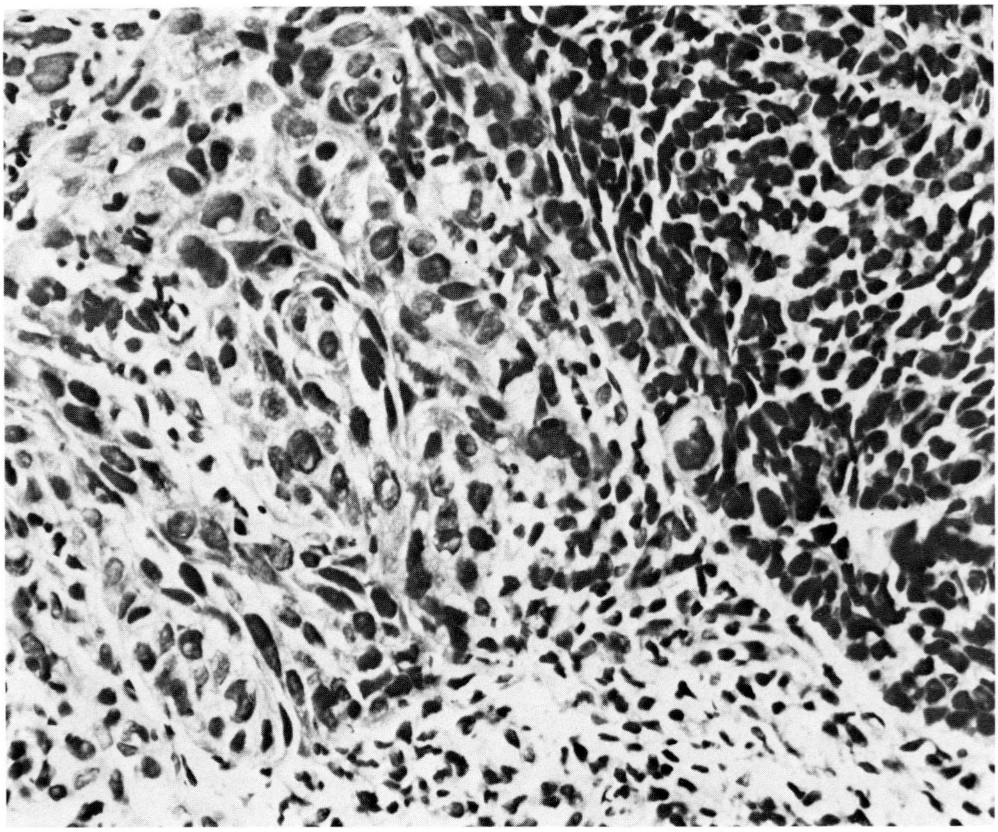

FIGURE 24. Combined small cell carcinoma. Note simultaneous squamous cell carcinoma adjacent to small cell carcinoma. (H.E.; magnification × 100.)

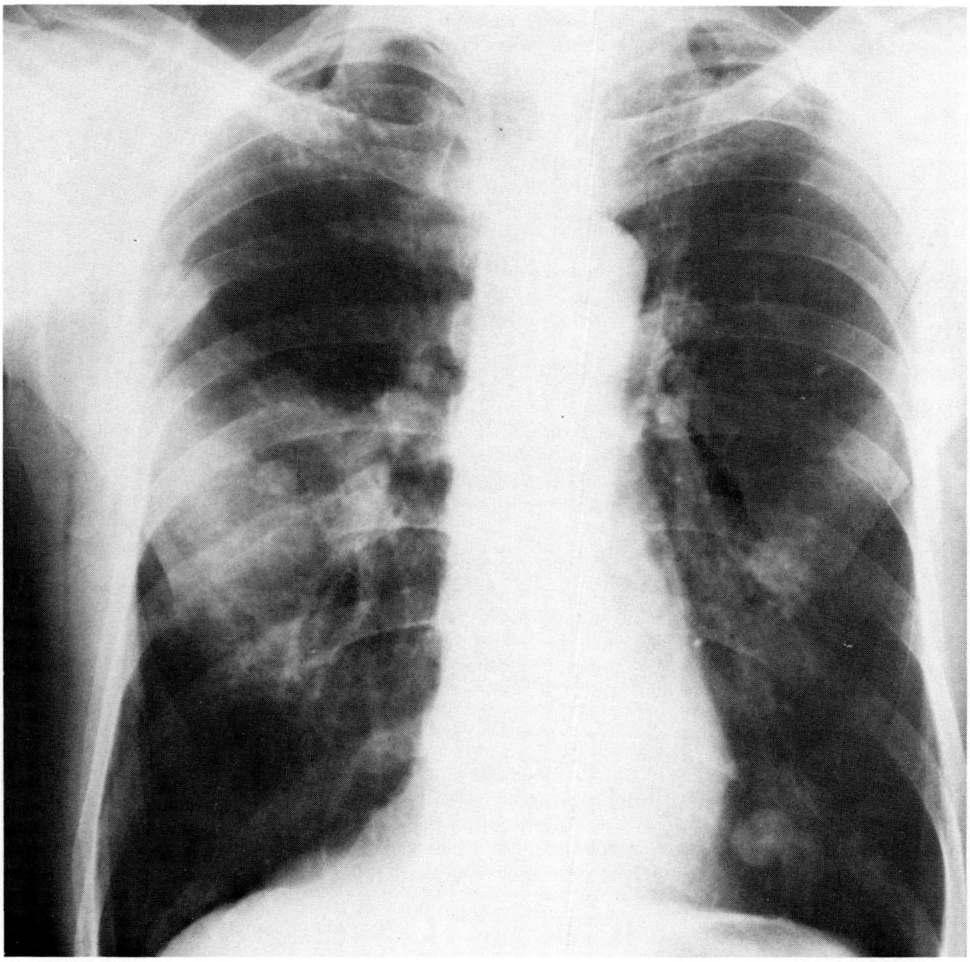

FIGURE 25. Chest roentgenogram showing multiple metastases from combined small cell carcinoma.

REFERENCES

1. **Lam, K. H.,** Extralaryngeal spread of cancer of the larynx: a study with whole-organ sections, *Head Neck Surg.,* 5, 410, 1983.
2. **Gérard-Marchant, R. and Micheau, C.,** Anatomie pathologique des épithéliomas laryngés, *Rev. Méd.,* 9, 547, 1968.
3. **Micheau, C., Luboinski, R., Sancho, H., and Cachin, Y.,** Modes of invasion of cancer of the larynx. A statistical, histological, and radioclinical analysis of 120 cases, *Cancer,* 38, 346, 1976.
4. **Willis, R. A.,** *The Spread of Tumor in the Human Body,* Churchill Livingston, London, 1934.
5. **Mazzarella, L. A., Pina, L. H., and Wolff, D.,** Asymptomatic metastasis to the larynx, *Laryngoscope,* 76, 1547, 1966.
6. **MacComb, W. S. and Fletcher, G. H.,** *Cancer of the Head and Neck,* Williams & Wilkins, Baltimore, 1967.
7. **Lam, K. H. and Wong, J.,** The preepiglottic and paraglottic spaces in relation to spread of carcinoma of the larynx, *Am.J.Otolaryngol.,* 4, 81, 1983.
8. **Bridger, G. P. and Nassar, V. H.,** Cancer spread in the larynx, *Arch.Otolaryngol.,* 95, 497, 1972.
9. **Bridger, G. P.,** Mucous gland involvement in cancer at the anterior commissure, *J.Otolaryngol.,* 3, 507, 1974.
10. **Olofsson, J.,** Growth and spread of laryngeal carcinoma, *Can.J.Otolaryngol.,* 3, 446, 1974.
11. **Friedmann, I. and Osborn, D. A.,** The larynx, in *Systemic Pathology,* Vol.1, 2nd ed., Symmers, W.St.C., Ed., Churchill Livingston, Edinburgh, 1976.
12. **van Nostrand, A. W. P. and Brodarec, I.,** Laryngeal carcinoma—modifications in surgical techniques based on an understanding of tumor growth characteristics, *J. Otolaryngol.,* 11, 186, 1982.
13. **Olofsson, J. and van Nostrand, A. W. P.,** Growth and spread of laryngeal and hypopharyngeal carcinoma with reflections on the effect of pre-operative irradiation. 139 cases studied by whole organ serial sectioning. *Acta Otolaryngol.,* Suppl. 308, 7, 1973.
14. **Shaw, H. J.,** Glottic cancer of the larynx, *J. Laryngol. Otol.,* 79, 1, 1965.
15. **Pressman, J. J., Simon, M. B. and Monel, C.,** Anatomical studies related to the dissemination of cancer of the larynx. *Trans. Am. Acad. Ophthalmol. Otolaryngol.,* 64, 628, 1960.
16. **Slezak, L.,** Histological serial block examination of 57 cases of laryngeal cancer, *Oncologia,* 20, 178, 1966.
17. **Günnel, F. and Baerthold, W.,** Zur Frage der Teilresektion bei Kehlkopfkrebsen. (Feingewebliche Untersuchungen an Stufenschnittserien), *Arch.Ohren-Nasen-Kehlkopfheilk,* 189, 195, 1967.
18. **Hommerich, K. W., Sauer, H. and Weede, W.,** Zur Wachstumstendenz von Larynxtumoren, *Arch.Ohren-Nasen-Kehlkopfheilk,* 199, 749, 1971.
19. **McDonald, T. J., DeSanto, L. W., and Weiland, L. H.,** Supraglottic larynx and its pathology as studied by whole laryngeal sections, *Laryngoscope,* 86, 635, 1976.
20. **Kirchner, J. A. and Som, M. L.,** Clinical and histological observations on supraglottic cancer, *Ann. Otol. Rhinol. Laryngol.,* 80, 638, 1971.
21. **Michaels, L. and Hassmann, E.,** Ventriculosaccular carcinoma of the larynx, *Clin.Otolaryngol.,* 7, 165, 1982.
22. **Lawson, W. and Biller, H. F.,** Cancer of the larynx, in *Cancer of the Head and Neck.* Suen, J. Y. and Myers, E. N., Eds., Churchill Livingston, N.Y., 1981.
23. **Harrison, D. F. N.,** The pathology and management of subglottic cancer, *Ann. Otol. Rhinol. Laryngol.,* 80, 6, 1971.
24. **Bauer, W. C., Edwards, D. L. and McGavran, M. H.,** A critical analysis of laryngectomy in the treatment of epidermoid carcinoma of the larynx, *Cancer,* 15, 263, 1962.
25. **Carter, R. L. and Tanner, N. S. B.,** Local invasion by laryngeal carcinoma—the importance of focal (metaplastic) ossification with laryngeal cartilage. *Clin. Otolaryngol.,* 4, 283, 1979.
26. **Kirchner, J. A.,** One hundred laryngeal cancers studied by serial section, *Ann. Otol. Rhinol. Laryngol.,* 78, 689, 1969.
27. **Kirchner, J. A., Cornog, J. L., Jr., and Holmes, R. E.,** Transglottic cancer: its growth and spread within the larynx, *Arch. Otolaryngol.,* 99, 247, 1974.
28. **Kirchner, J. A.,** Two hundred laryngeal cancers: patterns of growth and spread as seen in serial sections, *Laryngoscope,* 87, 474, 1977.
29. **Pillsbury, H. C. and Kirchner, J. A.,** Clinical vs. histopathologic staging in laryngeal cancer, *Arch.Otolaryngol.,* 105, 157, 1979.
30. **Pittam, M. R. and Carter, R. L.,** Framework invasion by laryngeal carcinomas, *Head Neck Surg.,* 4, 200, 1982.

30a. **Glanz, H. K.,** Carcinoma of the Larynx. Growth, p-classification and grading of squamous cell carcinoma of the vocal cords, in *New Aspects of Fundamental Problems in Laryngology and Otology, Advances in Oto-Rhino-Laryngology* , Vol. 32, Pfaltz, C. R., Ed., Karger, Basel, 1984.
31. **McGavran, M. H., Bauer, W. C., and Ogura, J. H.,** The incidence of cervical lymph node metastases from epidermoid carcinoma of the larynx and their relationship to certain characteristics of the primary tumor. A study based on the clinical and pathological findings in 96 patients treated by primary en bloc laryngectomy and radical neck dissection, *Cancer,* 14, 55, 1961.
32. **Pearson, B. W.,** Laryngeal microcirculation and pathways of cancer spread, *Laryngoscope,* 85, 700, 1975.
33. **Carter, R. L.,** Direct bone invasion by squamous carcinomas of the head and neck, *Clin.Otolaryngol.,* 5, 85, 1980.
34. **Carter, R. L.,** Some aspects of the metastatic process, *J.Clin.Pathol.,* 35, 1041, 1982.
35. **Cummings, C. W.,** Incidence of nodal metastases in T2 supraglottic carcinoma, *Arch.Otolaryngol.,* 99, 268, 1974.
36. **Meyer-Breiting, E. and von Ilberg, C.,** Spread and mode of metastases of supraglottic laryngeal carcinoma, *ORL,* 41, 288, 1979.
37. **Ogura, J. H., Biller, H. F., and Wette, R.,** Elective neck dissection for pharyngeal and laryngeal cancers, *Ann. Otol. Rhinol. Laryngol.,* 80, 646,1971.
38. **Gudziol, HJ. and Beleites, E.,** Über die Häufigkeit regionärer Metastases beim supraglottischen Karzinom, *Laryngol. Rhinol. Otol.,* 62, 35, 1983.
39. **O'Keefe, J. J.,** Evaluation of laryngectomy with radical neck dissection, *Laryngoscope,* 69, 914, 1959.
40. **Smith, R. R., Caulk, R. M., Russell, W. O., and Jackson, C. L.,** End results in 600 laryngeal cancers using the American Joint Committee's proposed method of stage classification and end results reporting, *Surg. Gynecol. Obstet.,* 113, 435, 1961.
41. **Bocca, E., Pignataro, O., and Mosciaro, O.,** Supraglottic surgery of the larynx, *Ann. Otol. Rhinol. Laryngol.,* 77, 1005, 1968.
42. **Som, M. L.,** Conservation surgery for carcinoma of the supraglottis, *J. Laryngol. Otol.,* 84, 655, 1970.
43. **Bocca, E., Pignataro, O., and Oldini, C.,** Supraglottic laryngectomy: 30 years of experience, *Ann. Otol. Rhinol. Laryngol.,* 92, 41, 1983.
44. **Ogura, J. H., Sessions, D. G., and Ciralsky, R. H.,** Supraglottic carcinoma with extension to the arytenoid, *Laryngoscope,* 85, 1327, 1975.
45. **Smith, R. R., Caulk, R., Frazell, E., Holinger, P. H., MacComb, W. S., Russell, W. O., Schulz, M. D., and Tucker, G. F.,** Revision of the clinical staging system for cancer of the larynx, *Cancer,* 31, 72, 1973.
46. **Shah, J. P., and Tollefson, H. R.,** Epidermoid carcinoma of the supraglottic larynx. Role of neck dissection in initial surgical treatment. *Am. J. Surg.,* 128, 494, 1974.
47. **Bocca, E.,** Supraglottic cancer, *Laryngoscope,* 85, 1318, 1975.
48. **Fayos, J. V.,** Carcinoma of the endolarynx: results of irradiation, *Cancer,* 35, 1525, 1975.
49. **Cachin, Y.,** Supraglottic carcinomas: the early cases, *Laryngoscope,* 85, 1617, 1975.
50. **Hansen, H. S.,** Supraglottic carcinoma of the aryepiglottic fold, *Laryngoscope,* 85, 1667, 1975.
51. **Taskinen, P. J.,** The early case of supraglottic carcinoma, *Laryngoscope,* 85, 1643, 1975.
52. **Coates, H. L., DeSanto, L. W., Devine, K. D., and Elveback, L. R.,** Carcinoma of the supraglottic larynx. A review of 221 cases, *Arch.Otolaryngol.,* 102, 686, 1976.
53. **Kircher, J. A. and Owen, J. R.,** Five hundred cancers of the larynx and pyriform sinus. Results of treatment of radiation and surgery, *Laryngoscope,* 87, 1288, 1977.
54. **Bryce, D. P.,** The management of laryngeal cancer, *J. Otolaryngol.,* 8, 105, 1979.
55. **DeSanto, L. W.,** The options in early laryngeal carcinoma, *N. Engl. J. Med.,* 306, 910, 1982.
56. **Pietrantoni, L. and Fior, R.,** Clinical and surgical problems of cancer of the larynx and hypopharynx. A review of 570 consecutive cases operated on in the Ear, Nose and Throat Clinic of the University of Milan between 1948 and 1954, with special regard to the problem of metastases, *Acta Otolaryngol.,* Suppl. 142, 6, 1958.
57. **Feind, C. R.,** The head and neck, in *The Lymphatics in Cancer,* Haagensen, C. D., Feind, C. R., Herter, F. P., Slanetz, C. A., Jr., and Weinberg, L. A., Eds., W. B. Saunders, Philadelphia, 1972.
58. **Lindberg, R.,** Distribution of cervical lymph node metastases from squamous cell carcinoma of the upper respiratory and digestive tracts, *Cancer,* 29, 1446, 1972.
59. **Feldman, D. E. and Applebaum, E. L.,** The submandibular triangle in radical neck dissection, *Arch. Otolaryngol.,* 103, 70, 1977.
60. **Rubenfeld, S. and Kaplan, G.,** Carcinoma of the larynx with distant lymphatic metastases, *Arch. Otolaryngol.,* 56, 255, 1952.
61. **Gnepp, D. R., Ferlito, A., and Hyams, V.,** Primary anaplastic small cell (oat cell) carcinoma of the larynx. Review of the literature and report of 18 cases, *Cancer,* 51, 1731, 1983.

62. **Kashima, H. K.,** The characteristics of laryngeal cancer correlating with cervical lymph node metastasis (analysis based on 40 total organ sections), *Can. J. Otolaryngol.,* 4, 893, 1975.
63. **Bauer, W. C.,** Varieties of squamous carcinoma. Biologic behavior, therapeutic implications and prognostic significance in the upper aerodigestive tract, in *The Relationship of Histology to Cancer Treatment,* Proc. 9th Annu. W. Coast Cancer Symp., Karger, Basel, 1974.
64. **Ferlito, A.,** Histological classification of larynx and hypopharynx cancers and their clinical implications. Pathologic aspects of 2052 malignant neoplasms diagnosed at the ORL Department of Padua University from 1966 to 1976, *Acta Otolaryngol.,* Suppl. 342, 1, 1976.
65. **Batsakis, J. G.,** 'Pseudosarcoma' of the mucous membranes in the head and neck, *J. Laryngol. Otol.,* 95, 311, 1981.
66. **Batsakis, J. G., Rice, D. H., and Howard, D. R.,** The pathology of head and neck tumors: spindle cells lesions (sarcomatoid carcinomas, nodular fasciitis, and fibrosarcoma) of the aerodigestive tracts, Part 14, *Head Neck Surg.,* 4, 499, 1982.
67. **Lambert, P. R., Ward, P. H., and Berci, G.,** Pseudosarcoma of the larynx. A comprehensive analysis, *Arch. Otolaryngol.,* 106, 700, 1980.
68. **Leventon, G. S. and Evans, H. L.,** Sarcomatoid squamous cell carcinoma of the mucous membranes of the head and neck: a clinicopathologic study of 20 cases, *Cancer,* 48, 944, 1981.
69. **Hyams, V. J.,** Spindle cell carcinoma of the larynx, *Can. J. Otolaryngol.,* 4, 307, 1975.
70. **Ferlito, A.,** Primary lymphoepithelial carcinoma of the hypopharynx, *J. Laryngol. Otol.,* 91, 361, 1977.
71. **Dockerty, M. B., Parkhill, E. M., Dahlin, D. C., Woolner, L. B., Soule, E. H., and Harrison, E. G., Jr.,** Tumors of the Oral Cavity and Pharynx, Atlas of Tumor Pathology, Section 4, Fascicle 10b, Washington D.C. Armed Forces Institute of Pathology, 1968.
72. **Micheau, C., Luboinski, B., Schwaab, G., Richard, J., and Cachin, Y.,** Lymphoepitheliomas of the larynx (undifferentiated carcinomas of nasopharyngeal type), *Clin. Otolaryngol.,* 4, 43, 1979.
73. **Toker, C. and Peterson, D. W.,** Lymphoepithelioma of the vocal cord, *Arch. Otolaryngol.,* 104, 161, 1978.
74. **Gerughty, R. M., Hennigar, G. R., and Brown, F.M.,** Adenosquamous carcinoma of the nasal, oral, and laryngeal cavities. A clinicopathologic survey of ten cases, *Cancer,* 22, 1140, 1968.
75. **Ferlito, A.,** Adenosquamous carcinoma of the larynx. A clinical and pathologic study. Report of four cases and review of the literature, *Acta Otorhinolaryngol. Belg.,* 30, 379, 1976.
76. **Pesavento, G., Ferlito, A., and Recher, G.,** Primary clear cell carcinoma of the larynx, *J. Clin. Pathol.,* 33, 1160, 1980.
77. **Ferlito, A., Friedmann, I., and Recher, G.,** Primary giant cell carcinoma of the larynx. A clinico-pathological study of four cases, *ORL,* 47, 105, 1985
78. **Ferlito, A., Caruso, G., Nicolai, P., Recher, G., and Silvestri, F.,** Primary small cell ('oat cell') carcinoma of the larynx and hypopharynx. A clinico-pathological study of 8 cases with a review of the literature, *ORL,* 43, 204, 1981.
79. **Goldman, N. C., Hood, I., and Singleton, G. T.,** Carcinoid of the larynx, *Arch. Otolaryngol.,* 90, 64, 1969.
80. **Gapany-Gapanavicius, B. and Kenan, S.,** Carcinoid tumor of the larynx, *Ann. Otol. Rhinol. Laryngol.,* 90, 42, 1981.
81. **Tamai, S., Iri, H., Maruyama, T., Kasahara, M., Akatsuka, S., Sakurai, S., and Murakami, Y.,** Laryngeal carcinoid tumor: light and electron microscopic studies, *Cancer,* 48, 2256, 1981.
82. **Carles, D., Devars, F., Traissac, L., Darasse, D., Rinaldo, J. F., and Richir, C. L.,** Carcinoïde primitif du larynx, *Ann. Pathol.,* 3, 65, 1983.
83. **Pages, A., Pigodel, Ch., and Ramos, J.,** Carcinoïde du larynx. Etude ultrastructurale et immunofluoresc-ence, *Ann. Pathol.,* 3, 59, 1983.
84. **Goldman, N. C., Katibah, G. M., and Medina, J.,** Carcinoid tumors of the larynx, in press.
85. **Whicker, J. H., Neel, H. B., Weiland, L. H., and Devine, K. D.,** Adenocarcinoma of the larynx, *Ann. Otol. Rhinol. Laryngol.,* 83, 487, 1974.
86. **Ferlito, A., Recher, G., and Bottin, R.,** Mucoepidermoid carcinoma of the larynx. A clinicopathological study of 11 cases with review of the literature, *ORL,* 43, 280, 1981.
87. **Crissman, J. D. and Rosenblatt, A.,** Acinous cell carcinoma of the larynx, *Arch. Pathol. Lab. Med.,* 102, 233, 1978.
88. **Ferlito, A.,** Acinic cell carcinoma of the minor salivary glands, *Histopathology,* 4, 331, 1980.
89. **Montes Noriega, B.,** Adenomas de laringe, *An. Otorrinolaringol. Ibero Am.,* 1, 98, 1974.
90. **Squires, J. E., Mills, S. E., Cooper, P. H., Innes, D. J., Jr., and McLean, W. C.,** Acinic cell carcinoma. Its occurrence in the laryngotracheal junction after thyroid radiation, *Arch. Pathol. Lab. Med.,* 105, 266, 1981.
91. **Biller, H. F. and Bergman, J. A.,** Verrucous carcinoma of the larynx, *Can. J. Otolaryngol.,* 4, 280, 1975.

92. **Biller, H. F. and Bergman, J. A.,** Verrucous carcinoma of the larynx (discussion), *Can. J. Otolaryngol.*, 4, 280, 1975.
93. **van Nostrand, A. W. P. and Olofsson, J.,** Verrucous carcinoma of the larynx. A clinical and pathologic study of 10 cases, *Cancer*, 30, 691, 1972.
94. **Ferlito, A., Antonutto, G., and Silvestri, F.,** Histological appearances and nuclear DNA content of verrucous squamous cell carcinoma of the larynx, *ORL*, 38, 65, 1976.
95. **Ferlito, A. and Recher, G.,** Ackerman's tumor (or verrucous carcinoma) of the larynx. A clinicopathological study of 77 cases, *Cancer*, 46, 1617, 1980.
96. **Fisher, H. R.,** Verrucous carcinoma of the larynx. A study of its pathologic anatomy, *Can. J. Otolaryngol.*, 4, 270, 1975.
97. **Kraus, F. T. and Perez-Mesa, C.,** Verrucous carcinoma. Clinical and pathological study of 105 cases involving oral cavity, larynx and genitalia, *Cancer*, 19, 26, 1966.
98. **Ferlito, A. and Caruso, G.,** Biological behavior of laryngeal adenoid cystic carcinoma. Therapeutic considerations, *ORL*, 45, 245, 1983.
99. **Shanon, E., Covo, J., and Loeventhal, M.,** Melanoma of the epiglottis. A case treated by supraglottic laryngectomy, *Arch. Otolaryngol.*, 91, 304, 1970.
100. **Shah, J. P., Huvos, A. G., and Strong, E. W.,** Mucosal melanomas of the head and neck, *Am. J. Surg.*, 134, 531, 1977.
101. **Batsakis, J. G., Regezi, J. A., Solomon, A. R., and Rice, D. H.,** The pathology of head and neck tumors: mucosal melanomas, Part 13, *Head Neck Surg.*, 4, 404, 1982.
102. **Vetters, J. M. and Toner, P. G.,** Chemodectoma of larynx, *J. Pathol.*, 101, 259, 1970.
103. **Hooper, R.,** Chemodectoma of the glomus laryngicum superior, *Laryngoscope*, 82, 686, 1972.
104. **Zachariah, K. J. and Shah, J. H.,** Chemodectoma of the larynx, *J. Laryngol. Otol.*, 86, 1213, 1972.
105. **Adlington, P. and Woodhouse, M. A.,** The ultrastructure of chemodectoma of the larynx, *J. Laryngol. Otol.*, 86, 1219, 1972.
106. **Fraidooni, H.,** La chimiothérapie dans un cas de chémodectome du larynx, *Ann. Otolaryngol.*, 93, 303, 1976.
107. **Justrabo, E., Michiels, R., Calmettes, C., Cabanne, F., Bastein, H., Horiot, J. C., and Guerrin, J.,** An uncommon apudoma: a functional chemodectoma of the larynx. Report of a case and review of the literature, *Acta Otolaryngol.*, 89, 135, 1980.
108. **Sneige, N., Mackay, B., Ordonez, N. G., and Batsakis, J. G.,** Laryngeal paraganglioma. Report of two tumors with immunohistochemical and ultrastructural analysis, *Arch. Otolaryngol.*, 109, 113, 1983.
109. **Pedrazzini, A., Pedrinis, E., Luscieti, P., Losa, G., and Cavalli, F.,** Ein Fall von metastasierendem Paragangliom des Larynx, *Schweiz. Med. Wschr.*, 113, 1363, 1983.
109a. **Ohsawa, M., Kurita, Y., Horie, A., and Kurita, K.,** Malignant chemodectoma (paraganglioma) of the larynx. A case report with electron microscopy and biochemical assay, *Acta Pathol. Jpn.*, 33, 1279, 1984.
110. **von Urfer, F.,** Myxolipom des Kehlkopfs, *Pract. Otorhinolaryngol.*, 8, 545, 1946.
111. **Kapur, T. R.,** Recurrent lipomata of the larynx and the pharynx with late malignant change, *J. Laryngol. Otol.*, 82, 761, 1968.
112. **Miller, D., Goodman, M., Weber, A., and Goldstein, A.,** Primary liposarcoma of the larynx, *Trans. Am. Acad. Ophthalmol. Otolaryngol.*, 80, 444, 1975.
113. **Velek, J. P.,** Liposarcoma of the larynx, *Trans. Am. Acad. Ophthalmol. Otolaryngol.*, 82, 569, 1976.
114. **Krausen, A. S., Gall, A. M., Garza, R., Spector, G. J., and Ansel, D. G.,** Liposarcoma of the larynx: a multicentric or a metastatic malignancy, *Laryngoscope*, 87, 1116, 1977.
115. **Tobey, D. N., Wheelis, R. F., and Yarington, C. T.,** Electron microscopy in the diagnosis of liposarcoma and fibrosarcoma of the larynx, *Ann. Otol. Rhinol. Laryngol.*, 88, 867, 1979.
116. **Ferlito, A.,** Primary pleomorphic liposarcoma of the larynx, *J. Otolaryngol.*, 7, 161, 1978.
117. **Setzen, M., Sobol, S., and Toomey, J. M.,** Clinical course of unusual malignant sarcomas of head and neck, *Ann. Otol. Rhinol. Laryngol.*, 88, 486, 1979.
118. **Frey-Schlottmann, M. L. and Stiens, R.,** Liposarkom im Hypopharynxbereich, *Arch.Otorhinolaryngol.*, 223, 419, 1979.
118a. **Gaynor, E. B., Raghausan, U., and Weisbrot, I. M.,** Primary myxoid liposarcoma of the larynx, *Otolaryngol. Head Neck Surg.*, 92, 476, 1984.
119. **Stout, A. P.,** Tumors featuring pericytes; glomus tumor and hemangiopericytoma, *Lab. Invest.*, 5, 217, 1956.
120. **Walike, J. W. and Bailey, B. J.,** Head and neck hemangiopericytoma, *Arch.Otolaryngol.*, 93, 345, 1971.
121. **Taguchi, K. et al.,** Hemangiopericytoma of the larynx. A case report, *Otolaryngology (Tokyo)*, 46, 21, 1974.
122. **Ferlito, A.,** Primary malignant hemangiopericytoma of the larynx (a case report with autopsy), *J.Laryngol. Otol.*, 92, 511, 1978.

123. **Moncade, J. and Demaldent, J. E.,** A propos de deux cas d'hémangiopéricytomes O.R.L., *Ann. Otolaryngol.*, 96, 789, 1979.
124. **Pesavento, G. and Ferlito, A.,** Haemangiopericytoma of the larynx. A clinico-pathological study with review of the literature, *J. Laryngol. Otol.*, 96, 1065, 1982.
125. **Hertzanu, Y., Mendelsohn, D. B., Kassner, G., and Hockman, M.,** Haemangiopericytoma of the larynx, *Br. J. Rad.*, 55, 870, 1982.
126. **Pratt, L. W. and Goodof, I. I.,** Hemangioendotheliosarcoma of the larynx, *Arch. Otolaryngol.*, 87, 484, 1968.
127. **Havens, F. Z. and Parkhill, E. M.,** Tumors of the larynx other than squamous cell epithelioma, *Arch. Otolaryngol.*, 34, 1113, 1941.
128. **Triplet, I., Vankemmel, B., and Madalain, M.,** Hémangioendothéliome malin du larynx avec métastases sous-cutanées, *Lille Méd.*, 19, 743, 1974.
129. **Ferlito, A., Nicolai, P., and Caruso, G.,** Angiosarcoma of the larynx. Case report, *Ann. Otol. Rhinol. Laryngol.*, 94, 1985.
130. **Jernström, P.,** Synovial sarcoma of the pharynx: report of a case, *Am. J. Clin. Pathol.*, 24, 957, 1954.
131. **Pricolo, V., and Cenci, N.,** Sinovioma maligno dell'ipofaringe, *Minerva Otorinolaringol.*, 7, 218, 1957.
132. **Gatti, W. M., Strom, G., and Orfei, E.,** Synovial sarcoma of the laryngopharynx, *Arch. Otolaryngol.*, 101, 633, 1975.
133. **Miller, L. H., Santaella-Latimer, L., and Miller, T.,** Synovial sarcoma of the larynx, *Trans. Am. Acad. Ophthalmol. Otolaryngol.*, 80, 448, 1975.
134. **Junien-Lavillauroy, C., Roux, O., Pasquier, R., and Charachon, R.,** Synovialosarcome du sinus périforme chez l'enfant, *Ann. Otolaryngol. Chir. Cervicofac.*, 95, 336, 1978.
135. **Labayle, J., Brocheriou, C., Paraire, F., Dumaine, A., Dahan, S., and Cuzin, O.,** A propos de 2 cas de synovialosarcoma cervical extra-articulaire, *Ann. Otolaryngol. Chir. Cervicofac*, 97, 461, 1980.
136. **Lockey, M. W.,** Rare tumors of the ear, nose and throat: synovial sarcoma of the head and neck, *S. Med. J.*, 69, 316, 1976.
137. **Chelloul, N. and Labayle, J.,** Les synovialoblastomes extra-articulaires parapharyngés. A propos d'une observation, *Sem. Hôp. Paris*, 53, 707, 1977.
138. **Martin, F., Behbehani, A., and Wiebecke, B.,** Zervikale Synovialsarkome im Kindesalter, *Laryngol. Rhinol. Otol.*, 58, 871, 1979.
139. **Geahchan, N. E., Lambert, J., Micheau, C., and Richard, J. M.,** Synovialome malin du larynx, *Ann. Otolaryngol. Chir. Cervicofac.*, 100, 61, 1983.
140. **Roth, J. A., Enzinger, F. M., and Tannenbaum, M.,** Synovial sarcoma of the neck: a followup study of 24 cases, *Cancer*, 35, 1243, 1975.
141. **Panh, M. H., Aftimos, G., Pasquier, B., Couderc, P., and Mazabraud, A.,** Les synovialosarcomes cervicaux extra-articulaires. Revue de la littérature à propos de deux observations, *Bull. Cancer*, 63, 309, 1976.
142. **Gapany-Gapanavicius, B., Behar, A. J., and Chisin, R.,** Synovial sarcoma of the hypopharynx, *Ann. Otol. Rhinol. Laryngol.*, 87, 356, 1978.
143. **Applebaum, E. L., and Mantravadi, R. P.,** Synovial sarcoma of the hypopharynx, *Otolaryngol. Head Neck Surg*, 91, 452, 1983.

143a. **Mohr, W. and Pirsig, W.,** Synoviales Sarkom des Larynx. Fallbeschreibung und kurze Literaturübersicht, *Laryngol. Rhinol. Otol.*, 63, 453, 1984.

143b. **Quinn, H. J., Jr.,** Synovial sarcoma of the larynx treated by partial laryngectomy, *Laryngoscope*, 94, 1158, 1984.

144. **Abramson, A. L. and Simons, R. L.,** Kaposi's sarcoma of the head and neck, *Arch. Otolaryngol.*, 92, 505, 1970.
145. **Ferlito, A.,** Histiocytic tumors of the larynx. A clinicopathological study with review of the literature, *Cancer*, 42, 611, 1978.
146. **Ferlito, A., Nicolai, P., Recher, G., and Narne, S.,** Primary laryngeal malignant fibrous histiocytoma. Review of the literature and report of seven cases, *Laryngoscope*, 93, 1351, 1983.
147. **Gorenstein, A., Neel, H. B., III, Weiland, L. H., and Devine, K. D.,** Sarcomas of the larynx, *Arch. Otolaryngol.*, 106, 8, 1980.
148. **Sirota, H. H.,** 1958, Quoted by **Hyams, V. J. and Rabuzzi, D. D.,** Cartilaginous tumors of the larynx, *Laryngoscope*, 80, 755, 1970.
149. **Bronzini, E.,** Condrosarcoma della laringe, *Ann.Laringol. Otol. Rinol. Faringol.*, 58, 497, 1959.
150. **Al-Saleem, T., Tucker, G. F., Jr., Peale, A. R., and Norris, C. M.,** Cartilaginous tumors of the larynx. Clinical-pathologic study of ten cases, *Ann. Otol. Rhinol. Laryngol.*, 79, 33, 1970.
151. **Hyams, V. J. and Rabuzzi, D. D.,** Cartilaginous tumors of the larynx, *Laryngoscope*, 80, 755, 1970.
152. **Frenzel, H.,** Kehlkopfekondrome und ihr Charakteristishes Rontgebild, *Mschr. Ohrenheilk*, 87, 281, 1953.

152a. **Ferlito, A., Nicolai, P., Montaguti, A., Cecchetto, A., and Pennelli, N.,** Chondrosarcoma of the larynx. Review of the literature and report of 3 cases, *Am. J. Otolaryngol.*, 5, 350, 1984.

153. **Sprinkle, P. M., Allen, M. S., and Brookshire, P. F.,** Osteosarcoma of the larynx (a true primary sarcoma of the larynx), *Laryngoscope*, 76, 325, 1966.
154. **Morley, A. R., Cameron, D. S., and Watson, A. J.,** Osteosarcoma of the larynx, *J. Laryngol. Otol.*, 87, 997, 1973.
155. **Dahm, L. J., Schaeffer, S. D., Carder, H. M., and Vellios, F.,** Osteosarcoma of the soft tissue of the larynx. Report of a case with light and electron microscopic studies, *Cancer*, 42, 2343, 1978.
156. **Haar, J. G., Chaudhry, A. P., Karanjia, M. D., and Milley, P. S.,** Chondroblastic osteosarcoma of the larynx, *Arch. Otolaryngol.*, 104, 477, 1978.
156a. **Remagen, W., Löhr, J. and von Westerbhagen, B.,** Osteosarkom des Kehlkopfes, *HNO*, 31, 366, 1983.
157. **Kleinsasser, O. and Glanz, H.,** Myogenic tumors of the larynx, *Arch. Otorhinolaryngol.*, 225, 107, 1979.
158. **DeLozier, H. L.,** Intrinsic malignant schwannoma of the larynx. A case report, *Ann. Otol. Rhinol. Laryngol.*, 91, 336, 1982.
159. **Busanny-Caspari Von, W. and Hammar, C. H.,** Zur Malignität der sogenannten Myoblastenmyome, *Zentralbl. Pathol.*, 98, 401, 1958.
160. **Ormerod, F. C. and Shaw, H. J.,** An account of morbidity and mortality associated with total laryngectomy, *J. Laryngol. Otol.*, 70, 433, 1956.
161. **Abramson, A. L., Parisier, S. C., Zamansky, M. J., and Sulka, M.,** Distant metastases from carcincoma of the larynx, *Laryngoscope*, 81, 1503, 1971.
162. **O'Brien, P. H., Carlson, R., Steubner, E. A., Jr., and Staley, C. P.,** Distant metastases in epidermoid cell carcinoma of the head and neck, *Cancer*, 27, 304, 1971.
163. **Probert, J. C., Thompson, R. W., and Bagshaw, M. A.,** Patterns of spread of distant metastases in head and neck cancer, *Cancer*, 33, 127, 1974.
164. **Merino, O. R., Lindberg, R. D., and Fletcher, G. H.,** An analysis of distant metastases from squamous cell carcinoma of the upper respiratory and digestive tracts, *Cancer*, 40, 145, 1977.
165. **Harrer, W. V. and Lewis, P. L.,** Carcinoma of the larynx with cardiac metastases, *Arch. Otolaryngol.*, 91, 382, 1970.
166. **Palmer, B. W. and Reynders, M.,** Cardiac metastases in carcinoma of the laryngopharynx, *Arch. Otolaryngol.*, 79, 172, 1964.
167. **Barton, R. P. E. and Taylor, P. C. A.,** Cardiac metastases from primary carcinoma of the larynx, *J. Laryngol. Otol.*, 93, 833, 1979.
168. **McAllister, H. A., Jr. and Fenoglio, J. J., Jr.,** Tumors of the Cardiovascular System, Atlas of Tumor Pathology, Second Series, Fascicle 15, Armed Forces Institute of Pathology, Washington, D.C., 1978.
169. **Cline, I. K.,** Cardiac lymphatic involvement by metastatic tumor, *Cancer*, 29, 799, 1972.
170. **Jordaens, L., Van Kerckvoorde, L., Brys, R., and De Keyser, R.,** A metastatic tumor to the heart, *Acta Cardiol.(Bruxelles)*, 38, 61, 1983.
171. **Vize, G.,** Laryngeal metastasis to the temporal bone causing facial paralysis, *J. Laryngol. Otol.*, 88, 175, 1974.
172. **Ferlito, A. and Di Bonito, L.,** Primary cancer of the larynx associated with primary lung cancer. Report of 21 cases, 14 with autopsy findings and 7 biopsies, *ORL*, 38, 230, 1976.
173. **Carter, R. L.,** Metastasis, in *Scientific Foundations of Oncology*, Smyngton, T. and Carter, R. L., Eds., Heinemann, London, 1976.
174. **Fisher, B. and Fisher, E. R.,** The interrelationship of hematogenous and lymphatic tumor cell dissemination, *Surg. Gynecol. Obstet.*, 122, 791, 1966.
175. **Hilgard, P., Beyerle, L., Hohage, R., Hiemeyer, V., and Kübler, M.,** The effect of heparin on the initial phase of metastasis formation, *Eur. J. Cancer*, 8, 347, 1972.
176. **Haagensen, C. D.,** The spread of cancer in the lymphatic system, in *The Lymphatics in Cancer*, Haagensen, C. D., Feind, C. R., Herter, F. P., Slanetz, C. A., Jr., and Weinberg, J. A., Eds., W. B. Saunders, Philadelphia, 1972.

Chapter 5

CLINICAL MANIFESTATIONS OF CANCER OF THE LARYNX

H. J. Shaw

TABLE OF CONTENTS

I. LARYNGEAL BOUNDARIES AND LOCAL ANATOMY

Superiorly the mucosa of the tongue base extends across the floor of the valleculae onto the anterior aspect of the epiglottis to form the superior boundary of the larynx. Laterally this then becomes drawn up into the linguoepiglottic folds.

The free-standing or suprahyoid epiglottis lies above the level of these folds, which are projected downwards on either side of the epiglottis as the lateral laryngeal margins and aryepiglottic folds. Between them lies the attached infrahyoid epiglottis anteriorly, the paired arytenoids inferiorly, and contained between them lies the aditus laryngis, bounded posteriorly by the interarytenoid mucosa. All of this mucous membrane and submucous connective tissue is liberally drained by lymphatics, and particular attention must be drawn to the preepiglottic space filled by loose connective tissue and lying between the infrahyoid epiglottis and the hyoid bone with the thyrohyoid membrane. It is an important site for direct spread of epiglottic cancer.

By contrast, the thin mucous membrane and dense layer of connective tissue known as the *conus elasticus*, descending from the true vocal cords into the subglottis, acts as a fibrous barrier and contains no lymphatic vessels, which accounts for the slow growth of cancer of the vocal cords and the uncommon event of metastatic spread.

It is important to bear in mind the relatively isolated anatomical compartments of the larynx, especially when considering lymphatic spread of tumor cells. Although there is a small amount of crossover in the superficial mucosal lymph vessels, for practical purposes, the two halves of the larynx are separate structures joined in the midline. In each half there is a submucosal supraglottic and a subglottic compartment effectively separated by the glottis. Lymph flow tends to be upward in each compartment, vessels leaving the larynx via the thyrohyoid and cricothyroid membranes, respectively.[2] The glottis remains a lymphatic-free barrier to tumor spread, especially from the supraglottis (Figure 1).

For practical purposes, the effective lateral walls and boundaries of the endolarynx are the twin alae of the thyroid cartilage. They form a natural barrier to the spread of cancer from within the larynx and contain the false cords or ventricular bands, the ventricles, the true vocal cords, the conus elasticus, and the immediate subglottic region. At the level of the true cords also lie the intrinsic laryngeal muscles, lateral to which lie the thyroid cartilage alae, and from which they are separated by the potential paraglottic space.[4] The latter often acts as an important and often cryptic pathway of spread for cancer and a locus of residual disease, particularly after irradiation. The inferior boundary of the larynx is strictly the mucosa of the subglottic space extending below the true cords for 5 to 10 mm before joining the trachea. Anatomically, however, the whole extent of the cricoid ring and its attachments form the lower limits of the larynx. It is essential to have a clear idea of these boundaries, the intrinsic anatomy, blood supply, lymphatic drainage, and innervation of the larynx in order to interpret satisfactorily the many signs and symptoms of laryngeal cancer.

II. SUBJECTIVE MANIFESTATIONS

The location and size of the tumor will mainly determine the presence and type of symptoms. Small swellings, or even those of some size, in areas such as the outer side of the aryepiglottic folds or around the epiglottis may produce no symptoms and may only be discovered accidentally on routine inspection of the larynx.

A. Dysphonia

This is the principal, early or late, and most frequent symptom of cancer within the larynx.[1] The character of the hoarseness is generally that of rough, husky speech in varying degree and gradually resulting in a much weakened voice which tires easily. In supraglottic and the uncommon true subglottic tumors, with no glottic involvement, the quality of the voice change is more subtle, often giving only a deeper timbre with less distinct speech. Equally important is the duration of dysphonia. A persistent and worsening hoarseness over a period of weeks or months is of greater significance than one which comes and goes. In addition, a voice which deteriorates again after a successful course of irradiation frequently indicates recurrence of tumor. Dysphonia that has been present for years is unlikely to be due to cancer.

B. Dyspnea

In contrast to dysphonia, this symptom usually accompanies only a late stage in the disease when the growing tumor increasingly obstructs the natural airway. It is also not uncommon with persistence of tumor, infection, or necrosis after full-course irradiation.

The onset is often very gradual and may be noticed at first by the patient only on exertion. Exceptionally, a small- or moderate-sized tumor may cause dyspnea in a patient already suffering from chronic cardiopulmonary disease or in which one vocal cord fixed in the midline has been paralyzed by some unrelated, long-standing condition.

C. Discomfort or Pain

It is common for patients with laryngeal cancer of any stage or site to experience a variable degree of discomfort in the region of the larynx, usually more frequent on swallowing or speaking. Pain in the larynx or neck, often radiating via the superior laryngeal nerve up to the ear and side of the head, is less common but characteristic of advanced glottic, transglottic, or supraglottic tumors.[3] It is also characteristic of persistent edema and soft tissue infection or perichondritis of the larynx during or following irradiation. Frequently, this is accompanied by the presence of residual tumor, usually deep within the laryngeal muscles and tissue planes, often difficult to identify by histological analysis of biopsy specimens. Laryngeal or other cancer metastatic to paratracheal or jugular lymphatics may also give rise to discomfort or pain related to the side of the neck or to the ear.

D. Dysphagia

In the sense of discomfort on swallowing, many supraglottic tumors may cause dysphagia. Advanced glottic or transglottic cancer may also give rise to similar disagreeable sensations. In addition, tumors, especially if grossly exophytic and also involving the pharynx, may give rise to real difficulties in swallowing solids, and with liquids some laryngeal spillover and cough may often be noticed.

III. OBJECTIVE MANIFESTATIONS

A. Local

The most frequent site of laryngeal cancer in the majority of ethnic groups is on the true vocal cord (50 to 60%). At this site the clinical appearance may vary from a single white patch of leukoplakia or keratosis, which is found to contain a small area of carcinoma *in situ* or early invasive tumor, to more extensive leukoplakia or to an extensive granular, heaped-up, ulcerating neoplasm involving the whole vocal cord. Both cords may also be involved. Spread to the opposite cord across the midline via the anterior commissure may be found, or extension vertically to produce a transglottic tumor with fixation of the involved cord and a bulky reduction of the natural airway. Cancer which originates in the supraglottic region (40 to 50%) more often arises directly as an area of granularity or local swelling and ulceration on the epiglottis or ventricular band. The same local appearances apply to the

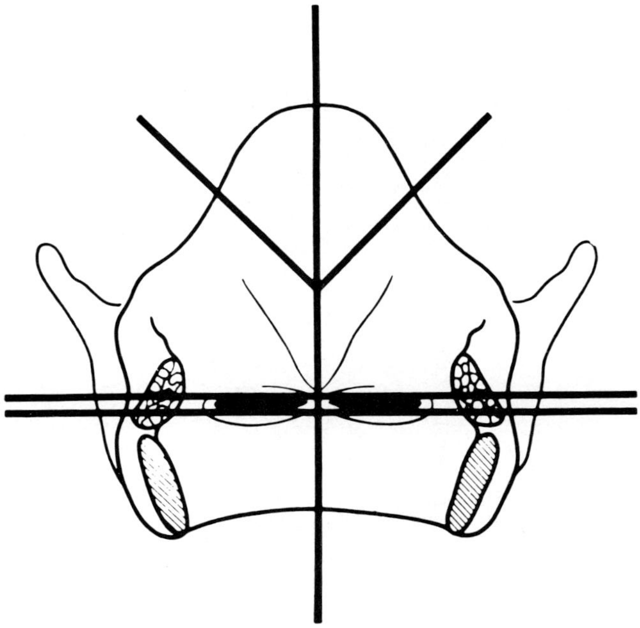

FIGURE 1. The four main submucosal lymphatic compartments on either side of the larynx. (From Pressman, J. J. and Simon, M. B., *Trans. Am. Acad. Ophthalmol. Otolaryngol.*, 64, 628, 1960, With permission.

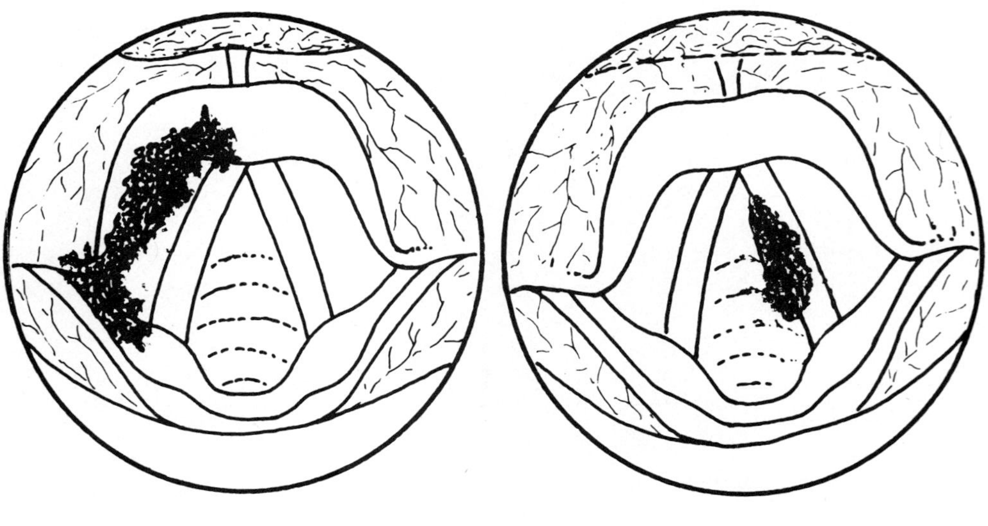

A B

FIGURE 2. Diagrams to show: (A) supraglottic cancer (T1b); (B)glottic cancer (T1a); (C)subglottic cancer (T1a).

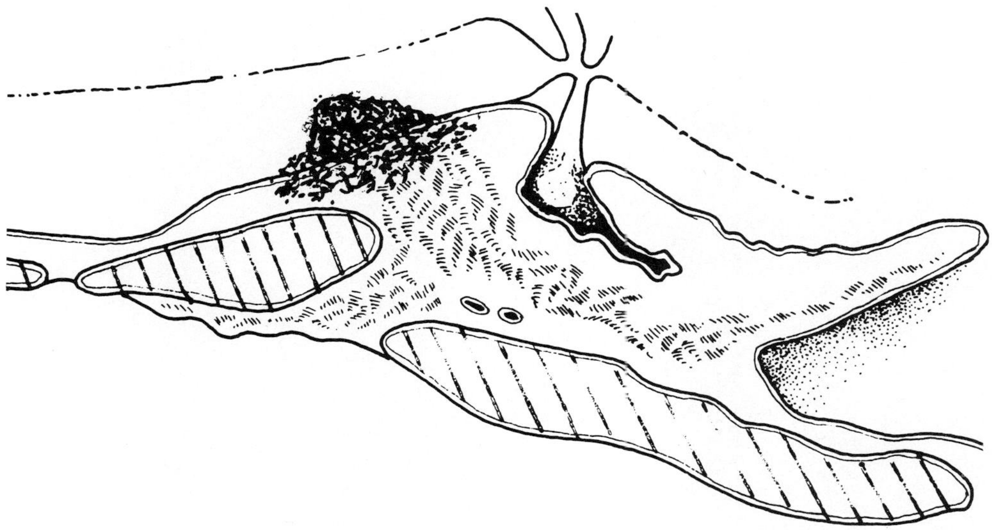

FIGURE 2C

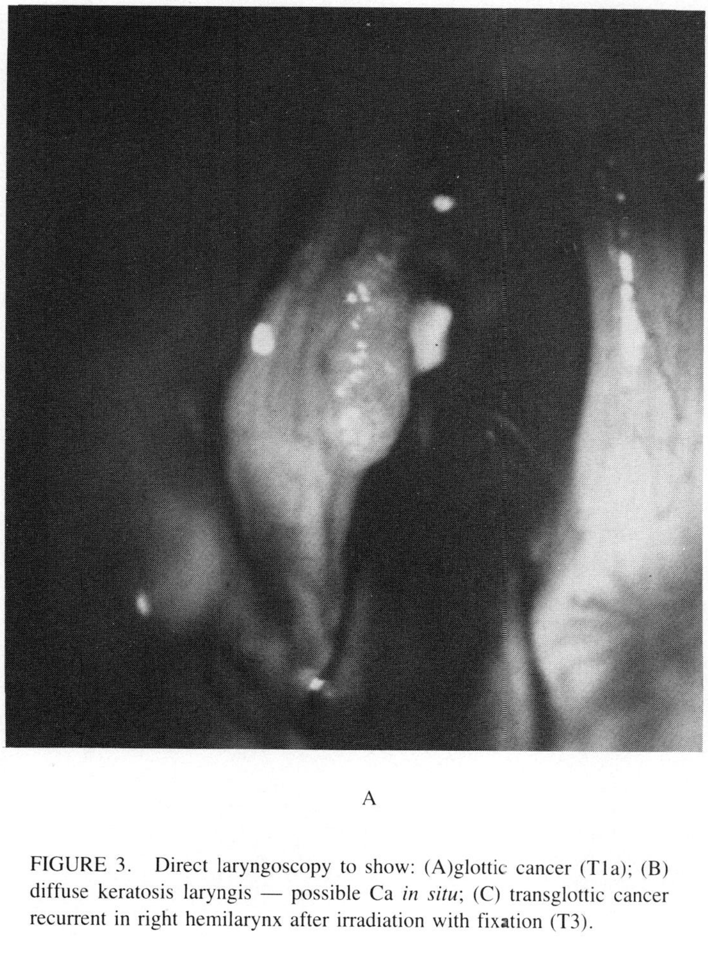

A

FIGURE 3. Direct laryngoscopy to show: (A)glottic cancer (T1a); (B) diffuse keratosis laryngis — possible Ca *in situ*; (C) transglottic cancer recurrent in right hemilarynx after irradiation with fixation (T3).

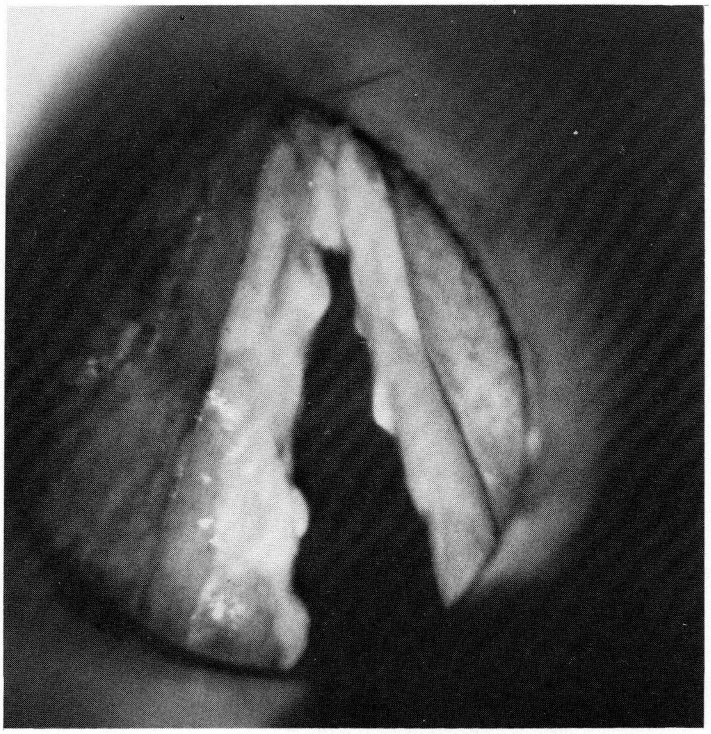

FIGURE 3B

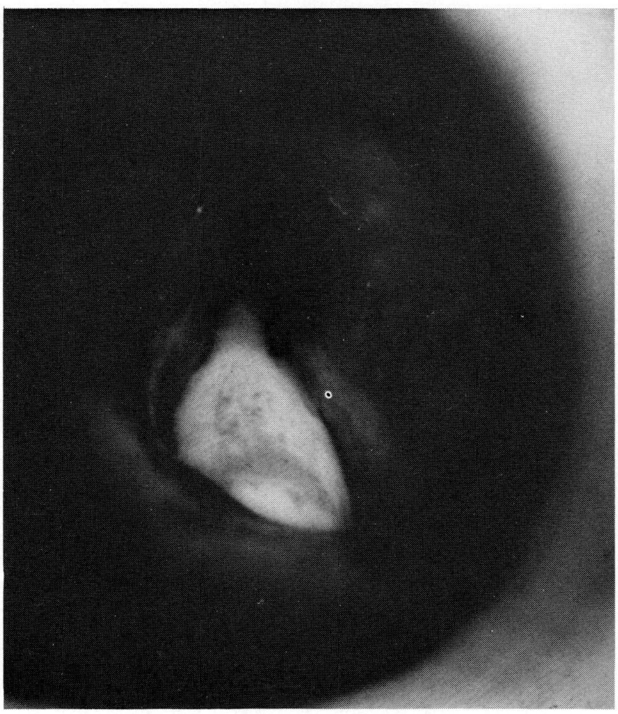

FIGURE 3C

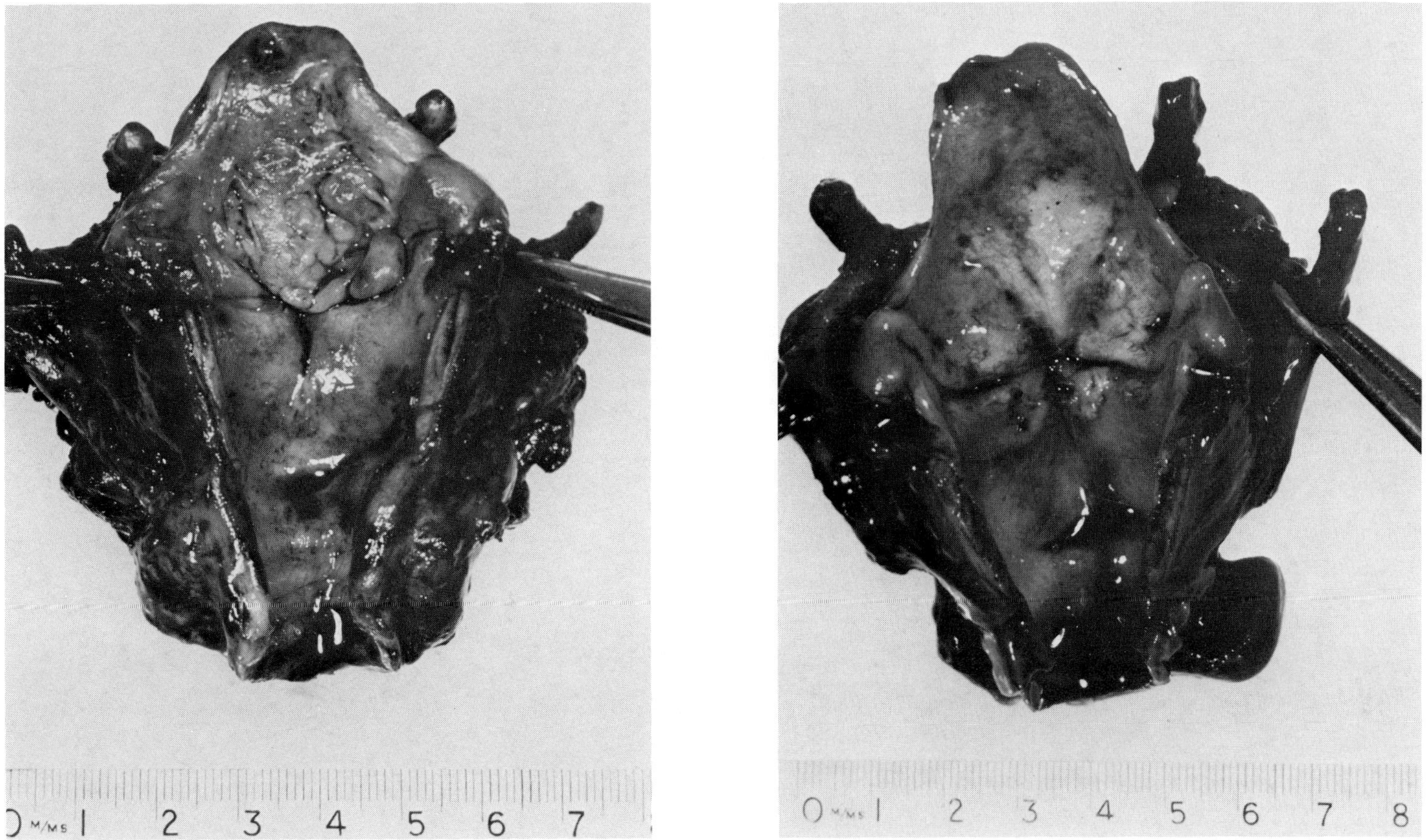

A B

FIGURE 4. Surgical specimens showing: (A) epiglottic cancer — extensive but not crossing the glottis (T3); (B)supraglottic cancer also extending to the vocal cords (T2); (C)glottic cancer following vertical partial laryngectomy after irradiation (T1a); (D)supraglottic cancer of ventricular band after horizontal partial laryngectomy and after irradiation (T2).

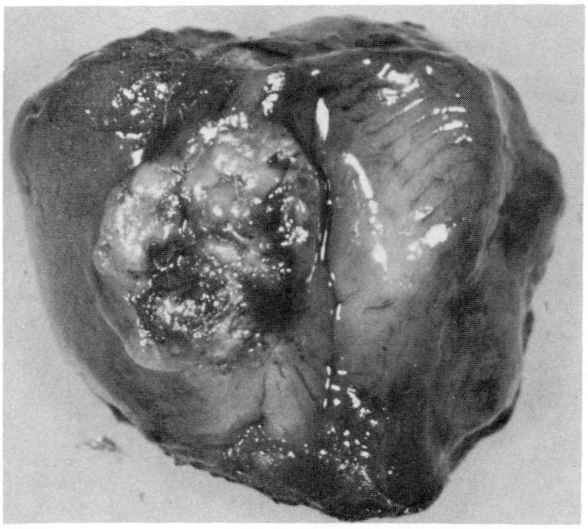

FIGURE 4C

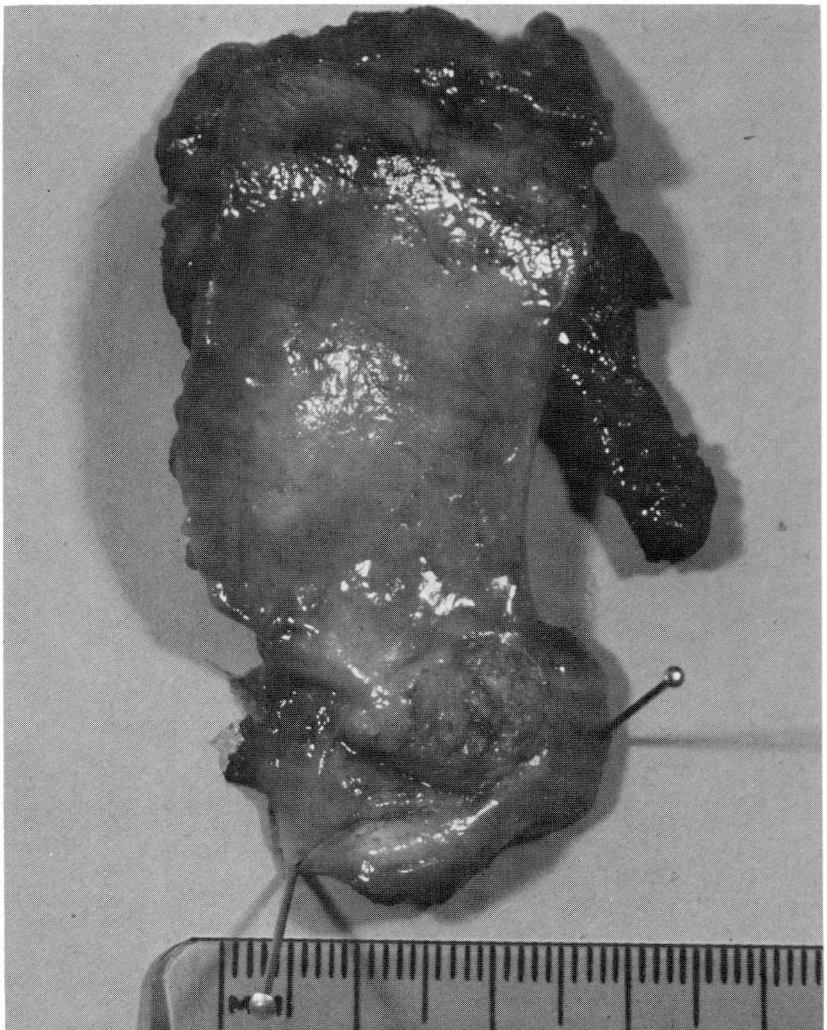

FIGURE 4D

very small minority of tumors (about 1%) arising in the true subglottic region. Owing to the difficulty of obtaining a view of the laryngeal ventricles and the subglottis by indirect laryngoscopy, tumors of these regions tend not to be recognized in their early stages when no more than a slight swelling of the covering ventricular band or vocal cord, sometimes with reduced mobility, can be identified. Careful direct laryngoscopy is usually essential for diagnosis in these cases. Occasionally, after full-course irradiation, diagnosis and confirmatory biopsy may even require vertical thyrotomy.

In advanced tumors, objective signs of disease may include intermittent hemorrhage with persistent cough and bloody sputum, external swelling of the laryngeal framework, and even fistula formation with skin involvement by tumor. These signs will usually be accompanied by a variety of severe subjective symptoms.

B. Regional

The visible and palpable manifestations of laryngeal cancer in the cervical region are commonly due to involvement of lymphatics, mainly of the internal jugular chain, but on occasions also of the prelaryngeal and pretracheal lymph nodes. The principal node groups affected are the subdigastric and upper jugular nodes, most frequently from supraglottic tumors. Glottic cancer rarely spreads to cervical nodes unless advanced and transglottic when upper and midjugular nodes are often involved. Subglottic tumors commonly involve prelaryngeal, paratracheal, and lower jugular nodes, often with extension into the mediastinum. The submaxillary and posterior triangle groups of nodes are seldom involved by laryngeal cancer and spread to the opposite side is uncommon unless the primary lesion has crossed the midline or in cases which have been previously irradiated.

Less commonly and perhaps more often associated with sarcoma of the larynx is swelling and displacement of the laryngeal cartilages by tumor growing directly through the thyroid cartilage or through the fascial membranes above or below this structure. Very occasionally, gross perichondritis of the thyroid cartilage following irradiation may present as a tender and painful swelling to one side of the midline. It is often also associated with persistent tumor.

C. Distant

Metastatic spread to any structures below the clavicles is uncommon even when the disease is advanced and then it is mainly associated with poorly differentiated squamous cancer. The mediastinum and lungs are the sites most frequently affected. Occasionally, metastases may be encountered in the long bones and also those of the spine and pelvis. Among distant soft tissues rarely involved, the liver, kidney, brain, and heart muscle have also been noted. Very rarely, skin deposits have been found.

IV. DOCUMENTATION

Although careful observation, description, drawing, and if possible, photography, of all laryngeal tumors by the investigator should require no emphasis, some further points need to be stated.

The first essential is to obtain a clear and accurate view of the lesion using whatever indirect or direct means of inspection is appropriate. Usually this will require a direct laryngoscopy under local or general anaesthesia which should then give an adequate view for inspection of the whole laryngeal anatomy. The extent and character of the tumor can be noted and the appropriate visual record made. At the same time a biopsy sample will usually be required for histological diagnosis.

Furthermore, it is important that anyone who undertakes the treatment of a patient with laryngeal cancer does not uncritically accept any submitted description or characterization of a lesion from a referring doctor. He must carry out his own complete examination, and the importance of this may also need to be explained to the patient, who may object to repeated investigations. Providing this discipline is maintained, two necessary pretreatment objectives are achieved. The tumor can be clinically staged and other important baseline data essential for future reference will have been recorded.

It is also of first importance that a standard method of description, classification, and visual recording be adopted within the institution concerned, preferably that proposed by International Organizations such as the UICC (1982) or by National Cancer Committees.

REFERENCES

1. **Negus, V. E. and Thomson, St.C,** *Diseases of the Nose and Throat,* 6th ed., Cassell, London, 1955.
2. **Pressman, J. J. and Simon, M. B.,** Submucosal compartments of the larynx, *Trans. Am. Acad. Ophthalmol. Otolaryngol.,* 64, 628, 1960.
3. **Shaw, H. J.,** *Diseases of the Ear, Nose and Throat,* 4th ed., Ballantyne, J. and Groves, J., Eds., Butterworth, London, 1979.
4. **Tucker, G. F.,** *Centennial Conference on Laryngeal Cancer,* Worksh. No. 1, Alberti, P. and Bryce, D. P., Eds., Appleton-Century-Crofts, N. Y., 1974, 11.
5. International Union against Cancer (U.I.C.C.). Report of Committee on T.N.M. Classification, World Health Organization, Geneva, 1982.

Chapter 6

DIAGNOSTIC PROCEDURES IN CANCER OF THE LARYNX

Jan Olofsson

TABLE OF CONTENTS

I. OUTPATIENT PROCEDURES

Mirror laryngoscopy is still the most commonly employed method of examining the larynx (Figure 1)* and may be complemented by the use of an operating microscope giving a magnified view of the larynx, which has proved to be useful in evaluating superficial lesions of the vocal cords. The microscope can also be equipped with a stroboscope, which may further increase the chance of diagnosing early and recurrent carcinomas.

The use of 90° optical instruments such as the Storz-Hopkins laryngoscope or the Wolf instruments (Figures 2 and 3) has become more and more popular as this method also allows photographic documentation and video recording. In some centers, the telescopic method has entirely replaced the mirror examination.

Cytologic smears may be taken during these procedures and biopsy specimens removed, which can be useful, especially in patients being at a high risk for general anesthesia (Figures 4A to D).

Another method is the use of flexible instruments (Figures 5A and B), which allows inspection of patients with an overhanging epiglottis. This method gives an excellent possibility for a close and easy inspection of the laryngeal surface of the epiglottis, ventricles, vocal cords, anterior commissure, and subglottis. A special laryngofiberscope may be used or a regular bronchofiberscope, which is more versatile. The fiberscope is introduced through the nose after decongestion and application of local anesthesia. When the scope has been introduced, 2 or 4% xylocain is instilled through the suction channel of the scope under inspection so that all surfaces will be anesthetized. Cytologic smears can be removed by the use of a small brush, and biopsies can be taken. Fiberscopic inspection of the larynx may be very useful, especially in the follow-up of irradiated patients, who cannot be inspected by mirror or telescopes, and can be performed as an outpatient procedure.

II. MICROLARYNGOSCOPY

The mirror laryngoscopy and telescopic examination cannot compete in accuracy with the direct laryngoscopy using the operating microscope — microlaryngoscopy — a method introduced in the 1960s by Kleinsasser.[1] Microlaryngoscopy has markedly improved our possibilities to diagnose early lesions as dysplasia, carcinoma *in situ*, and superficial carcinoma, which is reflected in the increased number of premalignant lesions diagnosed in relation to invasive carcinomas.[2] The microlaryngoscopy has improved the possibilities of procuring representative biopsy specimens and to perform endolaryngeal surgery, which has been well documented in the literature. Some practical and technical details are of importance. The head should be well extended, lying on a level with the back. Teeth protectors should be used at least for the upper gum, but better for both gums if the patient is not edentulous as the laryngoscopes will press with force, especially on the upper teeth.

The large laryngoscopes used for microlaryngoscopy should not be introduced until an inspection has been made of the valleculae, piriform sinuses, postcricoid region, and the laryngeal inlet using a regular laryngoscope such as the Holinger laryngoscope (Figure 6). Otherwise, lesions in these areas may be overlooked.

Intubation anesthesia, jet technique, or the HFPPV (High Frequency Positive Pressure Ventilation) may be used. In most adult patients the intubation tube does not interfere with the procedure and gives a controlled airway (Figure 7). For children, one of the other methods may be used.

The microlaryngoscopy is complemented by inspection using 90° optical instruments for examining the undersurface of the vocal cords and the anterior commissure area (Figure 8).

* **All figures are found at the end of the text.**

This technique may also add information about the lower margin of an epiglottic tumor covering the anterior commissure, which is of importance for the decision if a horizontal supraglottic laryngectomy can be performed (Figure 28C). By marking the level of the vocal cord on the optical instrument, a more exact estimation of the subglottic extension may be obtained as a complement to the laryngographic examination. The ventricles may be inspected — at least a part of them — by elevating the false vocal cords by small hooks.

The microlaryngoscopic technique has improved our possibilities for routine laryngeal photography (Figures 7, 9, and 10).[3] A good laryngeal picture is very informative and invaluable for teaching purposes as well as in the management of the patients as it assists in the interdisciplinary discussion with, e.g., the therapeutic and diagnostic radiologists, and aids in the follow-up. Movie and video recording are also possible. For teaching purposes, a video monitor may always be stationed within the operating theater.

A. Premalignant Lesions

Premalignant lesions are most commonly diagnosed on the vocal cords, where they cause discomfort and hoarseness, the main symptoms causing the patient to seek medical advice. Laryngeal biopsies disclose hyperplasia, keratosis, dysplasia, and carcinoma *in situ* in nearly 20% of all laryngeal patients in many reports.[4-6] As mentioned above, the microlaryngoscopic technique has increased the number of premalignant lesions diagnosed in comparison to invasive carcinomas.[2] In addition, the wider recognition of hoarseness as the most important sign for vocal cord lesions has also increased the probability for an early diagnosis. From the screening examination performed by Steiner[7] and the post-mortem examinations by Auerbach and associates,[8] it appears that the proportion of silent, premalignant lesions is large and that screening examinations may be recommended for high-risk groups.

The microlaryngoscopic appearance of 'premalignant' lesions may vary considerably from a greyish-white thickening of the mucosa-leukoplakia (Figure 11), which sometimes may be elevated and warty-adult papillomatosis (Figures 14 to 16) to a reddish, somewhat edematous lesion-erythroplasia (Figures 17 and 18). Both types of lesions may be present at the same time, especially in patients with 'chronic laryngitis' (Figure 18). Biopsy specimens have to be removed from both types of lesions as the erythroplasia often represents a severe dysplasia-carcinoma *in situ* or an invasive carcinoma (Figure 17). The final diagnosis must always be based upon the histological examination. Localized lesions (Figures 11, 14, and 15) can be removed entirely, mounted, and orientated on a piece of paper for at least step-serial sectioning (Figures 12 and 13). A careful histological examination is important as the histology may vary considerably despite a similiar microlaryngoscopic appearance.

B. Smear Cytology

Different aids can be applied to improve the diagnostic accuracy, such as the use of smear cytology, toluidine blue vital stain, and improvement in the histologic diagnosis by performing DNA measurements. Especially in diffuse lesions it may be difficult to obtain representative biopsy specimens and in these cases smear cytology may be an aid for correct diagnosis, which is further elaborated upon in a separate chapter. In a prospective study, the reliability of laryngeal smear cytology was evaluated in comparison with the histologic diagnoses in 520 microlaryngoscopic examinations.[9,10] The sensitivity of the direct method (smear taken at the microlaryngoscopic procedure) in the detection of severe dysplasia — carcinoma *in situ* and invasive carcinoma — was 83% (59/71) and 93% (137/147), respectively. A false negative smear was more common after previous radiotherapy. The specificity of the cytologic technique in detecting histopathologically benign lesions was 80% (210/264). A smaller series with sampling by an indirect technique (Figures 3 and 4C) gave about the same result. It has to be stressed, however, that a cytologic examination can only be a complement to the histological diagnoses on which all therapeutic descisions have to be based. A negative clinical and histologic finding, combined with a positive cytologic reading, necessitates a search for a primary tumor somewhere else within the upper aerodigestive tract.

C. Toluidine Blue Vital Staining

Supravital staining methods have been used for many years as an adjunct in the diagnosis of premalignant and malignant lesions. Schiller, in 1928,[11] used Lugol's iodine solution (iodine and potassium iodide) for diagnosing carcinoma of the cervix uteri. Toluidine blue, which is an acidophilic metachromatic dye belonging to the thiazine group, selectively stains acid components as sulfate, carboxylate, and phosphate radicals as DNA and RNA. Toluidine blue is usually considered a nuclear stain. Dysplastic and anaplastic cells contain quantitatively more nucleic acids than normal cells and are therefore more heavily stained.[12] Toluidine blue penetrates to a depth of two to ten cell layers. The mechanism of the staining may be a penetration in the intercellular channels, which are wider in carcinomatous epithelium than in normal mucosa, which is supported by the findings of Strong et al.[13] However, other researchers found intense staining of the nuclei and a weaker staining of the cytoplasm, while the intercellular spaces were found to be both stained and unstained.[14]

Toluidine blue has been used in a number of organs. Richart[15] found a more than 93% agreement between distribution of 'intraepithelial neoplasia' as assessed by colpomicroscopy and stained areas. A good correlation was also found by Niebel and Chomet,[16] Shedd et al.,[17] Myers,[18] and Iwano et al.[19] using toluidine blue for the oral cavity, by Tarkkanen et al.[20] in the diagnosis of bronchogenic carcinoma, and by Wang[21] for staining of esophageal epithelium.

The use of toluidine blue in the larynx has been very much discussed due to false positive and false negative staining reactions.[22] However, Strong et al.[23] recommended the use of toluidine blue as an adjunct in the diagnosis of premalignant and early malignant laryngeal lesions. This is in line with our own findings in a prospective study where we compared the results of toluidine blue staining with the histologic examination in 272 biopsy specimens from the vocal cords.[24] Of the malignant specimens, 91% (135/148) had a positive staining reaction (Figures 19 and 20); 9% (13/148) did not stain at all, and most of these (11) had a clinically easily detectable keratosis. However, only 52% (64/124) of the benign lesions did not stain. Thus, 48% (60/124) had a 'false positive' staining reaction due to the presence of ulceration, granulation tissue, papillary keratosis, etc. The proportion of false positive staining reactions decreased with the intensity of the staining reactions. False positive stainings in the benign group were significantly more numerous in the patients who had received radiotherapy. Toluidine blue vital staining is easy to perform during microlaryngoscopy and may be an aid in the diagnosis of laryngeal lesions. Care must be taken not to traumatize the mucosa when introducing the intubation tube and the laryngoscope. We have to remember that toluidine blue vital stain can never replace a biopsy from a clinically suspect area.

III. HISTOPATHOLOGICAL EXAMINATION

The specimens (excised mucosa) should be mounted and orientated and examined by at least step-serial sectioning to minimize the risk of overlooking an invasive carcinoma (Figure 13). The therapeutic decision has to be based on the histological examination. However, the squamous lesion is the pathological entity whose evaluation involves the largest subjective component.[25] The nomenclature is poorly defined and inconsistently applied as was evident at the Centennial Conference on Laryngeal Cancer held in Toronto in 1974.[26] Therefore, it is necessary that the clinician and pathologist communicate with each other so that the clinician is well aware of the nomenclature used by the pathologist and that the pathologist knows the therapeutic consequences of his diagnosis. Kleinsasser[27] and later, Delemarre[28] and Lubsen[29] have used a three-graded classification for "premalignant" lesions which seems to be quite adequate for clinical purposes. This classification is also in line with the one suggested in Toronto in 1974.[26] The degree of atypia should be the basis of the classification used and is also considered the most important histological criterion,[30-32] and has the advantage that it permits an objective evaluation by the use of photometry which, up until now, has been used mainly as a research tool (Figure 21).[33,34] It is important to distinguish between well- and moderately low-differentiated forms of severe dysplasia-carcinoma *in situ* as it seems to be the well-differentiated forms that present the greatest difficulty in diagnosis and is most likely to recur and to lead to invasive carcinoma.[35-37]

As there is an increased risk that patients with hyperplasia, keratosis, and moderate dysplasia may develop more severe forms of dysplasia or invasive carcinoma, all these patients must be followed regularly and a sharp look-out should be kept for signs of carcinoma. It is also important to perform an excision of the entire lesion, when possible, to have the greatest chance for a correct diagnosis and as a preventive measure.[2]

IV. PROBLEMS IN DIAGNOSIS AND CLASSIFICATION

There are problems involved not only in the diagnosis of premalignant and early malignant lesions, but also in the correct assessment and classification of carcinomas, despite the fact that the larynx can be fairly easily inspected and palpated. The purpose of the classification is to be able to select the most appropriate treatment for the patients and to be able to compare the treatment results reported from different centers. A careful clinical examination as described above is the base for a correct classification, but has to be complemented by radiological examinations, which is mandatory for classification according to the rules laid down by the UICC.[38] Carcinoma of the vocal cords is often diagnosed at an early stage (Figures 22 to 24), as the patient seeks medical advice because of hoarseness. Supraglottic carcinomas are usually larger when diagnosed (Figures 29 and 30) as the symptoms are more diffuse as irritation, dysphagia, and cough. Subglottic carcinomas are often advanced when diagnosed and often grow circumferentially, causing stridor, which may necessitate a tracheostomy. Hoarseness is a late symptom and indicates glottic extension of the tumor.

The initial diagnosis is usually made at mirror laryngoscopy or telescopic examination. Radiological examinations should then be performed prior to microlaryngoscopy to avoid difficulties in assessing the radiographic findings due to edema following biopsies.

V. RADIOLOGICAL EXAMINATIONS

The aims of the radiological examinations (Figure 25) are to assess the superficial extent of the tumors and especially the lower margin, but also the deep invasion. Soft tissue plain films, tomography, laryngography, xerography, and computed tomography are the different radiographic methods used.

A. Soft Tissue Plain Films

Lateral plain films have been used since the turn of the century for studying the ossified parts of the laryngeal cartilages and later to study pathologic changes.[39-41] Coutard[42] stressed the use of this examination to decide the treatment in patients with laryngeal carcinoma. Important advances in the technique were made by Baclesse.[43,44] High-voltage technique using heavy filtration reduced the overprojection of the spine in A-P views.[45,46]

B. Tomography

Tomography reduces the disturbances of the skeletal structures, was introduced by Gunsett[47] and Leborgne,[48] and has been the most commonly applied radiological examination of the larynx. Linear tomography has been recommended as it requires the shortest exposure time.[46,49]

C. Laryngography

Examination with positive-contrast laryngography was introduced in 1926 by Iglauer.[50] Powers[51-53] and associates further improved and popularized the laryngographic technique. The application of laryngography and cinelaryngography is well described by Landman.[54]

D. Xerography

Xerography is used in some centers and gives good information about the ossified parts but there is a risk for misinterpretations.[55] Xerography also gives information about the laryngeal soft tissues.[49,56] A high dose is necessary and xeroradiography has apparently no advantages over laryngography.[57]

E. Computed Tomography

Computed tomography (CT) has provided us with a method to evaluate the deep extent of laryngeal tumors that has been a major obstacle before for correct classification of laryngeal carcinomas.[58,59]

F. Evaluation and Use of the Different Radiographic Methods

Laryngography has been shown to provide important information about superficial tumor extent and involvement of the area around the anterior commissure (Figures 26B and 29B), the inferior surface of the vocal cords (Figures 26A and 27A), and the ventricles (Figure 27A).[60,61] At the Centennial Conference on Laryngeal Carcinoma in Toronto in 1974,[62] the glottic region was defined to include the free margin and the horizontal surface of the vocal cords and the commissures. Therefore, a correct classification requires a detailed mapping of these areas. Slight subglottic extension may be difficult to delineate by plain films and tomograms, which often only portray the tumors as a thickening of the vocal cord, if at all, whereas laryngograms enable the extent of the tumors to be more reliably assessed and especially the lower margin of the tumor to be clearly visualized (Figures 26 and 27). Even a small involvement of the undersurface of the vocal cord may be assessed. Major subglottic extent with flattening of the subglottic angle may be equally well assessed by all conventional radiographic techniques.[60]

A correct assessment of the ventricles and the inferior part of the epiglottis is important if contemplating a horizontal supraglottic laryngectomy. However, there is a risk of both false positive and false negative radiological findings and the final decision between total or partial laryngectomy must be performed at the time of operation (Figure 28).

The anterior commissure is the anterior midline between the vocal cords, measuring only a few millimeters in height.[62,63] Subglottic extension is a frequent finding in tumors involving the anterior commissure. Then there is a risk of extralaryngeal spread by extension through the cricothyroid membrane.[63] There is also a great risk of early invasion of the thyroid cartilage, mainly due to the close proximity between mucosa and cartilage in the anterior commissure. The lateral laryngogram demonstrates the areas below and above the anterior commissure (Figures 26B and 29B). More marked anterior subglottic extension can be demonstrated in plain films. The laryngogram should be exposed when the vocal cords are completely abducted, which is at the end of an inspiration. If the cords are adducted, an incorrect representation of the anterior commissure will be obtained and may be misinterpreted. The use of 90° optical instruments during the microlaryngoscopic procedure adds further information concerning the anterior commissure area and the subglottis (Figure 28C). The laryngography as well as the use of optical instruments are of great value when dealing with exophytic epiglottic carcinomas.

Invasion of the thyroid cartilage is most common at the anterior midline with its close proximity between mucosa and cartilage.[63] More extensive invasion of the cartilage may be assessed by lateral soft tissue plain films showing a disappearance of the normal figure eight configuration.[61] More accurate assessment of deep invasion and cartilage destruction can be obtained by the use of computed tomography.[64-67]

Clinically, fixation is a severe sign and indicates cartilage invasion and/or spread outside the larynx of the tumor in about 50% of the cases.[59] The irregular ossification of the thyroid cartilage has made the assessment of invasion difficult, at least when using "conventional" radiographic methods.

Computed tomography depicts the larynx in the transverse plane and is indicated for tumors having a risk for cartilage invasion such as T3 and large T2 carcinomas and tumors involving the anterior commissure (Figures 27B, 29C, and 30). Evidence of cartilage invasion will change the classification to T4 and most probably indicates an increased radioresistance. Posterior extension of tumors lateral to the arytenoid cartilage with widening of the thyroarytenoid space is usually well visualized on CT — information of importance for the decision about partial vertical laryngectomy. It also indicates for the surgeon that the mucosa of the piriform sinus on the affected side should be removed entirely at the total laryngectomy. Otherwise, there is a risk of leaving tumor cells behind and a recurrence above the stoma will occur.

CT also adds important information when dealing with supraglottic carcinomas, both concerning invasion of the preepiglottic space and lateral extension and invasion of the cartilage (Figures 28 to 30).

CT is considered a complement in the radiographic diagnosis of laryngeal carcinoma and does not replace laryngography, which gives better information concerning mucosal extension.

VI. EXAMINATION OF THE NECK

Palpation of the neck should always be performed at a routine ENT examination. Palpable nodes in the neck changes the classification and staging of laryngeal carcinoma (UICC).[38] The nodes may be moveable, homo-, contra-, or bilateral, or fixed (Figure 31). Fine-needle aspiration cytology adds further information about the nodes, but a negative aspiration cytology does not exclude metastases and the classification is based on the findings at the clinical examination. CT, when performed for assessment of the laryngeal carcinoma, may add further information about the nodes in the neck, too.

VII. CHEST X-RAY

An initial chest X-ray is mandatory when dealing with head and neck carcinomas. Metastases to the lungs may be present but there is also a risk of a second primary in the lung due to common etiologic factors (Figure 32).

VIII. MULTIPLE PRIMARIES

There are a number of reports that emphasize the risk of synchronous and metachronous second and third primaries in patients with head and neck carcinomas.[68-75] A high incidence of second primary respiratory tract neoplasms has been reported in patients with laryngeal carcinomas. A second primary within the respiratory tract was found in 6.5% of patients with glottic carcinomas and in 12.2% of patients with supraglottic carcinomas, and more than 50% of these were located within the lungs (as reported by Wagenfeld et al.).[68,69] We[70] found 9% second primaries in patients treated for laryngeal carcinoma (24/270). Metachronous tumors were most frequent (21) and the index tumor occurred most often in the larynx (17). The second primary was in the lungs in nine and in the oral cavity, hypopharynx, or esophagus in six. The raised incidence of second primary malignancies in anatomic related areas subject to the same influences is in line with the concept of "field cancerization". Panendoscopies have therefore been advocated in patients with head and neck cancer and may yield a high incidence of simultaneous primary carcinomas.[72-75]

IX. PREVENTIVE MEASURES

All exogenic carcinogenic agents should be removed when a carcinoma is diagnosed. The patients who continue to smoke are at a higher risk of developing a recurrent tumor than those who quit smoking.[76] Excessive consumption of alcohol may also be a factor of importance. The doctors have a great responsibility to inform their patients about the risk of continuous exposure to carcinogenic agents.

X. FOLLOW-UP

The patients treated by radiotherapy or surgery for laryngeal carcinoma should be followed regularly. A repeat microlaryngoscopy should be performed with photographic documentation (Figure 24B) 2 to 3 months after radiotherapy. Mirror laryngoscopy or telescopic inspection (Figures 23C and 28E) and palpation of the neck should then be performed every 2nd to 3rd month for the 1st year, depending on the tumor, every 3rd month during the 2nd year, every 4th month for the following 3 years, and every 6th month up to at least 10 years following treatment. Chest X-ray is performed every year and should perhaps be complemented by sputum cytology in patients considered treatable if a primary lung carcinoma is detected.

Impaired mobility or fixation of the vocal cord after previous radiotherapy should be considered an indication of a recurrent tumor until proven otherwise.

Irradiation-induced carcinomas are not common, but cannot be neglected in patients treated at a younger age.[77-79] These tumors are often diagnosed decades after the radiation therapy was administered. Patients that have undergone radiotherapy therefore have to be followed for their lifetime.

I agree entirely with Professor Douglas Bryce[80] that all patients with laryngeal cancer should be treated and followed at oncologic centers with all diagnostic and therapeutic expertise and facilities available.

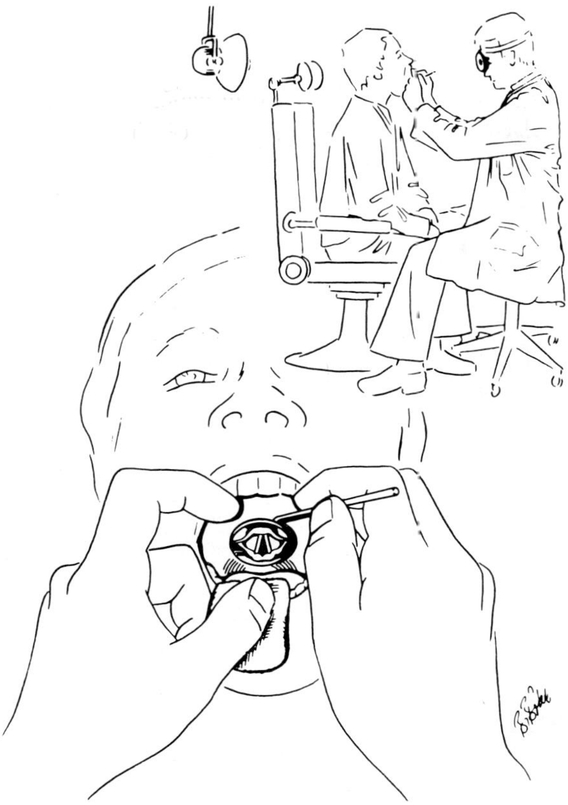

FIGURE 1. Mirror laryngoscopy.

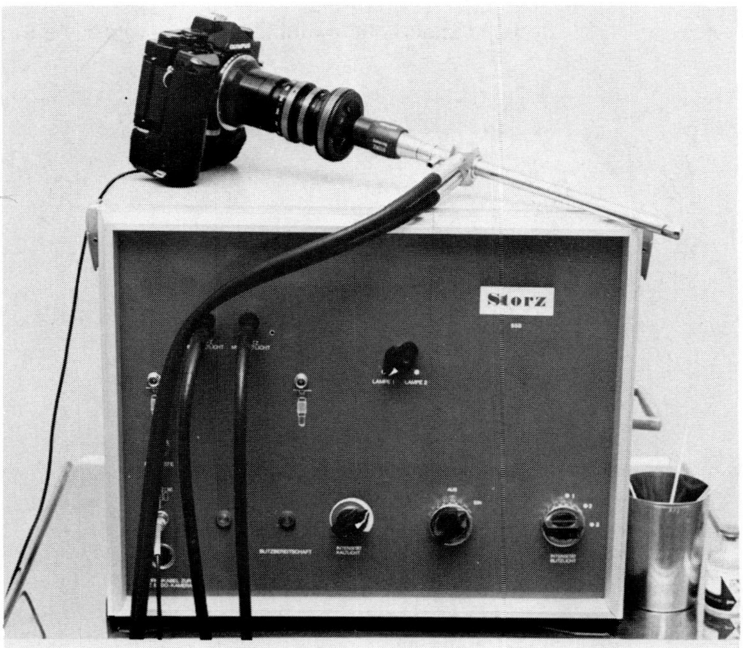

FIGURE 2. Storz-Hopkins' telescopic equipment with an Olympus camera attached. Kodak Ectachrome 400 ASA film is used.

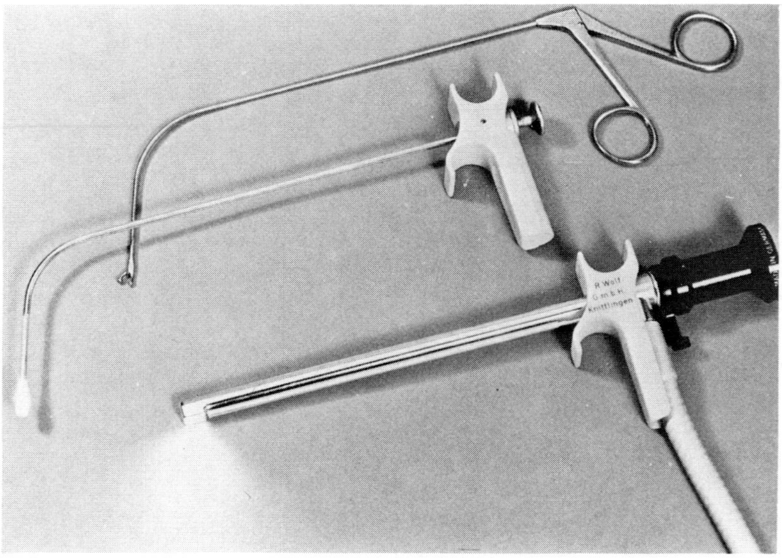

FIGURE 3. The Wolf telescope and the sampling device for indirect smear cytology and a cup forceps for biopsies.

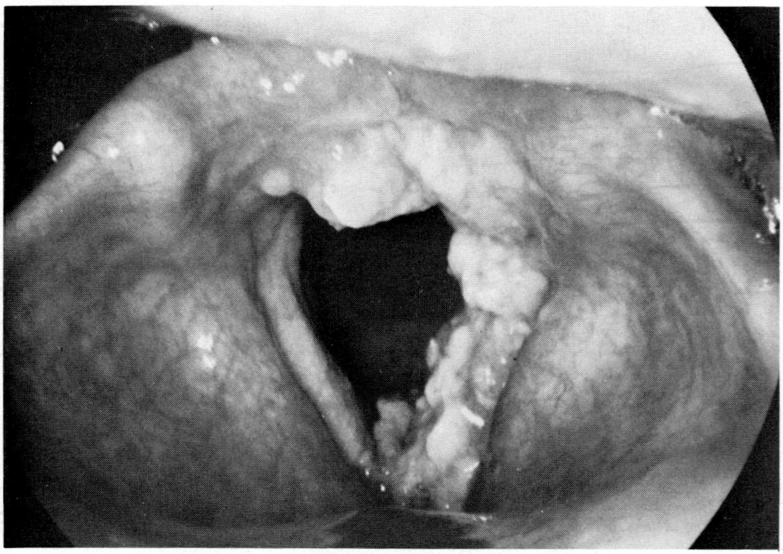

A

FIGURE 4. Extensive glottic carcinoma. Telescopic photographs. (A) Carcinoma of the left vocal cord with involvement of the anterior and posterior commissures; (B) adducted vocal cords illustrating the normal mobility of the vocal cords; (C) cytologic sampling by indirect technique; (D) biopsy specimens removed by indirect technique.

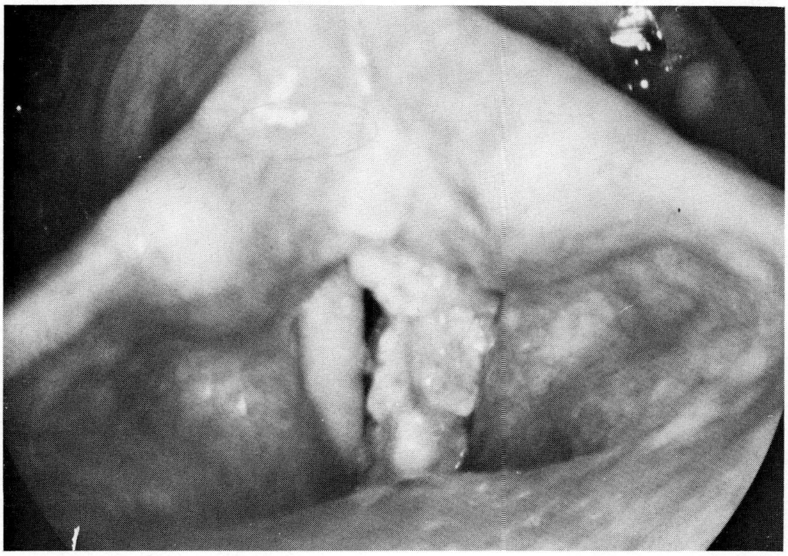

FIGURE 4B

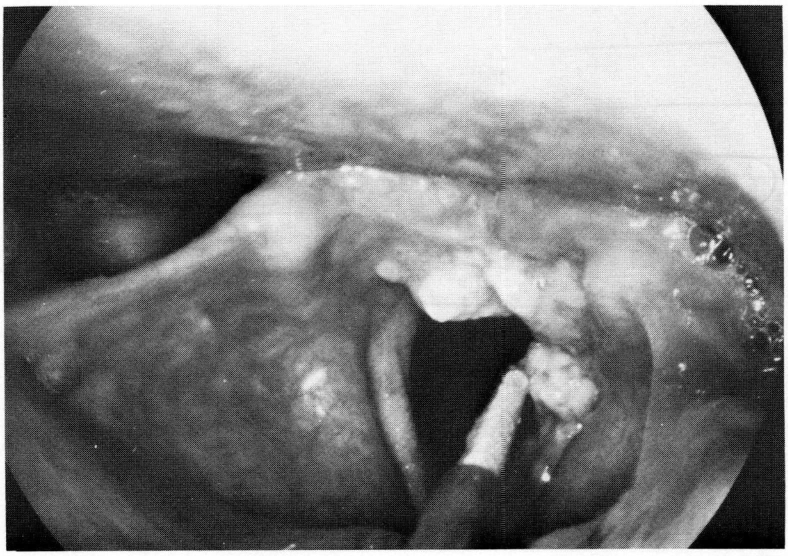

FIGURE 4C

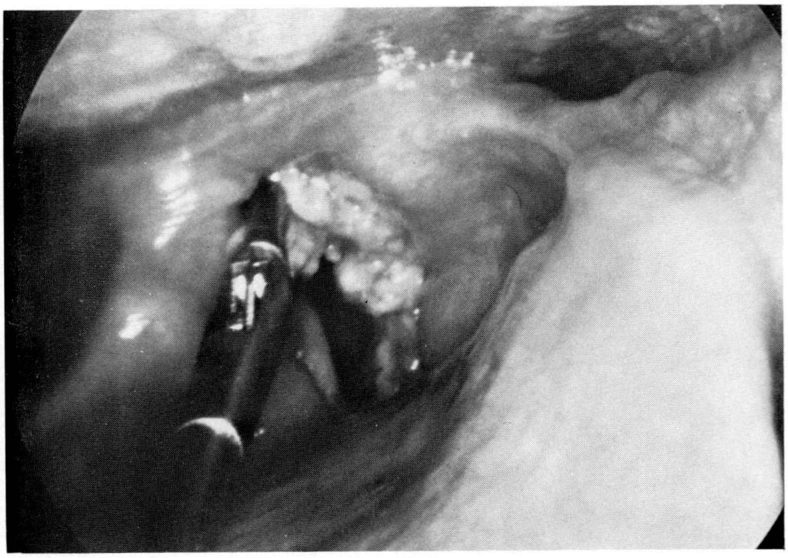

FIGURE 4D

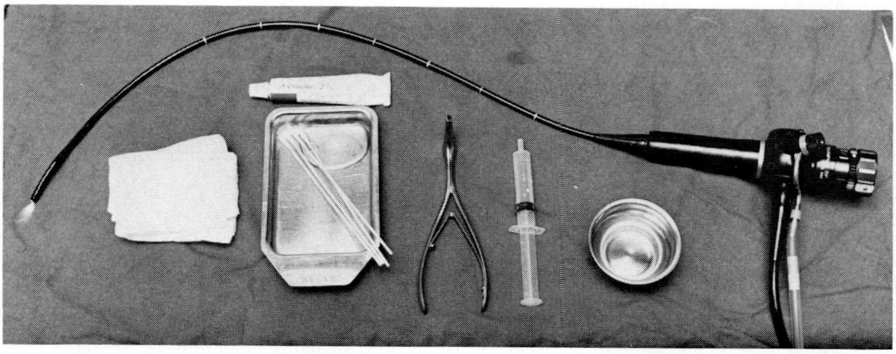

A

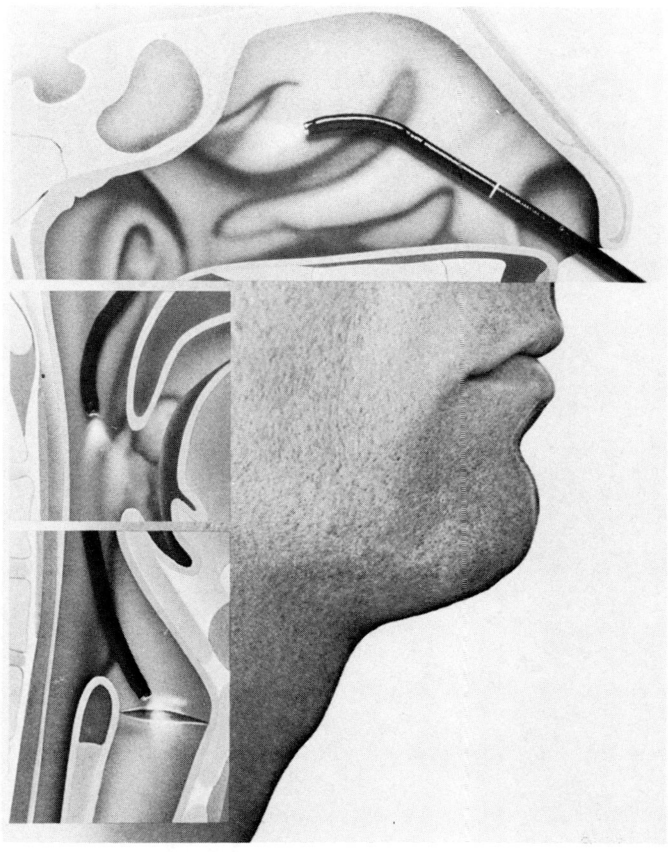

B

FIGURE 5. Inspection by flexible scope. (A) Bronchofiberscope. Xylocain viscous 2% is applied within the nasal cavities by the use of the cotton pins before the scope is introduced. Xylocain 2% is instilled through the suction channel of the fiberscope; (B) examination procedure (By permission of the Olympus Co.).

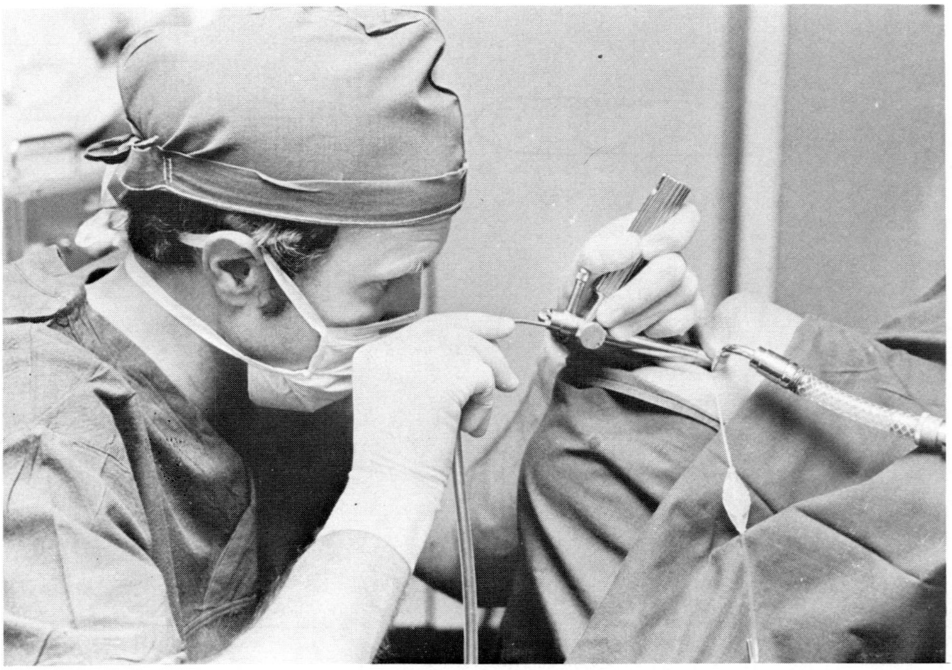

FIGURE 6. Inspection by a regular laryngoscope should always precede the microlaryngoscopy so as not to overlook pathologic processes in the valleculae, piriform sinuses, and post-cricoid region.

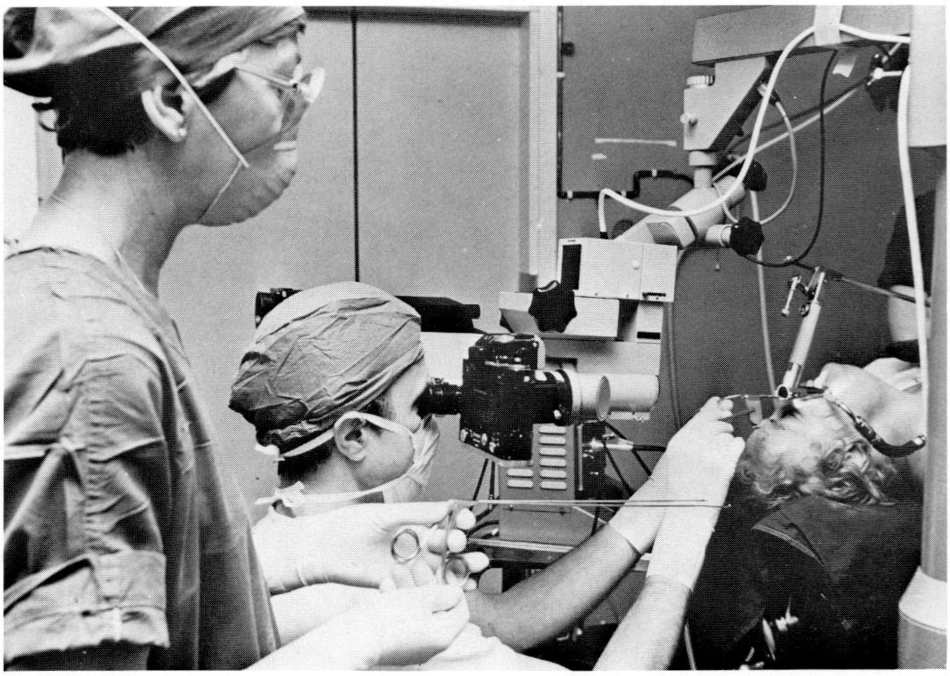

FIGURE 7. Microlaryngoscopy. Both camera and videocamera attached. The patient is intubated and a Portex tube 6.0 or 6.5 is used.

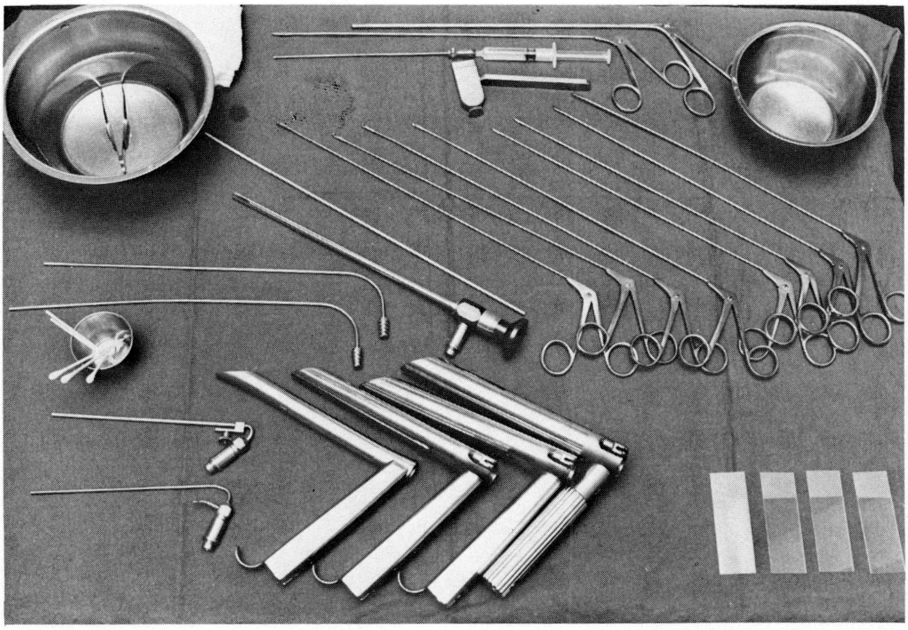

FIGURE 8. Instruments used at a regular microlaryngoscopy. Note the 90° optical instrument used for inspection of the subglottis, anterior commissure, and ventricles, and the glasses for the smear cytology.

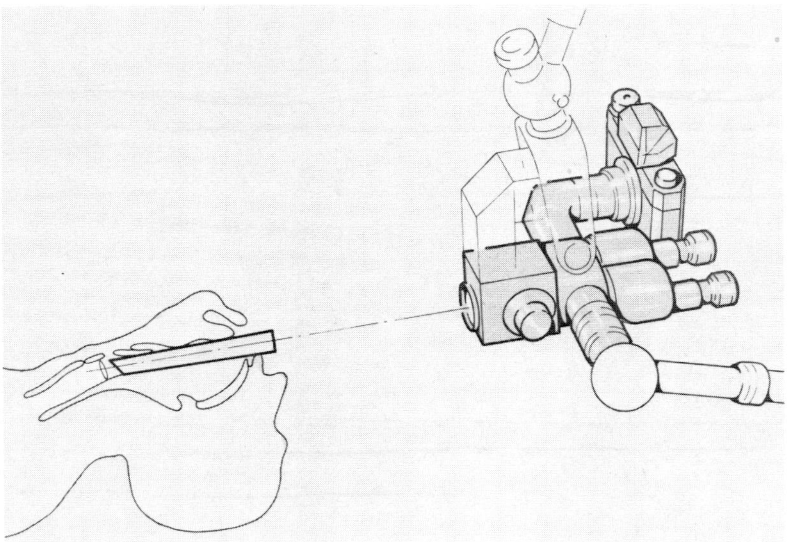

FIGURE 9. An exact alignment of the optical axes of the microscope and the laryngoscope is a necessity to achieve a good photographic documentation.

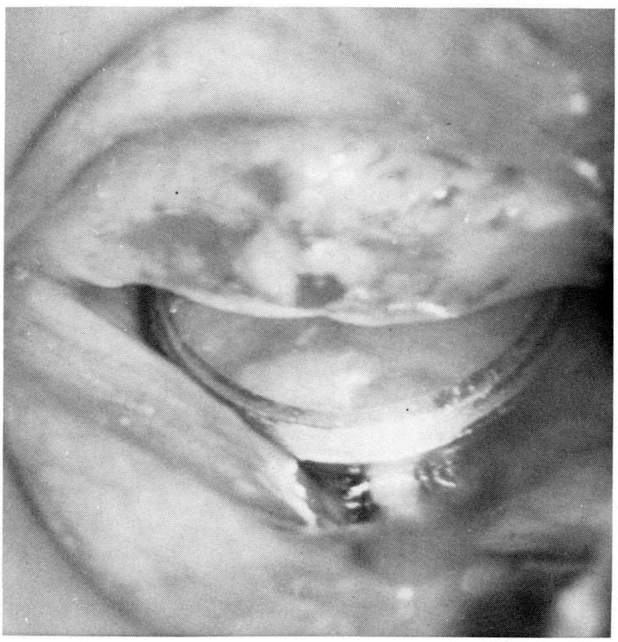

FIGURE 10. Inspection of the undersurface of the vocal cord by the use of a mirror.

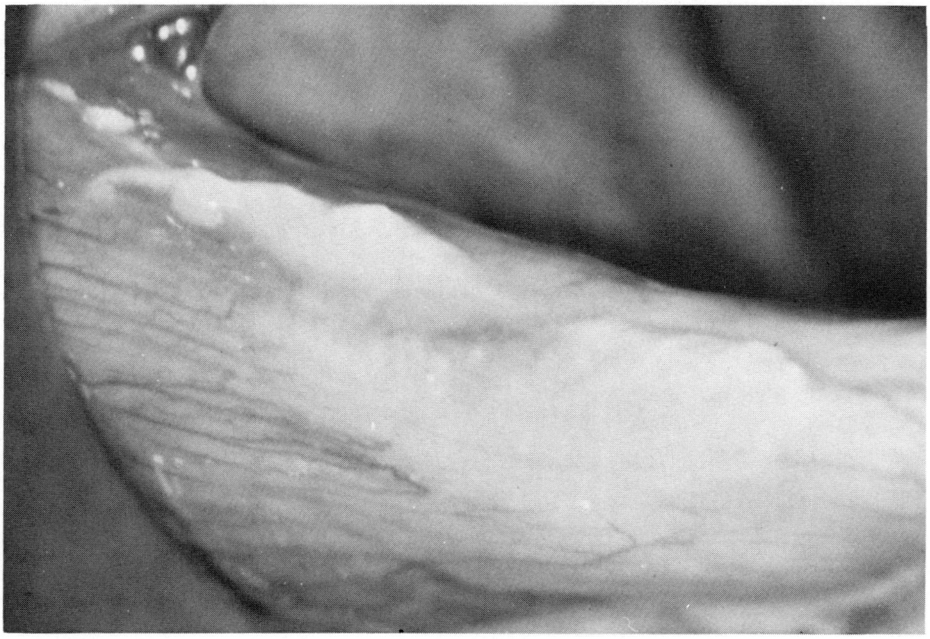

FIGURE 11. Keratosis of the left vocal cord. Histologically no atypia.

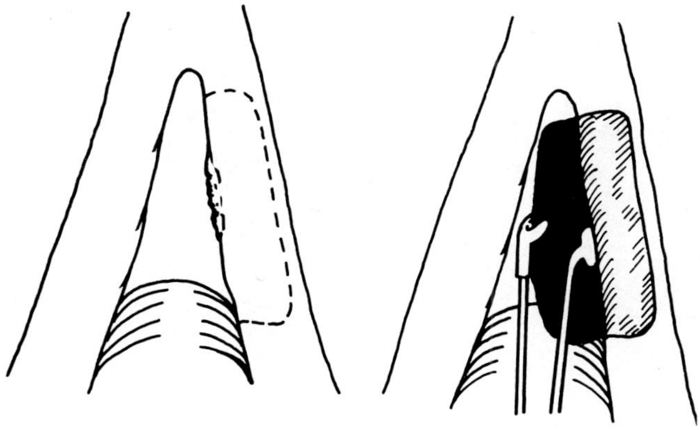

FIGURE 12. Localized lesions may well be removed by excision or stripping.

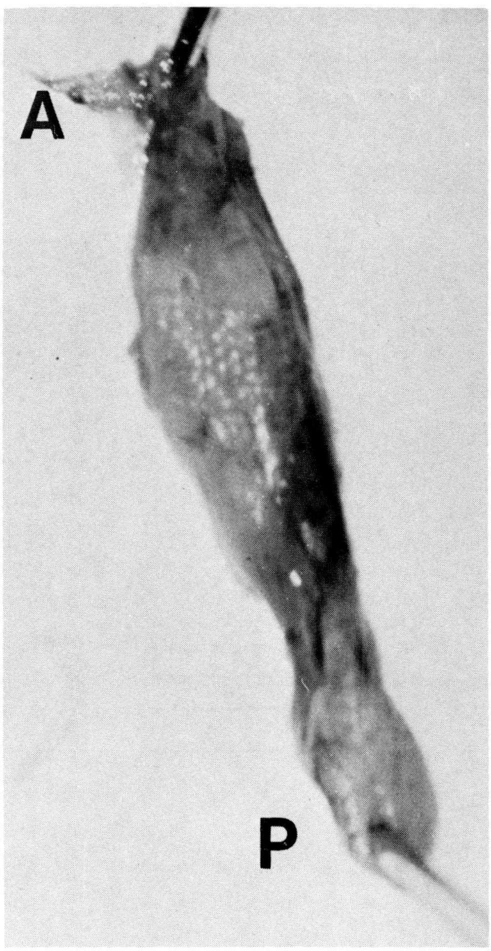

FIGURE 13. The excised mucosa should be mounted on a piece of paper and orientated for at least step-serial sectioning. A: anterior; P: posterior.

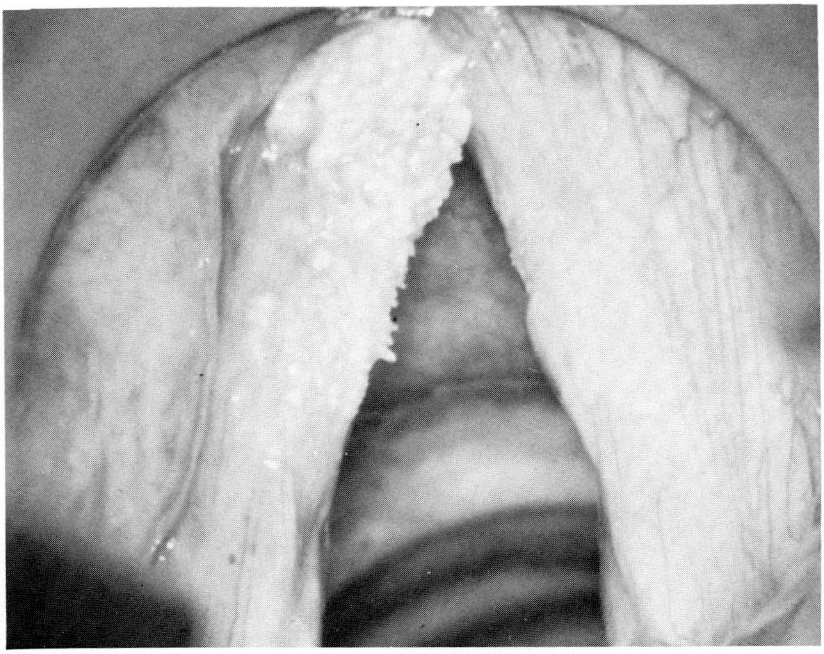

A

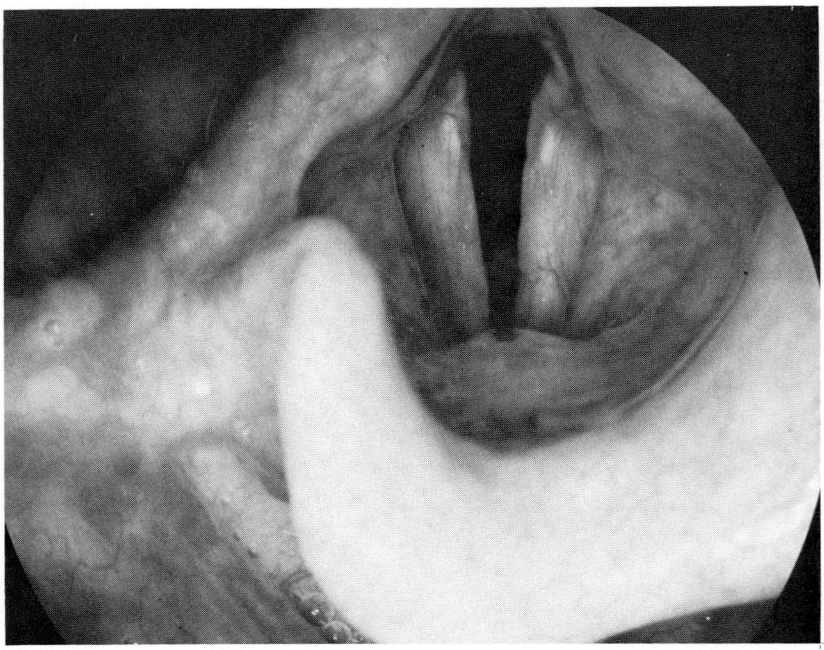

B

FIGURE 14. Microlaryngscopy. (A) Papillary lesion—adult papillomatosis of the left vocal cord with mild dysplasia. A slight thickening is also present of the right vocal cord. The lesions were excised; (B) telescopic view 9 years later showing normal-looking vocal cords.

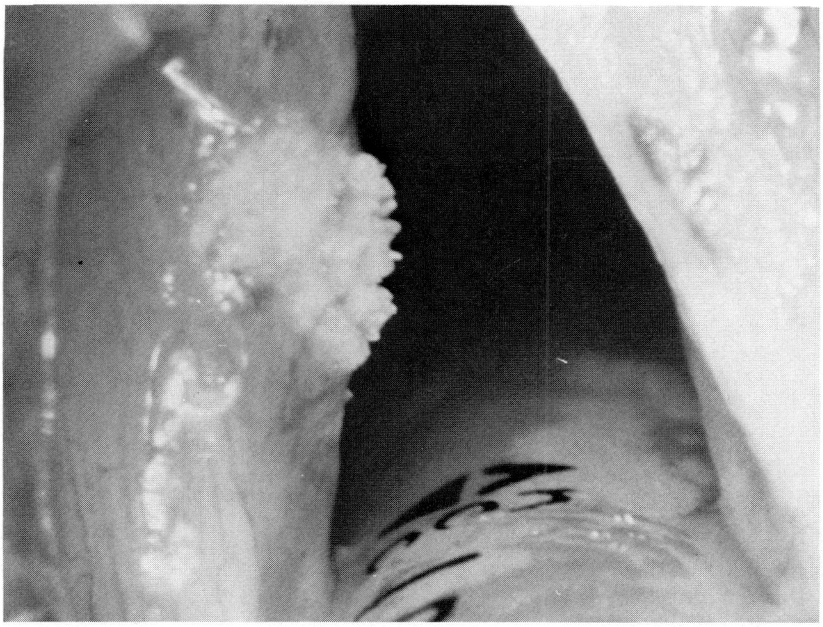

A

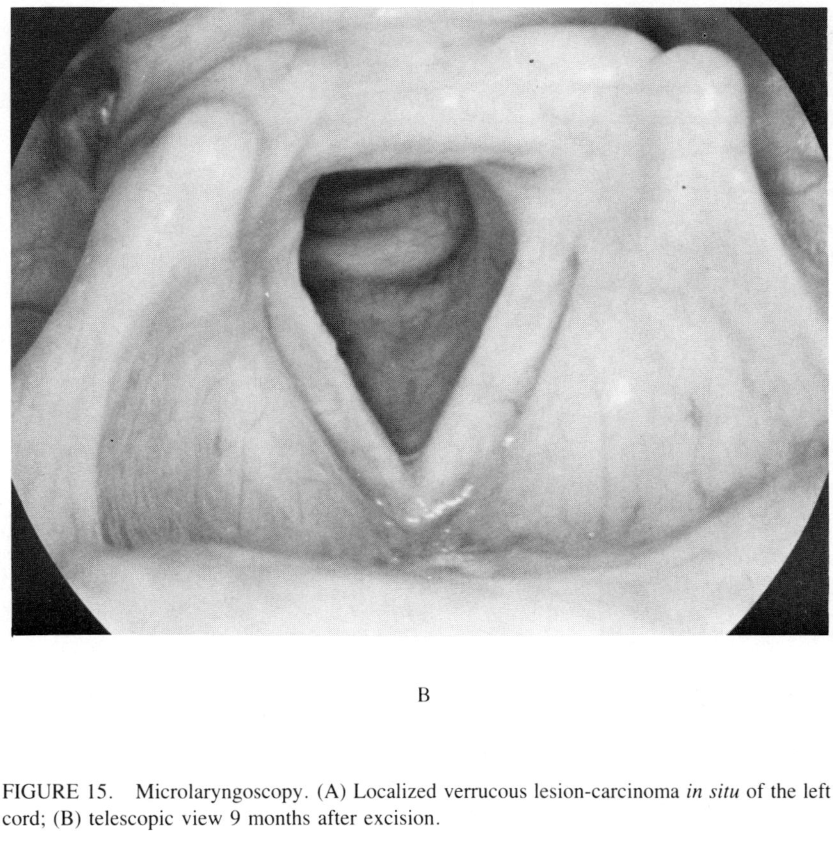

B

FIGURE 15. Microlaryngoscopy. (A) Localized verrucous lesion-carcinoma *in situ* of the left cord; (B) telescopic view 9 months after excision.

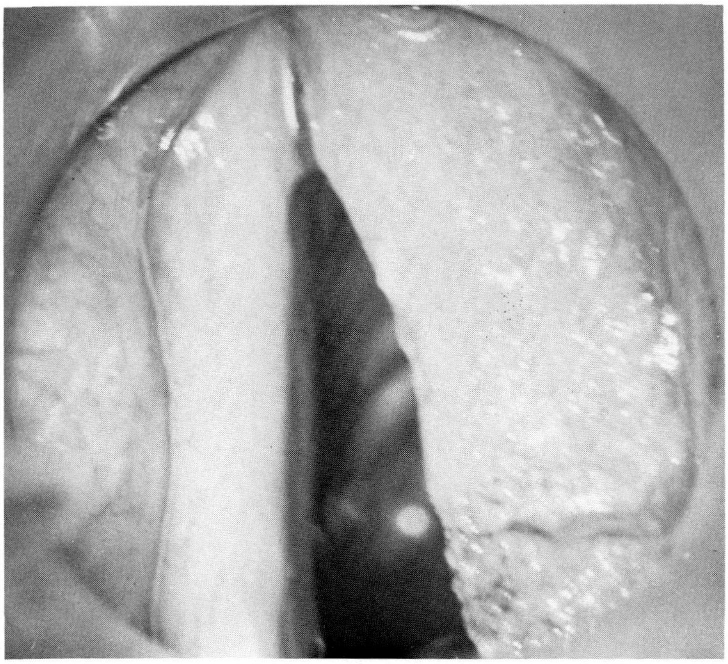

FIGURE 16. Microlaryngoscopy. Diffuse granulated-papillary lesion of the right vocal cord-hyperplasia with moderate dysplasia histologically. Smear cytology indicated carcinoma, which was diagnosed at a repeat biopsy 7 months later.

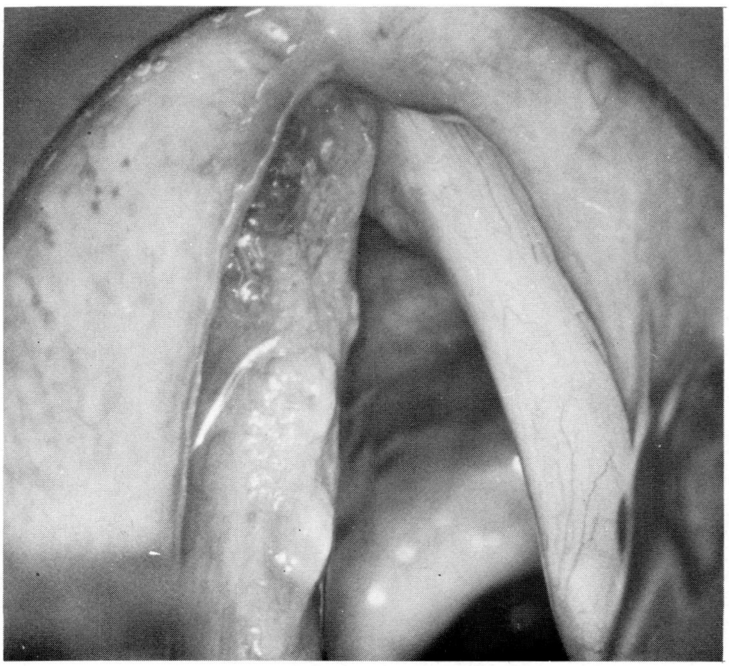

FIGURE 17. Microlaryngoscopy. Leukoplakia posteriorly and erytroplakia anteriorly on the left vocal cord. Biopsy specimens showed moderate dysplasia from the leukoplakia and invasive carcinoma from the erytroplakia. Multiple biopsies have to be taken to obtain representative histology from diffuse lesions, that can not be totally excised.

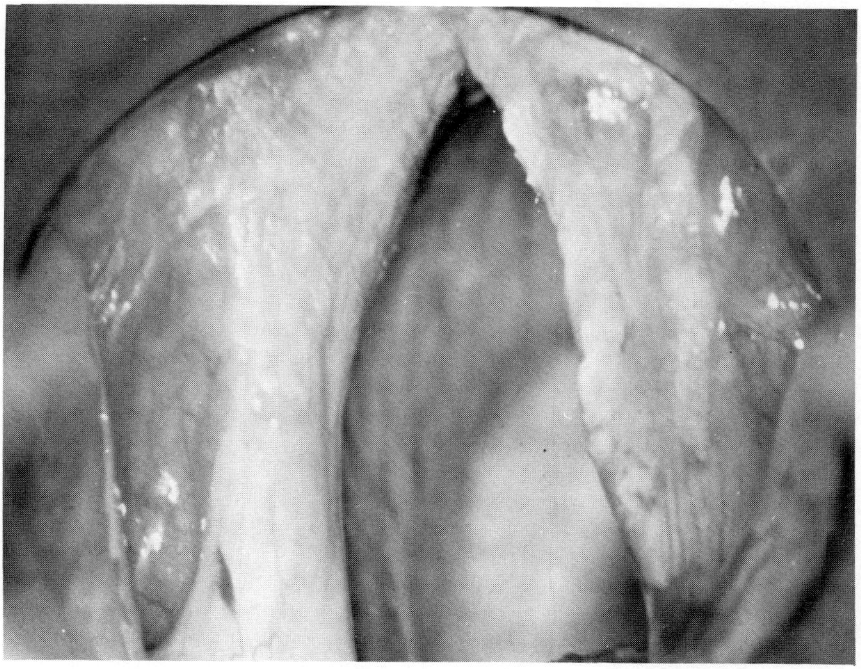

FIGURE 18. Microlaryngoscopy. Diffuse lesions of both vocal cords with both leukoplakias and erytroplakias. Multiple biopsies were taken and in some an early invasive carcinoma was diagnosed. This patient received radiotherapy and there are no signs of recurrence 10 years later.

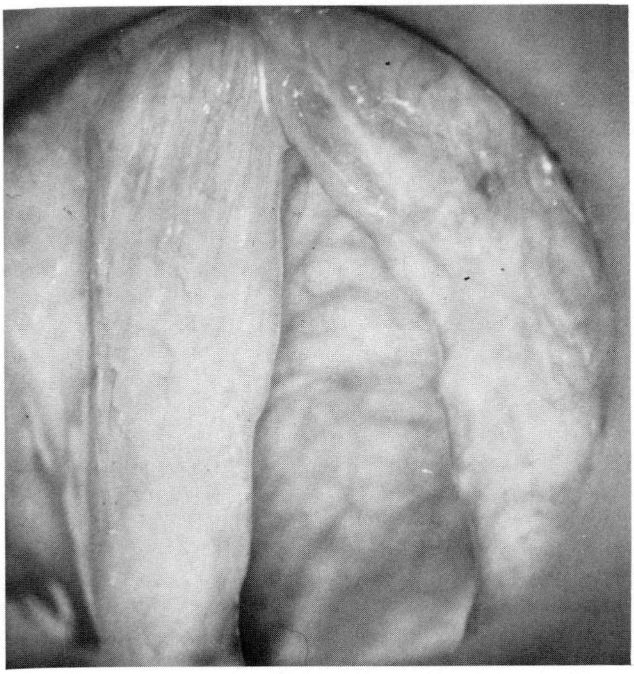

A

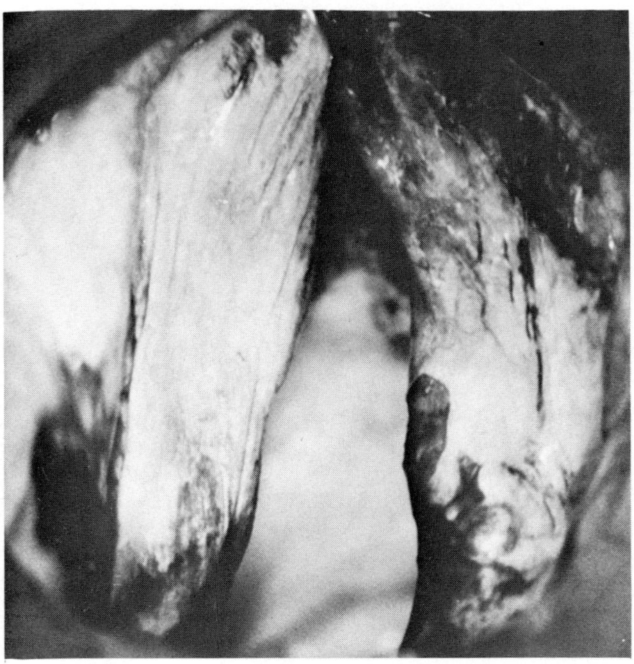

B

FIGURE 19. Microlaryngoscopy. (A) Slightly irregular mucosa of the right vocal cord; (B) toluidine blue staining showed increased staining in front of the right vocal process, which histologically was shown to be an invasive carcinoma.

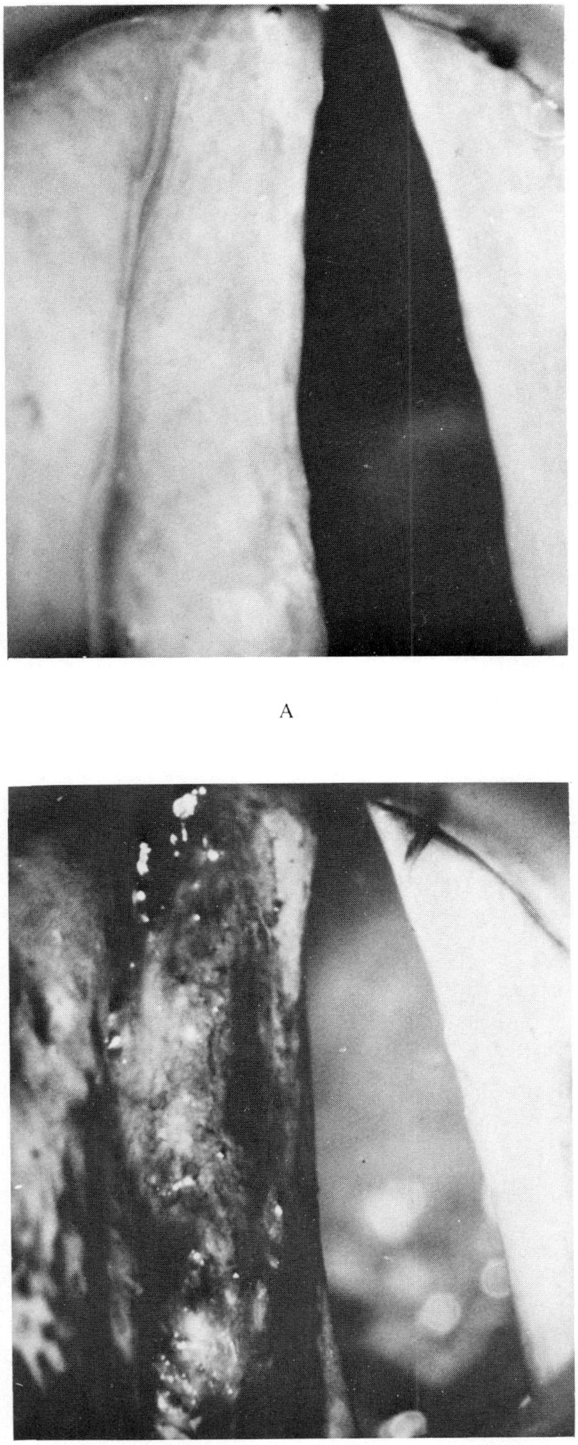

A

B

FIGURE 20. Microlaryngoscopy. Slightly thickened and granulated mucosa of the left vocal cord (A) with intense staining by toluidine blue (B). Histologic examination showed invasive carcinoma.

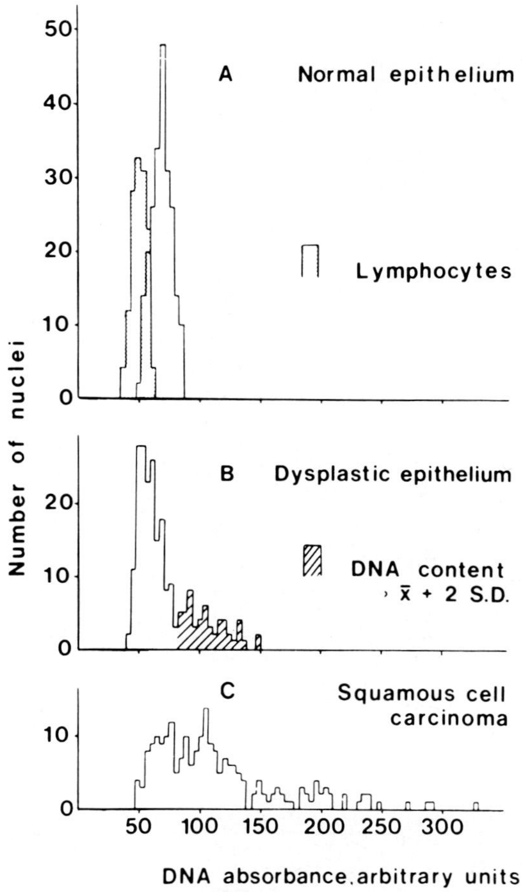

FIGURE 21. Scanning photometric measurements disclose differences in the nuclear DNA content of the different epithelia as shown in this frequency histogram. (From Gröntoft, O., Hellquist, H., Olofsson, J., and Nordström, G., *Acta Otolaryngol.*,86, 473, 1978. With permission.)

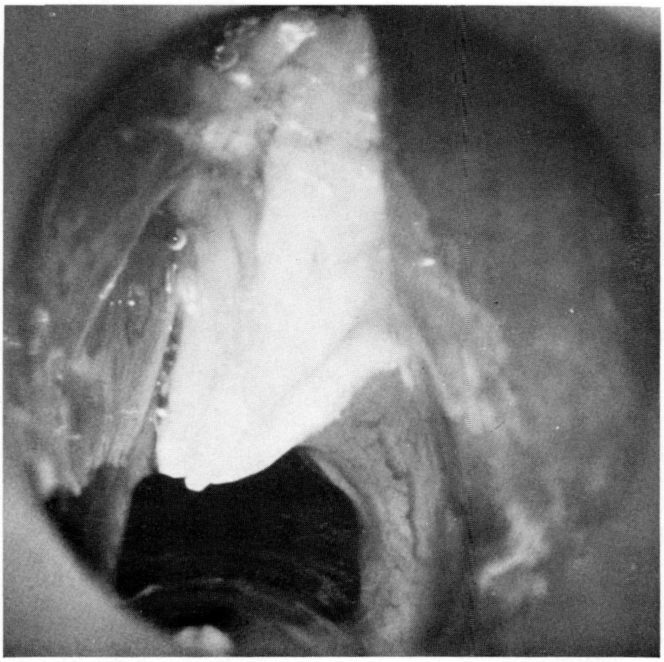

FIGURE 22. Verrucous carcinoma involving the anterior part of the right vocal cord and the anterior commissure. This tumor could be managed endoscopically by excision and the use of laser.

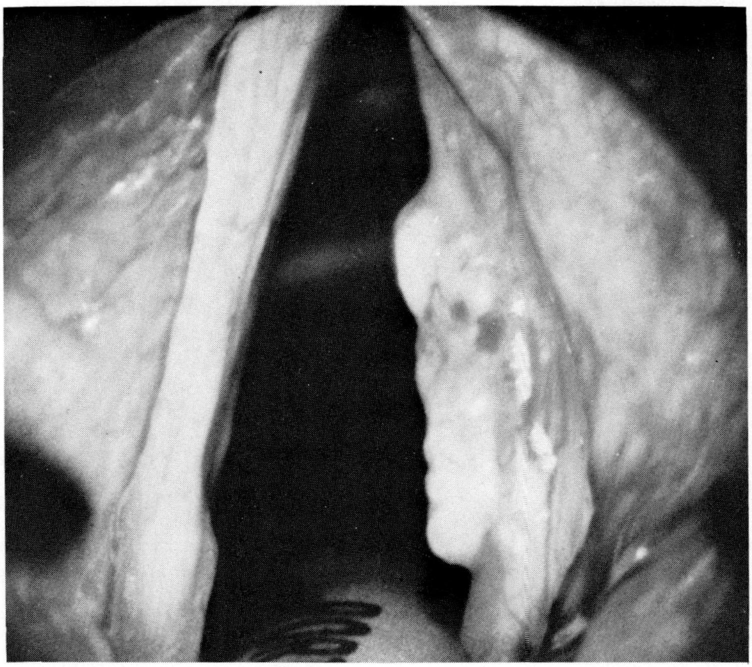

A

FIGURE 23. Microlaryngoscopy. (A and B) Glottic carcinoma of the right vocal cord. A better view is obtained by tilting the tumor and vocal cord upwards by the tip of the suction tube; (C) telescopic photograph 10 years later following radiotherapy showing smooth vocal cords with teleangiectasies.

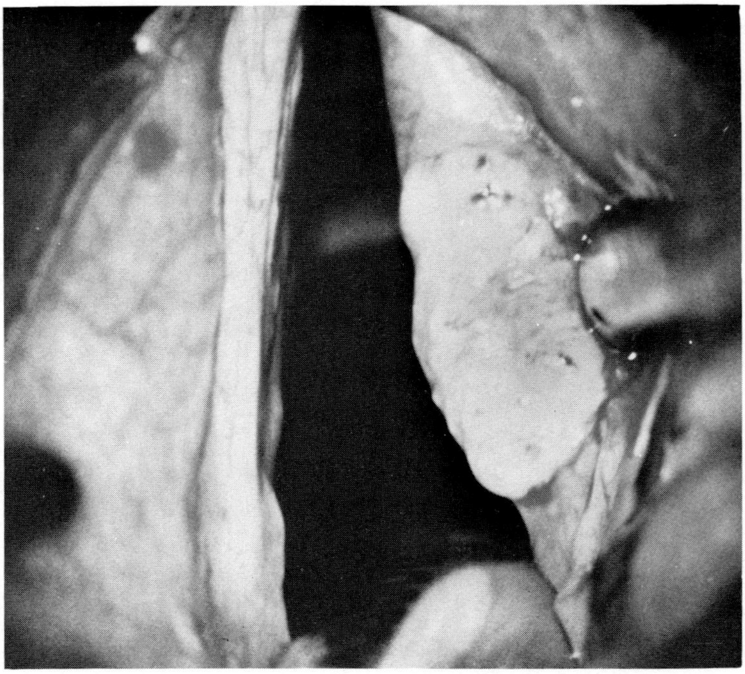

FIGURE 23B

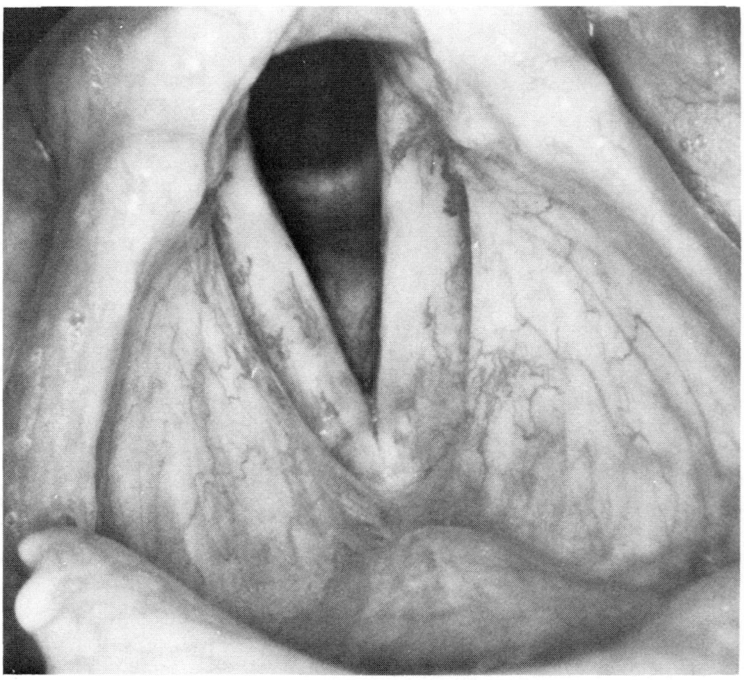

FIGURE 23C

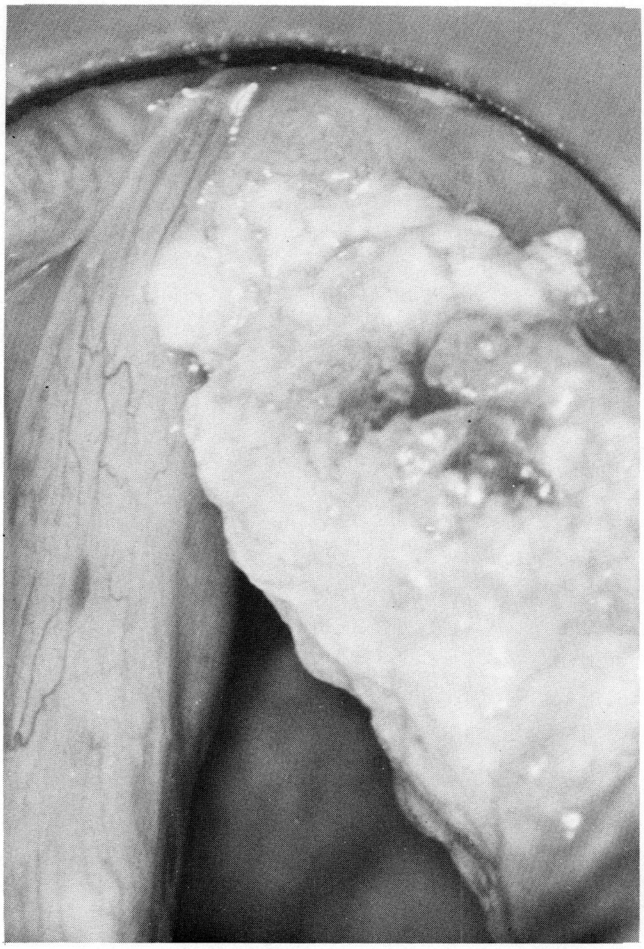

A

FIGURE 24. Microlaryngoscopy. Exophytic carcinoma of the right vocal cord (A); 4 months following radiotherapy there are no signs of residual disease (B).

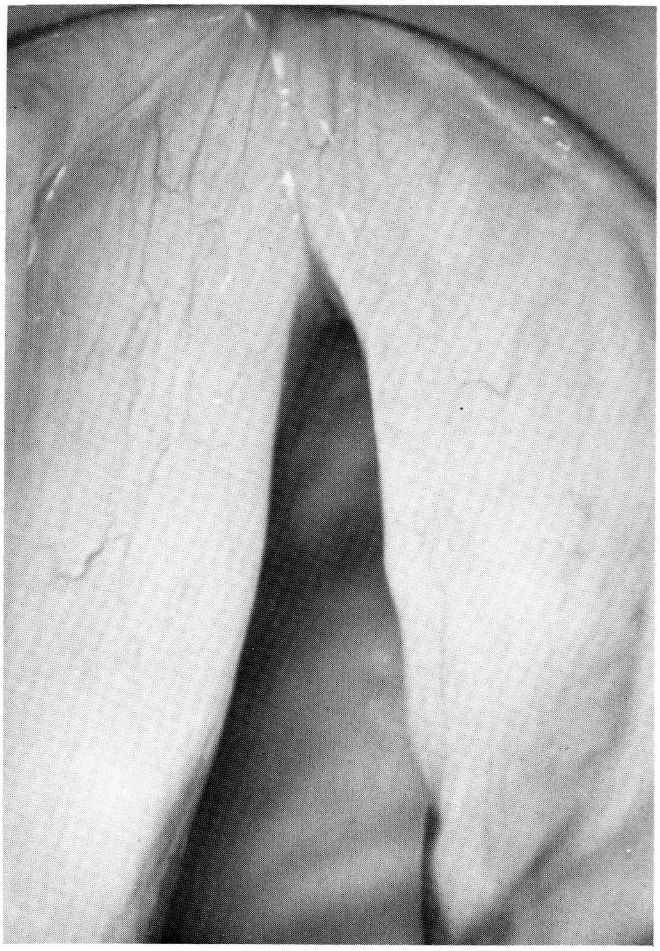

FIGURE 24B

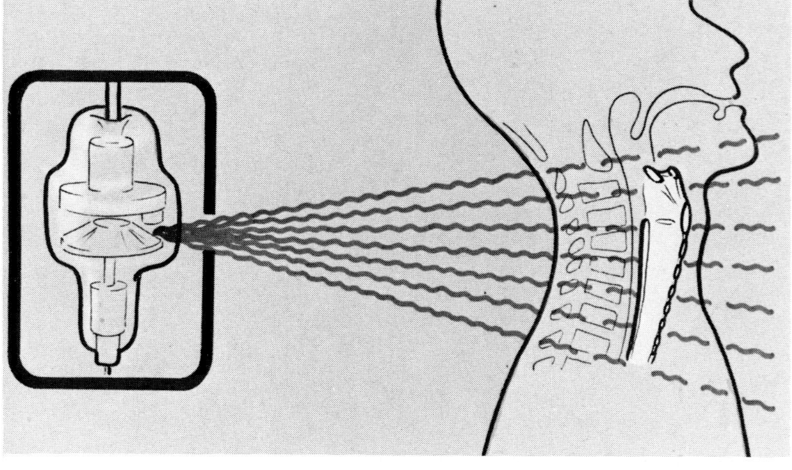

FIGURE 25. Radiologic examination adds important information about vertical tumor extension. CT also gives information about deep invasion with cartilage destruction and spread outside the larynx. Radiology is mandatory for classification according to UICC.

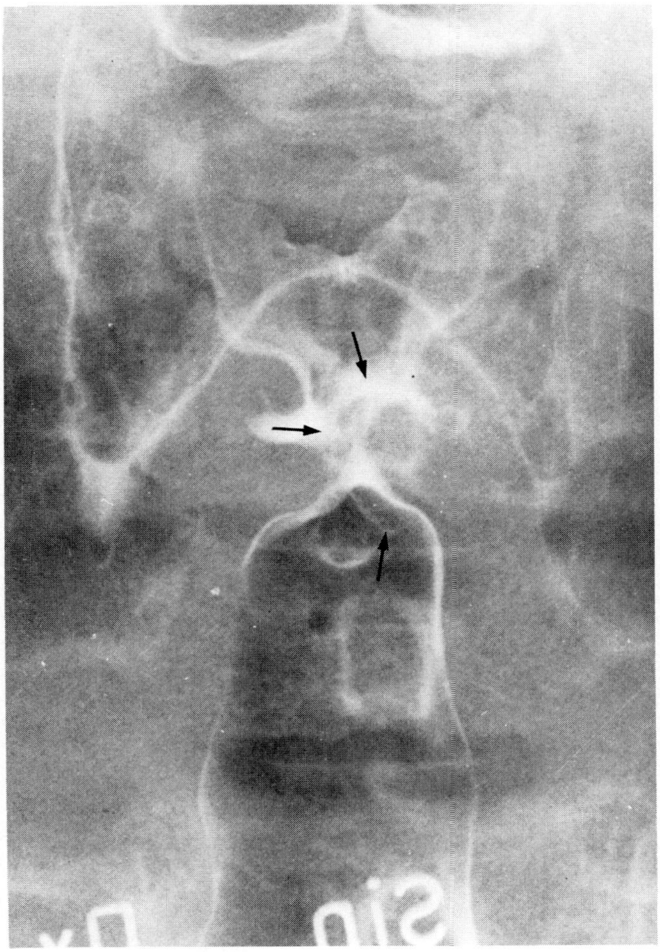

A

FIGURE 26. Glottic carcinoma with involvement of the anterior commissure and with subglottic extension. (A) Laryngogram, p.a.view. Tumor (arrows) of the left vocal cord with subglottic extension; (B) laryngogram, lateral view. Involvement of the anterior commissure and with subglottic extension as marked by arrows; (C) Microlaryngoscopy.

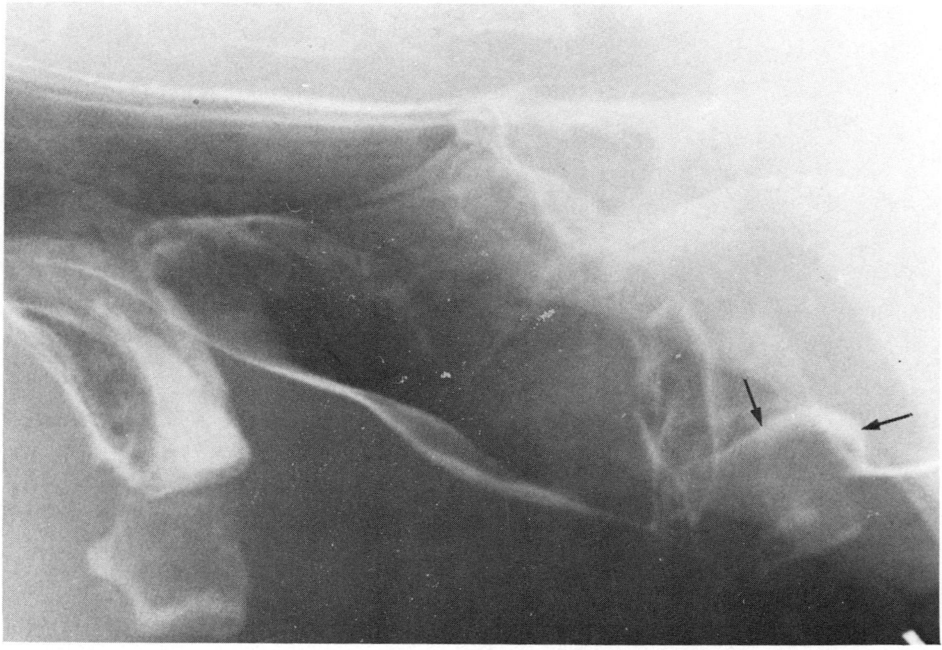

FIGURE 26B

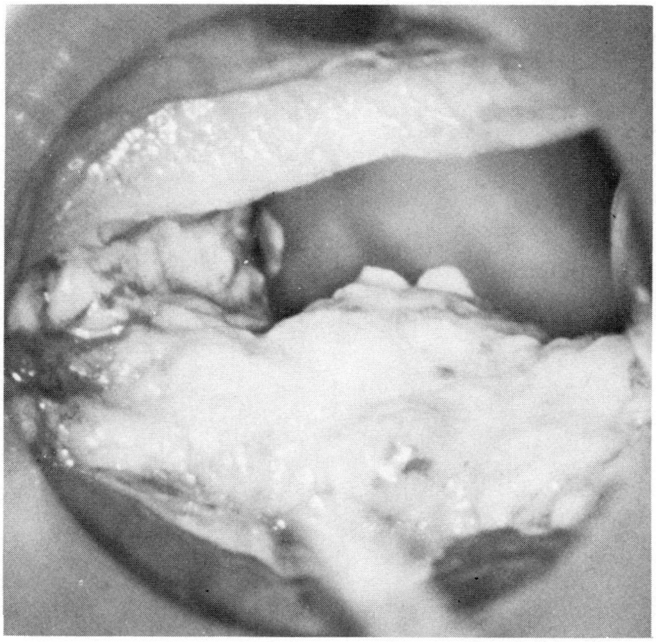

FIGURE 26C

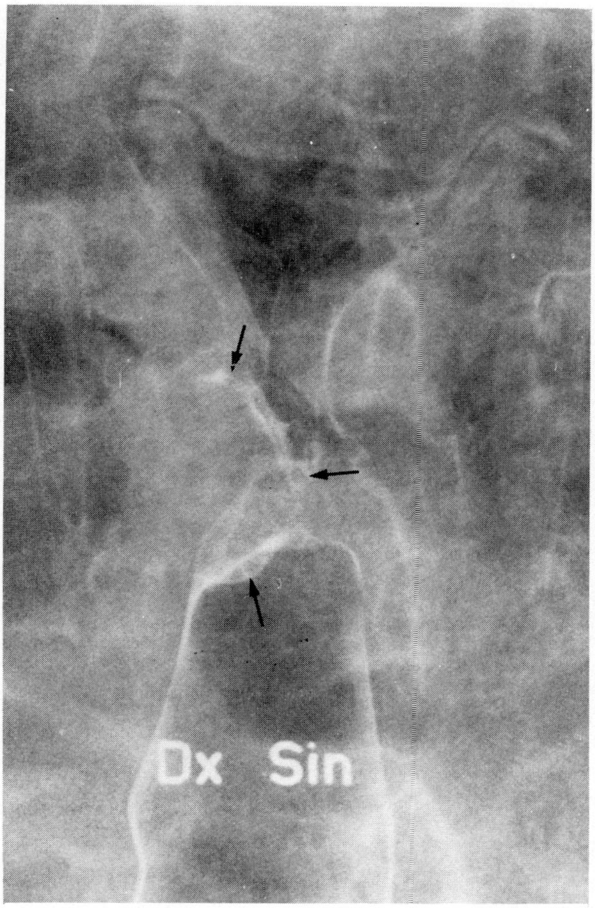

A

FIGURE 27. Glottic—sub- and supraglottic carcinoma. (A) Laryngogram, p.a.view. Tumor (arrows) of the right vocal cord with sub- and supraglottic extension; (B) CT — scan through the vocal cords. Suspect destruction of the thyroid cartilage anteriorly and spread to a prelaryngeal node to the left of the midline (arrows); (C) microlaryngoscopy. Exophytic tumor of the full length of the right vocal cord with involvement of the anterior commissure and with subglottic extension.

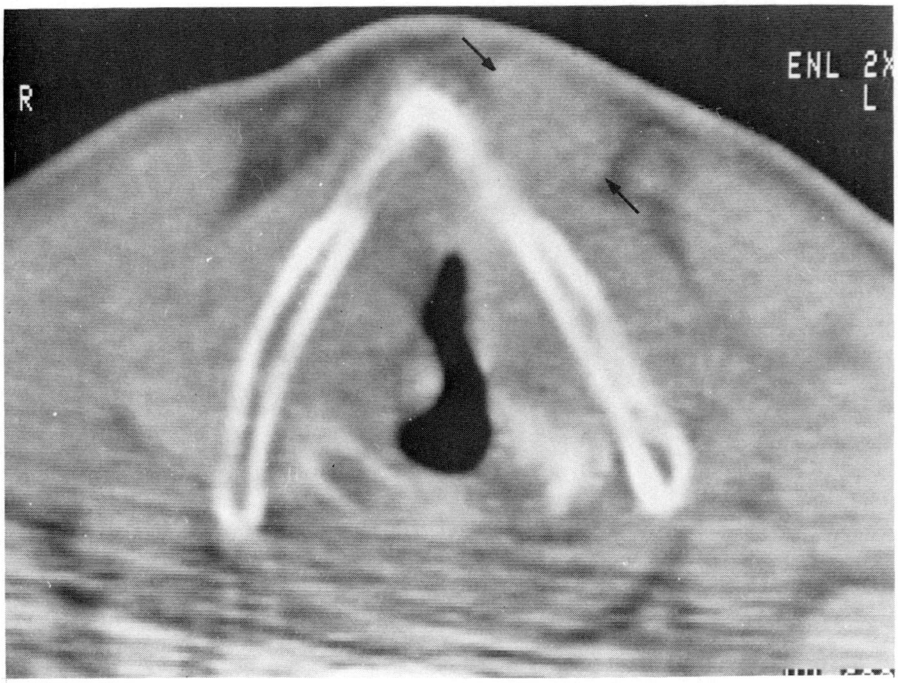

FIGURE 27B

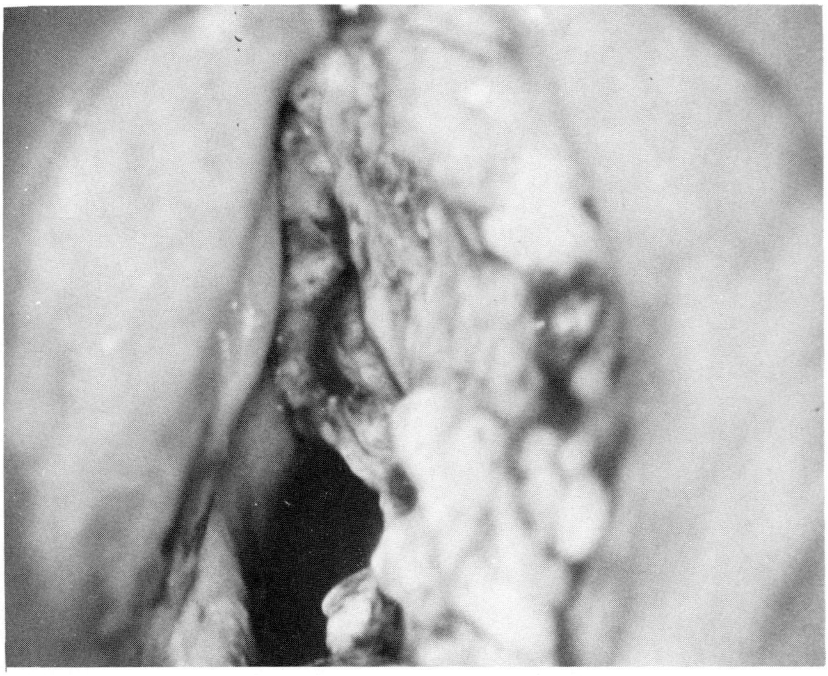

FIGURE 27C

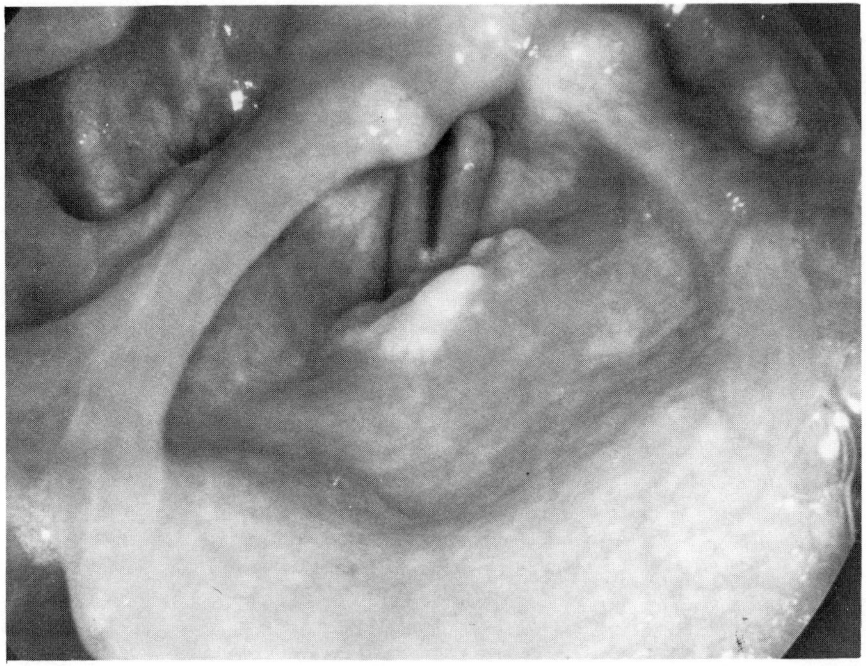

A

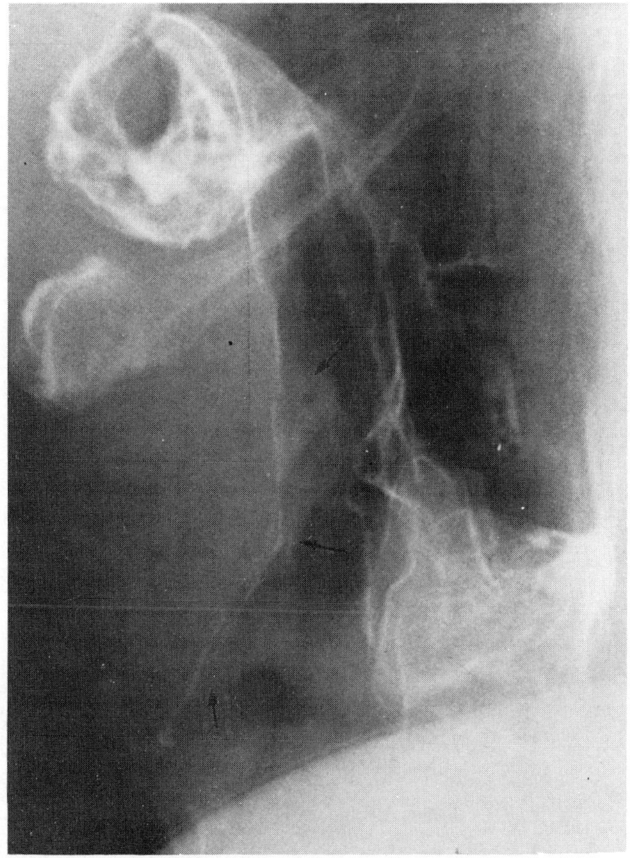

B

FIGURE 28. Carcinoma of the epiglottis amenable to horizontal supraglottic laryngectomy. (A) Telescopic view of the localized tumor on the laryngeal surface of the epiglottis; (B) laryngogram, lateral view. The tumor (arrows) leaves a free margin caudally to the anterior commissure; (C) photograph using a 90° optical instrument at the microlaryngoscopy, demonstrating the free margin down to the anterior commissure in line with the laryngogram; (D) CT — invasion of the preepiglottic space but no invasion of the thyroid cartilage; (E) telescopic view after preoperative radiotherapy and a horizontal supraglottic laryngectomy.

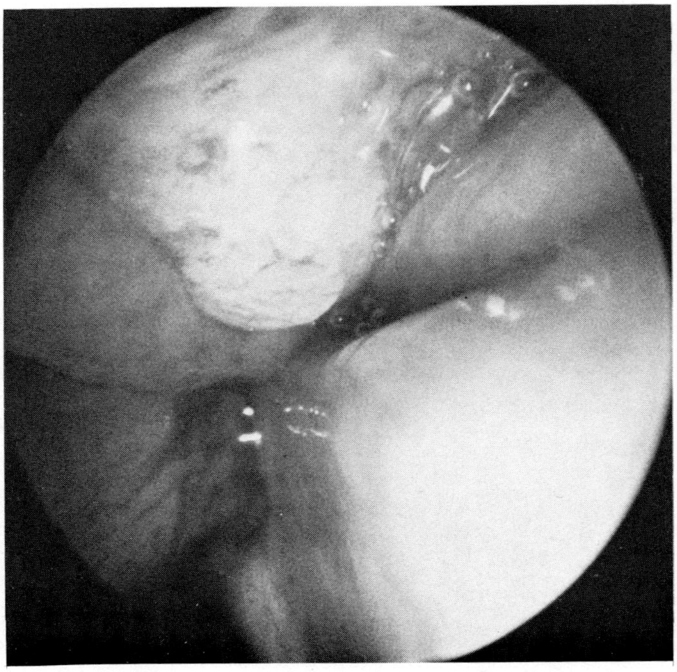

FIGURE 28C

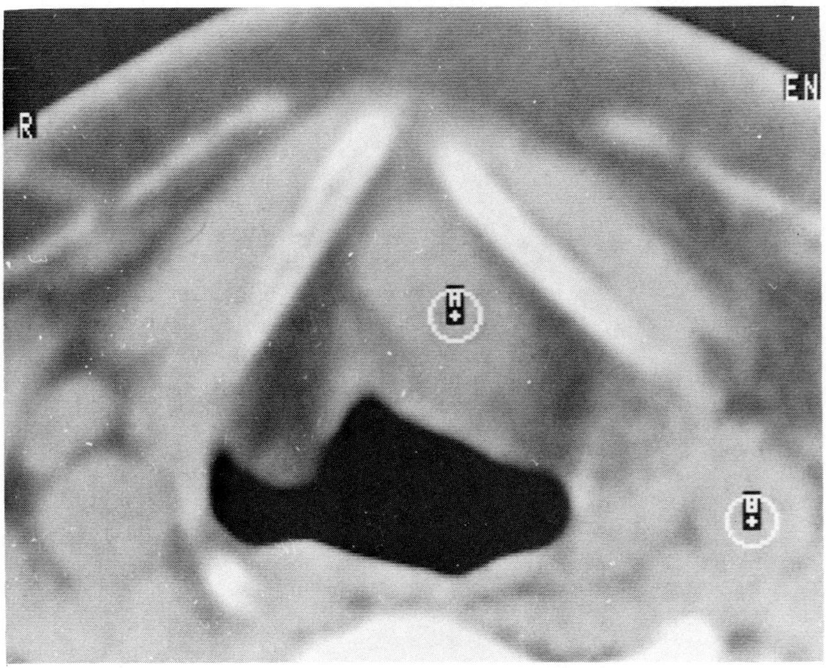

FIGURE 28D

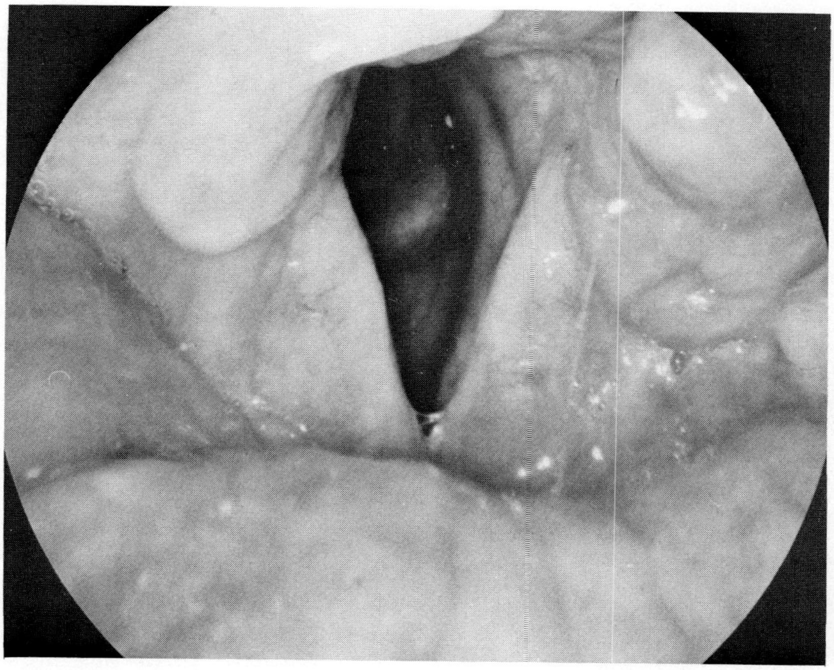

FIGURE 28E

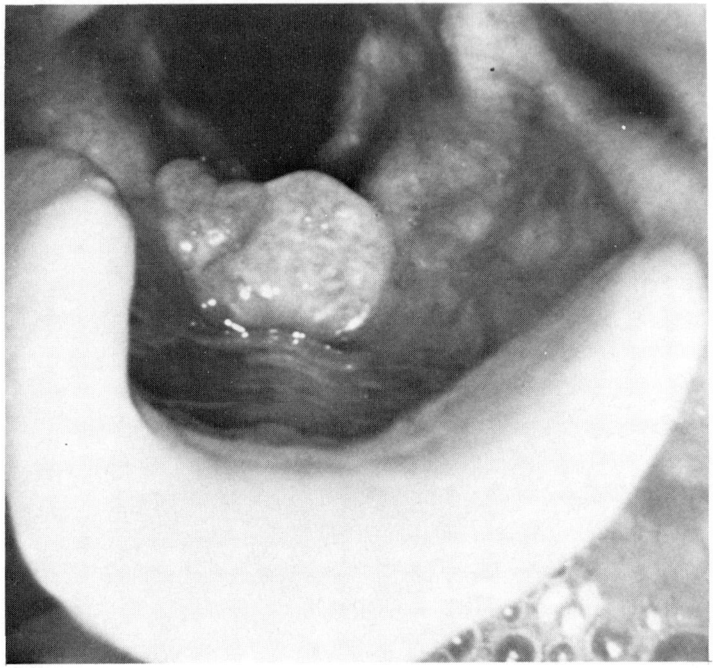

A

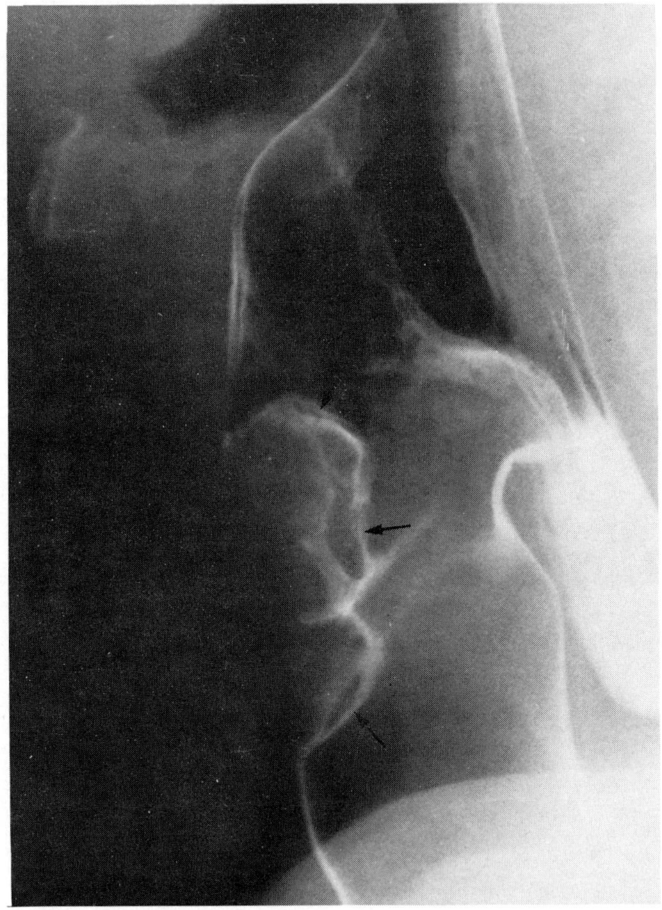

B

FIGURE 29. Supraglottic carcinoma with anterior glottic-subglottic extension. (A) Telescopic photograph. Exophytic tumor on the laryngeal surface of the epiglottis above the anterior commissure; (B) laryngogram, lateral view. Exophytic tumor with supraglottic, glottic, and subglottic involvement(arrows); (C) CT — scan below the vocal cords with suspect destruction of the thyroid cartilage anteriorly; (D) microlaryngoscopy.

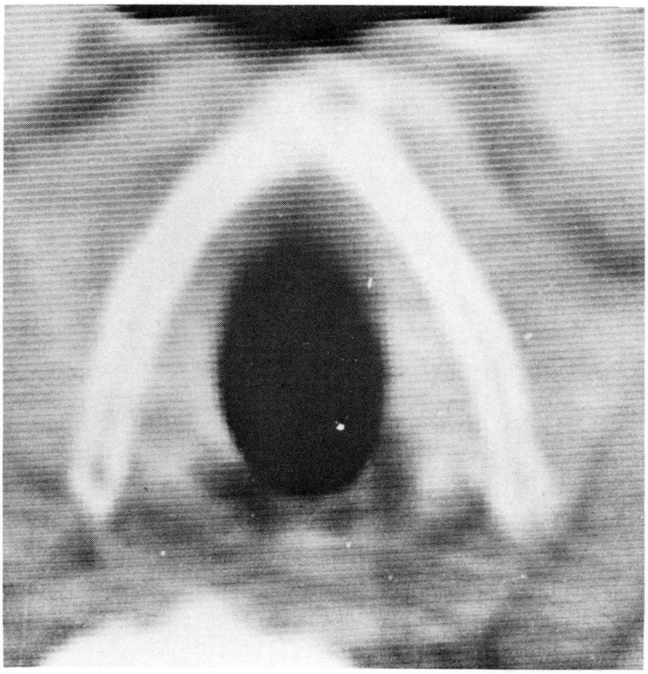

FIGURE 29C

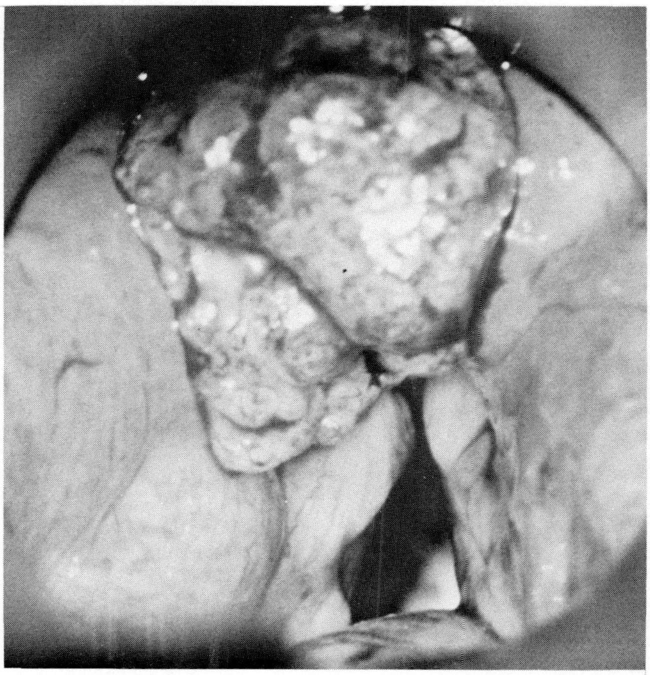

FIGURE 29D

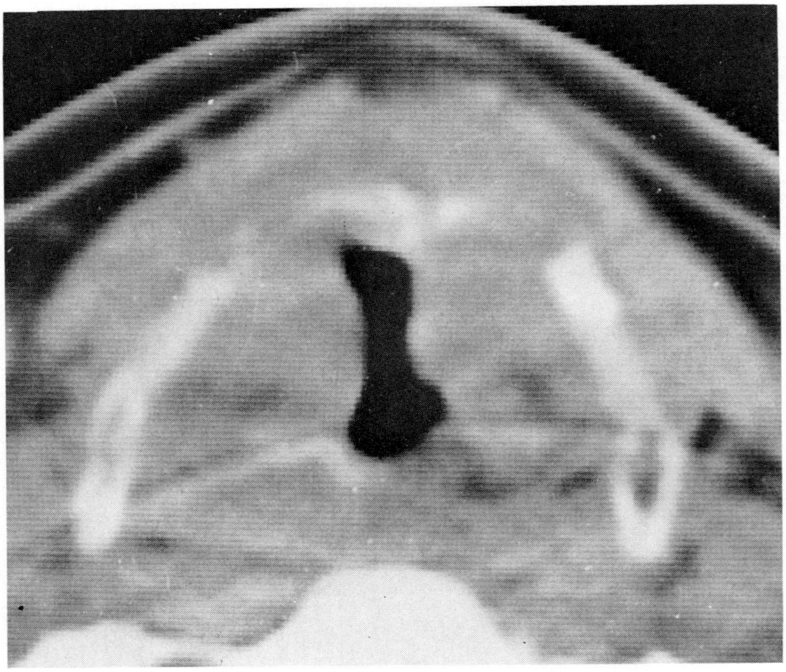

FIGURE 30. Supraglottic carcinoma with massive destruction of the thyroid cartilage. CT — scan through the false vocal cords.

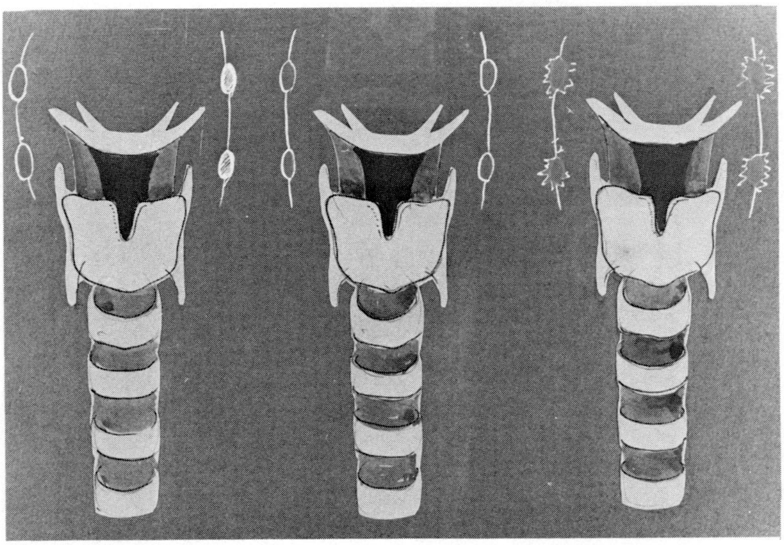

FIGURE 31. Nodal involvement; homolateral, bilateral, or fixed nodes.

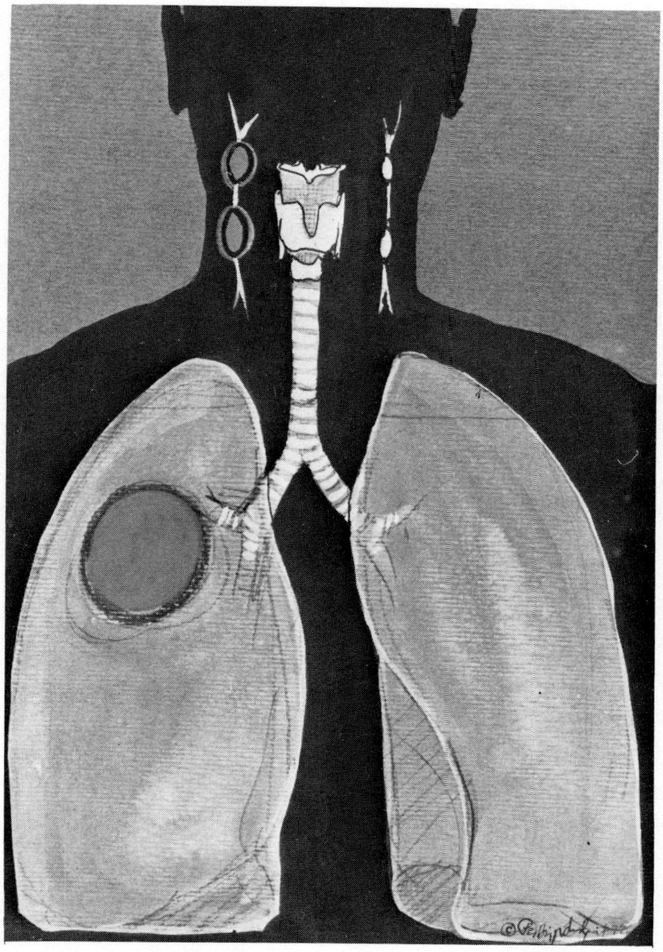

FIGURE 32. Chest X-rays should be performed at least every year to diagnose metastases and second primaries.

REFERENCES

1. **Kleinsasser, O.,** Mikrolaryngoskopie und endolaryngeale Mikrochirurgie, *Technik und Typische Befunde,* F. K. Schattauer, Stuttgart, 1968.
2. **Kleinsasser, O.,** Mikrolaryngoskopie und endolaryngeale Mikrochirurgie, *Technik und Typische Befunde,* F. K. Schattauer, Stuttgart, 1976.
3. **Olofsson, J. and Ohlsson, T.,** Techniques in microlaryngoscopic photography, *Can. J. Otolaryngol.,* 4, 770, 1975.
4. **Kleinsasser, O.,** Mikrolaryngoskopie und endolaryngeale Mikrochirurgie. II. Rückblick auf 2500 Fälle, *HNO,* 22, 69, 1974.
5. **Michaels, L.,** Laboratory diagnosis of laryngeal disease, *Laryngoscope,* 85, 1689, 1975.
6. **Crissman, J. D.,** Laryngeal keratosis and subsequent carcinoma, *Head Neck Surg.,* 1, 386, 1979.
7. **Steiner, W.,** Krebsfrüherkennung in Mund, Rachen und Kehlkopf. Ergebnisse des Erlanger Vorsorgetests, *Dtsch. Ärztebl-Ärtzl. Mitt.,* 73, 3159, 1976.
8. **Auerbach, O., Hammond, E. C., and Garfinkel, L.** Histologic changes in the larynx in relation to smoking habits, *Cancer,* 25, 92, 1970.
9. **Lundgren, J., Olofsson J., Hellquist, H. B., and Strandh, J.,** Exfoliative cytology in laryngology: comparison of cytologic and histologic diagnoses in 350 microlaryngoscopic examinations — a prospective study, *Cancer,* 47, 1336, 1981.
10. **Lundgren, J., Olofsson, J., Hellquist, H., and Strandh, J.,** The role of smear cytology in laryngeal diagnosis, *J. Otolaryngol.,* 11, 371, 1982.
11. **Schiller, W.,** Zur klinischen Frühdiagnose des Portiokarzinoms, *Zentralbl. Gynaekol.,* 30, 1886, 1928.
12. **Caspersson, T. and Santesson, L.,** Studies on protein metabolism in the cells of epithelial tumors, *Acta Radiol.,* 46(Suppl.), 17, 82, 1942.
13. **Strong, M. S., Vaughan, C. W., and Incze, J. S.,** Toluidine blue in the management of carcinoma of the oral cavity, *Arch. Otolaryngol.,* 87, 527, 1968.
14. **Sigurdson, Å. and Willén, R.,** Toluidine blue in diagnosing malignancy of the epithelial mucosa, *Swed. Dent. J.,* 68, 117, 1975.
15. **Richart, R. M.,** A clinical staining test for the in vivo delineation of dyplasia and carcinoma *in situ, Am. J. Obstet. Gynecol.,* 86, 703, 1963.
16. **Niebel, H. H. and Chomet, B.,** In vivo staining test for delineation of oral intraepithelial neoplastic change: preliminary report, *J. Am. Dent. Assoc.,* 68, 801, 1964.
17. **Shedd, D. P., Hukill, P. B., and Bahn, S.,** In vivo staining properties of oral cancer, *Am. J. Surg.,* 110, 631, 1965.
18. **Myers, E. N.,** The toluidine blue test in lesions of the oral cavity, *CA.,* 20, 134, 1970.
19. **Iwano, T., Yanagizawa, T., and Iwayanagi, T.,** An in vivo staining test using toluidine blue for oral cytodiagnosis, *Shikwa Gaku,* 65, 66, 1965.
20. **Tarkkanen, J., Paavolainen, M., and Saksela, E.,** Toluidine blue staining in the endoscopic diagnosis of carcinoma of the bronchus, *Ann. Clin. Res.,* 4, 7, 1972.
21. **Wang, G-Q.,** Endoscopic diagnosis of early oesophageal carcinoma, *J. R. Soc. Med.,* 74, 502, 1981.
22. **Koburg, E. and Steinbach, E.,** Toluidinblau-Vitalfärbung zur Früherkennung und Abgrenzung maligner Kehlkopftumoren, *Arch. Klin. Exp. Ohr. Nas. Kehlkopfheilkd.,* 194, 320, 1969.
23. **Strong, M. S., Vaughan, C. W., and Incze, J.,** Toluidine blue in diagnosis of cancer of the larynx, *Arch. Otolaryngol.,* 91, 515, 1970.
24. **Lundgren, J., Olofsson, J., and Hellquist, H.,** Toluidine blue. An aid in the microlaryngoscopic diagnosis of glottic lesions?, *Arch. Otolaryngol.,* 105, 169, 1979.
25. **Miller, A. H. and Batsakis, J. G.,** Premalignant laryngeal lesions, carcinoma *in situ,* superficial carcinoma-definition and management, *Can. J. Otolaryngol.,* 3, 515, 1974.
26. Centennial conference on laryngeal cancer, Workshop No 2, Premalignant laryngeal lesions, carcinoma in situ, superficial carcinoma-definition and management, Miller, A. H. and Batsakis, J. G., chairmen, *Can. J. Otolaryngol,* 3, 515, 1974.
27. **Kleinsasser, O.,** Die Klassifikation und Differentialdiagnose der Epithelhyperplasien der Kehlkopfschleimhaut auf Grund histomorphologischer Merkmale. II. Mitteilung, *Z. Laryngol. Rhinol. Otol.,* 42, 339, 1963.
28. **Delemarre, J. F. M.,** De Betekenis van de Plaveiselcellige Hyperplasie van het Larynxepitheel, Academisch Proefschrift, Amsterdam, 1970.
29. **Lubsen, H.,** De Plaveiselcellige Hyperplasie van de Larynx en het Papilloma Inversum van de Neus en de Neusbijholten, Academish Proefschrift, Amsterdam, 1980.
30. **Kleinsasser, O.,** Über den Krankheitsverlauf bei Epithelhyperplasien der Kehlkopfschleimhaut und die Enstehung von Karzinomen. IV. Mitteilung, *Z. Laryngol. Rhinol. Otol.,* 42, 541, 1963.
31. **Fechner, R. E.,** Laryngeal keratosis and atypia, *Can. J. Otolaryngol.,* 3, 516, 1974.

32. **Batsakis, J. G.,** ''Leukoplakia'', ''keratosis'' and intraepithelial squamous cell carcinoma of the head and neck, in *Tumors of the Head and Neck. Clinical and Pathological Considerations,* 2nd ed., Williams & Wilkins, Baltimore, 1979, 121.
33. **Gröntoft, O., Hellquist, H., Olofsson, J., and Nordström, G.,** The DNA content and nuclear size in normal, dysplastic, and carcinomatous laryngeal epithelium. A spectrophotometric study, *Acta Otolaryngol.,* 86, 473, 1978.
34. **Hellquist, H., Olofsson, J., and Gröntoft, O.,** Carcinoma *in situ* and severe dysplasia of the vocal cords. A clinicopathological and photometric investigation, *Acta Otolaryngol.,* 92, 543, 1981.
35. **Fisher, H. R. and Miller, A. H.,** Carcinoma *in situ* of the larynx: a ten year study of its histopathological classification, prognosis and treatment, *Ann. Otol.,* 67, 695, 1958.
36. **Elman, A. J., Goodman, M., Wang, C. C., Pilch, B., and Busse, J.,** In situ carcinoma of the vocal cords, *Cancer,* 43, 2422, 1979.
37. **Hellquist, H., Lundgren, J., and Olofsson, J.,** Hyperplasia, keratosis, dysplasia and carcinoma *in situ* of the vocal cords — a follow-up study, *Clin. Otolaryngol.,* 7, 11, 1982.
38. UICC (Union Internationale Contre le Cancer), *TNM Classification of Malignant Tumors,* 3rd ed., Geneva, 1982.
39. **Scheier, M.,** Weitere Mitteilungen über die Anwendung der Röntgenstrahlen in der Rhino- und Laryngologie, *Fortschr. Röntgenstr.,* 1, 59, 1899.
40. **Scheier, M.,** Über die Ossification des Kehlkopfs, *Arch. Mikr. Anat.,* 59, 220, 1901.
41. **Thost, A.,** Der normale und kranke Kehlkopf des Lebenden im Röntgenbild. (Archiv und Atlas der normalen und pathologischen Anatomie in typischen Röntgenbildern.), *Fortschr. Röntgenstr.,* Ergänzungsband 31, 1913.
42. **Coutard, H.,** Note préliminaire sur la radiographie du larynx normal et du larynx cancéreux, *J. Belge. Radiol.,* 13, 287, 1924.
43. **Baclesse, F.,** Carcinoma of the larynx. Radiotherapy of laryngeal cancer. Clinical, radiological and therapeutic study. Follow-up of 341 cases treated at the Fondation Curie, from 1919 to 1940, *Br. J. Radiol. Suppl.,* 3, 1, 1949.
44. **Baclesse, F.,** *Tumeurs Malignes du Pharynx et du Larynx,* (Étude anatomo-topographique et radiographique), 2nd ed.,Masson Cie, Paris, 190, 664, 1960.
45. **Maguire, G. H.,** The larynx: simplified radiological examination using heavy filtration and high voltage, *Radiology,* 87, 102, 1966.
46. **Hemmingsson, A.,** Roentgenologic methods in examination of the larynx. Comparative phantom investigations in the frontal projections. *Acta Radiol. Diagn.,* 12, 673, 1972.
47. **Gunsett, A.,** Uber die Anwendungsmöglichkeit der Planigraphie bei Erkrankungen des Kehlkopfinneren, insbesondere beim Karzinom des Endolarynx, *Fortschr. Röntgenstr.,* 56, 705, 1937.
48. **Leborgne, F.,** Tomographic study of cancer of the larynx, *Am. J. Roentgenol.,* 43, 493, 1940.
49. **Samuel, E.,** Xerography or conventional radiography for laryngeal examination?, *Can. J. Otolaryngol.,* 4, 59, 1975.
50. **Iglauer, S.,** Use of injected iodized oil in roentgen-ray diagnosis of laryngeal, tracheal and bronchopulmonary conditions, *JAMA,* 86, 1879, 1926.
51. **Powers, W. E., McGee, H. H., and Seaman, W. B.,** Contrast examination of the larynx and pharynx, *Radiology,* 68,169,1957.
52. **Powers, W. E., Holtz, S., Ogura, J., Ellis, B. L., and McGavran, M. H.,** Contrast examination of the larynx and pharynx. Accuracy and value in diagnosis, *Am. J. Roentgenol.,* 86, 651, 1961.
53. **Powers, W. E., Holtz, S., and Ogura, J.,** Contrast examination of the larynx and pharynx. Inspiratory phonation, *Am. J. Roentgenol.,* 92, 40, 1964.
54. **Landman, G. H. M.,** *Laryngography and Cinelaryngography,* Excerpta Medica, Amsterdam, 1970.
55. **Nathan, M. D., Sagel, S. S., Gall, A. M., Griffith, R. C., and Ogura, J. H.,** Diagnostic accuracy of xeroradiographic assessment of extent of carcinoma of the larynx, *Trans. Am. Acad. Ophtalmol. Otolaryngol.,* 84, 609, 1977.
56. **Di Guglielmo, L. and Cherubino, M.,** Laringe, in *La Xeroradiografia in Otorinolaringoiatria,* 32 Raduno gruppo alta Italia (Pavia, 29 novembre 1975), Di Guglielmo, L. and Cherubino, M., Eds., Società italiana di otorinolaringologia e patologia cervico-faciale, Pavia, 1975, 23.
57. **Hemmingsson, A. and Löfroth, P. O.,** Xeroradiography and conventional radiography in examination of the larynx, *Acta Radiol. Diagn.,* 17, 723, 1976.
58. **Olofsson, J. and van Nostrand, A. W. P.,** Growth and spread of laryngeal and hypopharyngeal carcinoma with reflections on the effect of preoperative irradiation. 139 cases studied by whole organ serial sectioning, *Acta Otolaryngol. Suppl.* 308, 1, 1973.
59. **Olofsson, J., Lord, I. J., and van Nostrand, A. W. P.,** Vocal cord fixation in laryngeal carcinoma, *Acta Otolaryngol.,* 75, 496, 1973.

60. **Olofsson, J. and Sökjer, H.,** Radiology and laryngoscopy for the diagnosis of laryngeal carcinoma, *Acta Radiol. Diagn.*, 18, 449, 1977.
61. **Olofsson, J. and Sökjer, H.,** Radiologic assessment of laryngeal carcinoma. A clinico-pathologic comparison based on whole-organ serial sections, *Acta Radiol. Diagn.*, 20, 789, 1979.
62. **van Nostrand, A. W. P.,** Classification, anatomy, growth and spread of laryngeal cancer, *Can. J. Otolaryngol.*, 3, 408, 1974.
63. **Olofsson, J.,** Specific features of laryngeal carcinoma involving the anterior commissure and the subglottic region, *Can. J. Otolaryngol.*, 4, 618, 1975.
64. **Archer, C. R., Yeager, V. L., Friedman, W. H., and Katsantonis, G. P.,** Computed tomography of the larynx, *J. Comp. Assist. Tomogr.*, 2, 404, 1978.
65. **Mancuso, A. A., Calcaterra, T. C., and Hanafee, W. N.,** Computed tomography of the larynx, *Rad. Clin. N. Am.*, 16, 195, 1978.
66. **Gregor, R. T., Lloyd, G. A. S., and Michaels, L.,** Computed tomography of the larynx: a clinical and pathologic study, *Head Neck Surg.*, 3, 284, 1981.
67. **Sökjer, H. and Olofsson, J.,** Computed tomography in carcinoma of the larynx and piriform sinus, *Clin. Otolaryngol.*, 6, 335, 1981.
68. **Wagenfeld, D. J. H., Harwood, A. R., Bryce, D. P., van Nostrand, A. W. P., and de Boer, G.,** Second primary respiratory tract malignancies in glottic carcinoma, *Cancer*, 46, 1883, 1980.
69. **Wagenfeld, D. J. H., Harwood, A. R., Bryce, D. P., van Nostrand, A. W. P., and de Boer, G.,** Second primary respiratory tract malignant neoplasm in supraglottic carcinoma, *Arch. Otolaryngol.*, 107, 135, 1981.
70. **Lundgren. J. and Olofsson, J.,** Multiple primary malignancies in laryngeal carinoma, *4th World Congr. Bronchoesophagol. Abst.*, 1983, 56.
71. **Ferlito, A.,** Double primary synchronous and metachronous cancer of the larynx and hypopharynx with dissimilar histology. Five case reports and review of the literature, *Arch. Otorhinolaryngol.*, 229, 107, 1980.
72. **Gluckman, J. L., Crissman, J. D., and Donegan, J. O.,** Multicentric squamous-cell carcinoma of the upper aerodigestive tract, *Head Neck Surg.*, 3, 90, 1980.
73. **McGuirt, W. F., Matthews, B., and Koufman, J. A.,** Multiple simultaneous tumors in patients with head and neck cancer. A prospective, sequential panendoscopic study, *Cancer*, 50, 1195, 1982.
74. **Incze, J., Vaughan, C. W., Lui, P., Strong, M. S., and Kulapaditharom, B.,** Premalignant changes in normal appearing epithelium in patients with squamous cell carcinoma of the upper aerodigestive tract, *Am. J. Surg.*, 144, 401, 1982.
75. **Atkinson, D., Fleming, S., and Weaver, A.,** Triple endoscopy. A valuable procedure in head and neck surgery, *Am. J. Surg.*, 144, 416, 1982.
76. **Rudin, R. and Sandberg, N.,** Ökad recidivfrekvens hos rökare med larynxcancer, *Med. Riksstämma*, 1972, 372.
77. **Baker, D. C. and Weissman, B.,** Postirradiation carcinoma of the larynx, *Ann. Otol.*, 80, 634, 1971.
78. **Glanz, H.,** Late recurrence or radiation induced cancer of the larynx, *Clin. Otolaryngol.*, 1, 123, 1976.
79. **Aanesen, J. P. and Olofsson, J.,** Irradiation-induced tumours of the head and neck, *Acta Otolaryngol.*, Suppl. 360, 178, 1979.
80. **Bryce, D. P.,** The management of laryngeal cancer, *J. Otolaryngol.*, 8, 105, 1979.

Chapter 7

THE RADIOLOGIC DIAGNOSIS OF CANCER OF THE LARYNX

Hannibal Sökjer

TABLE OF CONTENTS

I. INTRODUCTION

The role of radiology in the diagnosis of laryngeal carcinoma has changed during the last few years; the detailed information supplied by microlaryngoscopy has reduced the importance of radiology, and it has even been questioned whether radiological examination is at all necessary in small laryngeal tumors.[1] On the other hand, therapy has become more differentiated, with an increasing interest in the partial laryngeal surgery with preservation of the voice and the airway, which in turn requires detailed mapping of the tumor spread. According to the rules laid down by the UICC,[2] a radiological examination is necessary for the classification of laryngeal carcinoma.

The surface extension of laryngeal carcinoma is well mapped by a combination of endoscopic and radiological examinations. The deep infiltration by the tumor, however, is often underestimated by such a combination. Computed tomography (CT) has greatly improved the possibilities of diagnosing deep infiltration. CT has also meant an improvement in the planning of radiotherapy.

The purpose of this chapter is to describe the different radiological procedures with their advantages and drawbacks. This description may serve as a basis for deciding the appropriate examination method for the individual patient.

For optimal use of the diagnostic resources, close cooperation between the laryngologist and the radiologist is necessary. Both have to be aware of the advantages and shortcomings of the different methods of examination. For each patient it is necessary to consider what kind of treatment is conceivable — radiotherapy only, a combination of radiotherapy and surgery in the form of partial or total laryngectomy, or primary surgery — and what kind of information is important to be able to make this choice.

A tentative diagnosis of laryngeal carcinoma is usually made at mirror laryngoscopy. To avoid disturbing edema, the radiological examinations should be performed before direct laryngoscopy and biopsy. The purpose of the radiological examination is to determine the superficial and deep spread of the tumor.

A radiological examination cannot be used to rule out carcinoma of the larynx. For this purpose laryngoscopy and biopsy should be relied on.

Lateral *plain films* were being used already at the turn of the century to visualize ossified parts of the laryngeal cartilages,[3,4] and a little later by Thost[5] to examine pathologic alterations of the larynx. Coutard[6] considered that such a radiographic examination could be of value for deciding the mode of treatment in laryngeal carcinoma. Important advances in lateral projection technique applied to the diagnosis of laryngeal carcinoma have been made by Baclesse.[7,8]

With the improvement of radiologic equipment in the 1930s, frontal projections were made possible. By means of a special technique — postero-anterior beam direction, short focus-to-film and object-to-film distances — informative frontal films could be obtained despite overshadowing by the cervical spine.[9]

A further reduction of the interference due to overprojection is obtained with a high-voltage technique using heavy filtration.[10] The merits of this method have been demonstrated by Hemmingsson.[11]

Tomography, which also reduces disturbances due to skeletal structures, has been used by Gunsett[12] and Leborgne,[13] and is probably the most commonly applied method for the radiographic examination of the larynx. Linear tomography is usually recommended because it requires the shortest exposure time.[11,14] A tomographic angle of between 20 and 44° would seem to be large enough,[15] but an angle of 55° or more has been recommended.[16]

Laryngography with a positive contrast medium was used in man for the first time by Iglauer,[17] and it has also been described by Jackson[18] and Lindgren.[9] Improved by Powers and associates,[19-21] who demonstrated its value, the method is now widely adopted. Landman[22] has presented a monography on the application of laryngography and cinélaryngography.

Xeroradiography, which can be combined with tomography, is used in some centers for examining the laryngeal soft tissues.[14,23,24] A high radiation dose is necessary, and the method has no advantages over laryngography.[25] In xeroradiography the ossified parts of the laryngeal cartilages are well visualized, and any tumor invasion can be judged, although there is a risk of misinterpretation.[26]

Computed tomography — The first reports of the use of CT in carcinoma of the larynx were published in 1977.[27] Because of the possibility that the method furnishes of visualization in the transverse plane and of demonstrating differences in soft tissue attenuation, it enables a more detailed mapping of laryngeal carcinoma to be made than the usual methods have permitted. In particular, CT adds information on deep infiltration, cartilage invasion, and spread outside the larynx.[28-30] It has been suggested that CT should be the radiological method of choice if any additional information is sought after microlaryngoscopy.[30-32] Others have found CT to be complementary to other radiological methods.[33,34]

Angiography performed with selective contrast injection into the superior thyroid artery has been used in laryngeal carcinoma in an attempt to detect deep tumor infiltration.[35] The technique is complicated, general anaesthesia is necessary, and the examination is less informative than CT.

II. EXAMINATION TECHNIQUE

To allow both a functional and morphological examination, the larynx should be examined during functional conditions. Exposures are usually made during quiet respiration, expiratory phonation, inspiratory phonation, the Valsalva maneuver (blowing against pursed lips), and straining against a closed glottis.

It is important to instruct the patient and to train him in these maneuvers before starting the examination.

A. Plain Film Examination

The patient should be in the upright position. Fluoroscopy is used to check that the patient performs the different maneuvers correctly. At the same time, the mobility of the cords may be checked. The position of the patient is adjusted so as to make the incident beam parallel to the vocal cords (Figure 1*). Anteroposterior (or p.a.) and lateral exposures are made at the end of a quiet inspiration, during expiratory phonation, during a Valsalva maneuver, and during inspiratory phonation. In the lateral projection the last maneuver is omitted and replaced by an exposure at 55 kV to show the ossified parts of the larynx (Figure 2) if xeroradiography is not used. The other exposures are made with a high-voltage technique (150 kV) together with a brass filter.[36]

B. Tomography

The patient is placed supine with his neck extended. Linear tomography is recommended, because it requires the shortest exposure time.[11,14] An exposure angle of around 30° should be used. Complex motion tomography gives better resolution, but the image is often deranged by movement of the larynx in patients with laryngeal carcinoma, especially if the airway is compromised.

Exposures should be made during quiet inspiration and expiratory phonation. Even with linear tomography the exposure time is usually too long to give diagnostic films during

* All figures appear at end of text.

inspiratory phonation. Lateral tomography could be replaced by lateral plain films or lateral xeroradiography.

C. Contrast Laryngography

A cooperative patient and good anesthesia are essential requirements for a contrast laryngography of high quality. To avoid hypersecretion, atropin is given as premedication. Sedation should not be used as a routine. Before the examination, the patient should be informed of the procedure and trained to perform the respiratory maneuvers. Fluoroscopy should be used for a check on the patient's performance and on the positioning. Scout films should be taken to check the exposure. These preparations are necessary to be able to carry the examination through as fast as possible once the contrast has been applied.

When we first started to perform laryngography in 1971, we used the method described by Landman.[22] The anesthetic and contrast were applied by a laryngologist using a mirror and a laryngeal cannula. The results were excellent but called for the presence of a laryngologist or a trained radiologist. To make the examination easy to perform and consequently simple to teach, we have tested different methods and now use the following.

Xylocain (4%,6 mℓ) is administered via a de Vilbiss nebulizer during 10 to 15 min. The anesthesia deteriorates if the time is prolonged. At fluoroscopy, a straight or curved 12 Charrière Rüsch-Metra bronchography catheter* is introduced via the nose. The catheter is lubricated with xylocain gel and the tip is place in the larynx, where it usually gets stuck at the anterior commissure. The introduction is facilitated if the patient extends his neck and phonates to open up the larynx. The anesthesia is supplemented by another 2 mℓ of 4% xylocain administered in 0.5-mℓ doses into the larynx through the catheter. The first dose usually elicits coughing. The following doses are given during inspiration and phonation in order to spread the anesthetic over the mucosa.

The total amount of xylocain administered exceeds the recommended maximum dose. It has been shown that the administration of 10 mℓ of 4% xylocain via a nebulizer does not lead to toxic blood concentration.[37] We have not seen any unfavorable effects of this type of anesthesia in around 100 laryngographies.

The patient is now given some 10 mℓ of contrast medium to swallow in order to coat the valleculae and the piriform sinuses. We use aqueous Dionosil® as contrast medium since oily Dionosil is not available in Sweden. Contrast (6 to 8 mℓ) is introduced into the larynx through the catheter. By letting the patient phonate during inspiration and expiration, the contrast is spread over the entire laryngeal mucosa. Some additional contrast may be deposited in the valleculae and the piriform sinuses on removing the catheter. The catheter is removed before any films are taken.

The patient now must not cough, talk, or swallow. Films are taken during the same maneuvers as for a plain film examination. We usually take the films in the following order. Frontal projection: quiet inspiration, phonation, Valsalva. Lateral projection: quiet inspiration, two exposures, phonation, Valsalva. Frontal projection again: inspiratory phonation, quiet inspiration, expiratory phonation. The films taken during inspiratory phonation are taken at the end of the examination as this maneuver sometimes elicits coughing. The last two films are taken as there is usually a thin and even coating of the mucosa at this time (Figure 3). Any pools of contrast have disappeared and small exophytic tumors are seen to better advantage.

The anterior commissure is usually best seen on films taken during quiet inspiration. Only if the cords are fully abducted is it possible to judge the status of the anterior commissure (Figure 4). Insufficient abduction will result in a false impression of tumor engagement

* Willy Rüsch GmbH and Co.KG, D-7050 Waiblingen, West Germany.

(Figure 5). It takes at least two, often more, exposures to make certain that the commissure is properly depicted.

Because of the anesthesia, the patient should not eat or drink for 2 to 3 hr after the procedure. To avoid bronchopneumonia, a physiotherapist should help the patient to drain the bronchial tree from the aspirated contrast medium.

A narrow airway is usually said to be a contraindication for contrast laryngography besides known allergy to iodine or to the anesthetic.

Since 1971 we have performed contrast laryngography in all patients with laryngeal carcinoma, over 250 patients. We have refrained from examining a few patients because of their old age, but never for any other reason. In these patients with a large tumor and a narrow airway, preparations have been made to take care of an acute airway obstruction, which has never occurred. The only complications have been a few cases of bronchopneumonia, which have responded promptly to antibiotics.

These good results may be related to the use of xylocain as anesthetic and aqueous Dionosil® as contrast medium.

D. Computed Tomography

The patient should be in the supine position with his neck extended. He should be instructed to breath quietly and not to swallow during the exposures. A lateral scout view is taken and an attempt is made to tilt the gantry to a plane parallel to the vocal cords. To check that this is the case, the scanning should start at the level of the cords to continue upwards to the hyoid bone and then from the cords downwards to the first tracheal ring (Figure 6).

Any metal tracheostomy cannula should be removed, if possible. Otherwise, the lower scans will not be useful. Intravenous contrast is not used as a routine. It may be of use to separate vessels from other soft tissues of the neck and in the study of tumors with a rich vascular network such as thyroid carcinoma.

The greatest problem in CT is movement artifacts, which are mainly created by interfaces between air and soft tissues (Figure 7). In avoiding movement, the instruction of the patient is one important factor. A short exposure time is another, which conflicts with a wish to obtain thin sections and high resolution. The examination has to be adapted to the individual patient.

We use a Philips Tomoscan 310 scanner. The routine is to examine the larynx with 6-mm thick sections. The scanning time is 4.8 sec. Any area of special interest is rescanned in 3-mm thick sections, with the same scanning time. In patients with a compromised airway, the scanning time could be reduced to 2.8 sec., which reduces the risk of movement artifacts but diminishes the resolution. In some patients with small tumors, the resolution may be increased by using a scanning time of 9.6 sec. In such cases, scanning during both phonation and inspiration may be successful, thus giving a dynamic examination.[32]

The scanning could also be made with the patient holding his breath. This, however, usually means that the cords are adducted, which reduces the possibilities of separating the soft tissues of the larynx from each other. The mobility of the cords may be estimated if the scanning is performed both during respiration and while the patient holds his breath.[37]

The appearances of the normal larynx on CT have been described by several authors[39-42] and are shown in Figure 6.

III. WHICH RADIOLOGICAL EXAMINATION IS THE BEST ONE?

Until the arrival of CT, it was commonly considered that laryngography provided the best possibility of evaluating laryngeal carcinoma.[19,20,22,43] For judging invasion of the cartilage, laryngography should be supplemented with a lateral, low-voltage plain film.[43,44]

Comparison of the diagnostic efficacy of various methods for evaluation of laryngeal carcinoma was done by Thornbury and Latourette, [45] who compared the findings at laryngography and high-voltage plain film examination in 15 patients. They found that laryngography was the more accurate for tumor delineation, but that the two methods were equally reliable in outlining the subglottic extension of the tumors. Hemmingsson [15] compared the reliability of the T-classification of the carcinomas in 35 patients. Using the laryngoscopic findings as a criterion, he found that laryngography enabled a more reliable classification to be obtained than did cinélaryngography, high-voltage plain films, or tomography.

Using gross observations on laryngectomy specimens as the basis, Ogura et al. [46] found that laryngography added important information to that gained by laryngoscopy.

A comparison between the radiographic appearances — a.p. tomography and lateral plain films — and the histologic findings in laryngeal sections was performed by Fletcher et al.[44] They selected nine cases to illustrate the possibilities for direct comparison afforded by whole organ sections and concluded that tomography added important information regarding subglottic tumor spread and the lateral plain films regarding epiglottic and thyroid cartilage invasion by the tumor.

Comparative studies between the efficacy of CT and laryngography have been presented by Mancuso et al.,[28] who conclude that laryngography tends to duplicate the findings at microlaryngoscopy and that CT — if a radiological examination is needed — is the examination of choice for laryngeal carcinoma. This view is supported by Archer et al., [30] who compared laryngography with CT in laryngectomized patients and found more false negative and false positive information at laryngography than at CT. It should be noted, though, that in these studies, patients with small tumors not subjected to operations were not included. Gregor et al. [33] compared CT with a.p. tomography and found the two examinations to be entirely complementary as they depict the larynx in two different planes. This view is supported by Parsons et al. [29]

We have carried out prospective comparative studies on radiography in laryngeal carcinoma since 1971.[47-49] The comparison has encompassed plain films, a.p.tomography, contrast laryngography, and, since 1978, computed tomography.[34] The radiological findings have been compared with those of microlaryngoscopy, palpation, biopsy and, in those patients undergoing laryngectomy, also with the histopathological findings in whole organ serial sections of the specimen. From these studies we have reached the following conclusions. Ordinary radiography gives important information regarding the craniocaudal extent of the tumor, whereas laryngoscopy probably gives the most reliable assessment of antero-posterior extension. Contrast laryngography may supply information not gained at microlaryngoscopy — information that may be important for the correct classification of small tumors. On a low-voltage plain film it may be possible to diagnose cartilage invasion. The surface extension of the tumor is well mapped with a combination of ordinary radiography and microlaryngoscopy. The deep spread, however, is often underestimated, and for mapping deep-extension CT should be used.

To compare the advantages of the different examination methods we may look at their capability of supplying information in different respects important to classification and treatment, such as:

Surface extension in the larynx	Anterior commissure Posterior commissure Laryngeal ventricle Subglottis
Deep infiltration within the larynx	Vocal cord fixation Preepiglottic space Paraglottic space Cartilage invasion
Spread outside the larynx	

A. Surface Extension in the Larynx

Subglottic spread often occurs if the tumor invades the *anterior commissure* and, owing to the close proximity of the mucosa to the thyroid cartilage, this is often invaded by a tumor, involving the anterior commissure. There is also a risk of spread outside the larynx by penetration of the cricothyroid membrane.[50] Invasion of the commissure has to be excluded before a decision is made to do a supraglottic horizontal laryngectomy.

The commissure and the area just below and above are best visualized on lateral laryngograms (Figures 4, 7, and 9). It is also seen at CT (Figures 6 to 9) and, if the tumor extends far subglottically below the commissure, on plain films too.

For correct visualization of the anterior commissure, the laryngograms must be exposed when the vocal cords are completely abducted — usually at the end of a quiet inspiration. If the anterior parts of the cords are abducted, an incorrect representation of the commissure will be obtained, which may lead to misinterpretation[43] For this reason, at least two lateral views should be taken during quiet inspiration in order to confirm a positive finding.

It may be difficult to detect and assess the involvement of the anterior commissure by laryngography.[20,46] In a study of our own[48] on 33 patients undergoing laryngectomy for laryngeal cancer, 17 glottic tumors had spread to the anterior commissure; 6 of these were diagnosed at plain film examination, 13 at contrast laryngography, and 15 at microlaryngoscopy. All 17 were diagnosed by a combination of laryngography and microlaryngoscopy. There was one false positive finding at microlaryngoscopy. These findings thus indicate that a highly reliable evaluation of the anterior commissure can be made at laryngography.

Tumor spread to the anterior commissure may also be diagnosed at CT (Figures 7 to 9).[39] The commissure is, however, only 1 to 2 mm high and the thickness of the CT slices usually exceeds that.[51] Again, the degree of abduction of the vocal cords may influence the appearance and lead to an erroneous conclusion. It is, however, usually possible to separate the two vocal cords from each other even if they are adducted anteriorly.[28,39] Whenever there is question whether the anterior commissure is invaded or not, contrast laryngography should be performed. This may be the case in small glottic tumors and in tumors of the epiglottis.

Tumor invasion of the *posterior commissure* is usually well shown at CT, but is only occasionally possible to diagnose at contrast laryngography.

A new definition of the *subglottic region* was adopted at the Centennial Conference on Laryngeal Carcinoma held in Toronto (1974), according to which it includes the undersurface of the vocal cords. The reason for this modification is that the undersurface of the vocal cords is covered by ciliated columnar epithelium, but the free margin by squamous epithelium. Moreover, the conus elasticus has proven to be an effective barrier to tumor spread. A correct classification may thus require detailed mapping of the undersurface of the cords. This is particularly important in the classification of small glottic tumors (T1 and T2). In these tumors, plain film examination and tomography do not add any information to that gained by microlaryngoscopy.[1] At contrast laryngography, however, the appearance of the mucosa and the lower limit of the tumor is usually clearly mapped (Figures 7 and 9). In these cases the laryngographic findings may change the classification from T1 to T2.[47,48] Minor subglottic spread may not be seen at CT.[29]

Major subglottic spread, with flattening of the subglottic angle, is shown equally well at plain film examination, tomography, and contrast laryngography (Figure 11).[45,48] It is usually seen at CT (Figures 7 and 10).

All radiographic methods may show subglottic spread beneath an intact mucosa, overlooked at endoscopy. There is, however, a risk of diagnosing postirradiation deformity and fibrosis as tumor growth (Figures 12 and 13).[48,52]

The *laryngeal ventricle* is most fully distended and thus best visualized during inspiratory phonation and cannot be reliably judged on the basis of plain films or tomography unless it is air-filled. Positive contrast will most often fill even a compressed ventricle and does give a better opportunity to diagnose any involvement. With all three methods and microlaryngoscopy there is, however, a substantial risk of a false positive diagnosis.[48] With CT, the border between the glottic and supraglottic regions is often not discernible and it may be impossible to tell whether the tumor crosses the ventricle or not.[28,29]

A correct assessment of the ventricle is particularly important to have in the case of supraglottic tumors where horizontal supraglottic laryngectomy is contemplated. In doubtful cases it would thus seem that the definitive evaluation of the ventricle and the choice between total and partial laryngectomy must be made during the course of the operation.

B. Deep Infiltration within the Larynx

CT has meant an improvement in the diagnosis of deep tumor spread. Ordinary radiography and clinical examinations usually indicate deep infiltration only by indirect signs, if at all. Loss of pliability of the epiglottis is one such sign; *vocal cord fixation* is another, often indicating tumor invasion of the laryngeal framework and spread outside the larynx.[53] When a supraglottic tumor obstructs the view, ordinary radiography may be superior to inspection in diagnosing fixation of the cord.[48]

The *paraglottic space* is the space lateral to the cords, above the conus elasticus. Superiorly it has no sharp border towards the preepiglottic space. Laterally it is separated from the thyroid cartilage by a thin layer of loose connective tissue that contains the intrinsic laryngeal vessels. At CT a thin zone of low attenuation has been seen along the inner border of the thyroid cartilage.[27,54,55] Obliteration of this zone has been said to indicate deep tumor invasion with the risk of spread to the cartilage. To our experience, the presence or absence of the zone is to be judged with caution. It may be absent even when the tumor is superficial, and its appearance will probably be different with different CT equipment[32] and is likely to be an artifact created by the image processing in the computer.

At CT, invasion of the paraglottic space is often not possible to diagnose directly as the attenuation of the tumor tissue does not differ sufficiently from that of the normal tissues (Figure 7). Sometimes, however, the tumor may be seen spreading in the paraglottic space and abutting the thyroid cartilage. This implies a risk of invasion, but to be able to diagnose cartilage invasion with certainty, the destruction has to be fairly large as the ossification of the thyroid cartilage may be incomplete and asymmetric (Figures 6 and 8).

If the tumor has spread posteriorly in the larynx, this may be seen as an increased distance between the thyroid wing and the arytenoid cartilage (Figures 10 and 13). This distance does not differ by more than 3 mm between the two sides of the normal larynx. This information is important and not achievable by any other radiological method, and it is seldom discernible at endoscopy. Tumor invasion of the cricoarytenoid joint is usually shown by CT (Figure 10).

When invasion of the *laryngeal cartilages* occurs, it is usually the ossified parts that are involved.[56,57]

The diagnosis of cartilage invasion on low-voltage plain films is said to be difficult because of the erratic ossification of the cartilages. Baclesse[7,8] showed that there is a predictable pattern of ossification, especially in men over 50 years of age, in whom the anterior parts of the thyroid cartilage form a ''figure-of-eight'' on a lateral low-voltage plain film (Figure 2). In the prospective study on 33 laryngectomized patients mentioned before,[48] 23 men had primary glottic carcinoma. Whole organ serial sectioning revealed that 12 of these tumors had invaded the laryngeal framework. In 6 of the 12 patients this invasion was diagnosed on a low-voltage lateral plain film and, to our surprise, there were no false positives. It should be noted, though, that these were all glottic carcinomas, which particularly tend to invade the anterior part of the thyroid cartilage. Supraglottic tumors may sometimes extend down across the anterior commissure, and then a risk of invasion of the anterior part of the thyroid cartilage exists.[58]

Obviously, a negative plain film finding does not rule out the possibility of cartilage invasion. The status of the rest of the laryngeal cartilages cannot usually be judged on plain film because of the erratic ossification.

Computed tomography improves the diagnosis of cartilage invasion.[51] Several factors will influence the accuracy of the diagnosis, such as the thickness of the cuts, the exposure time, movement artifacts, and the extent and symmetry of ossification. The thinner the sections, the smaller need the invasion be to be discernible.[59] Any movement artifacts will deteriorate the possibilities of a correct diagnosis.[59] In the choice between thin sections and long exposure time vs. thick sections and short exposure time, the latter is often the best choice. The dilemma is that the larger the tumor is, the higher is the risk for cartilage invasion, the more compromised is the patient's airway, and the greater is the risk of movement artifacts on CT. Sometimes it is possible to diagnose cartilage invasion only when the tumor has spread outside the larynx. This may be diagnosed if the normal appearances of the extralaryngeal muscles and fascial planes are deranged (Figure 15). In these cases tissue with the same attenuation as the tumor will be seen outside the larynx (Figure 10). The tumor may also cause deformity of the cartilage (Figure 15), which suggests invasion. In the arytenoid cartilages, tumor invasion may result in both osteolysis and osteosclerosis.[60]

The *preepiglottic space* (PES) lends itself excellently to CT examination, as it normally contains fat which has an entirely different attenuation than tumor tissue. Invasion of the PES is thus easily seen at CT (Figure 14).

C. Spread Outside the Larynx

It is usually possible to diagnose oropharyngeal spread at palpation under general anesthesia. As has been said before, the craniocaudal extent of tumor is well assessed by radiological methods, and both oropharyngeal and tracheal spread is well shown on plain films and at laryngography. Oropharyngeal spread is well shown at CT (Figure 15), and postcricoid spread may be diagnosed on a barium swallow.

Computed tomography is indispensible for detecting spread anterior and lateral to the laryngeal framework, through the thyroid or cricoid cartilages, or through the thyrohyoid membrane, which is common in piriform sinus carcinoma, or through the cricothyroid membrane (Figure 16), which is common for carcinomas crossing the anterior commissure. It is impossible to detect tumor spread in these directions by any other means than CT, unless it is visible on plain films or extensive enough to be palpable.

At CT, enlarged nodes of the neck will be detected, whereas metastatic nodes of normal size will not. In piriform sinus carcinoma it may sometimes be impossible to separate the primary tumor from a lymph node metastasis adjacent to the larynx. Sometimes, intravenous contrast may be used to differ nodes from vessels. It is not possible to differ an inflammatory cause of the enlargement from a malignant one.

The neck is readily accessible to palpation. At palpation, the texture of nodes of normal size may indicate malignancy. Palpation, possibly supplemented by fine-needle aspiration biopsy, is usually the best way to diagnose tumor spread to the lymph nodes.[61]

At the level of the hyoid bone the two submandibular glands are seen. They may be asymmetric and should not be mistaken for metastatic nodes.

IV. WHICH EXAMINATION METHOD SHOULD BE CHOSEN IN THE INDIVIDUAL SITUATION?

Patients with small tumors are usually treated with radiotherapy. Careful mapping of the mucosal extent of tumor is important for the classification. Microlaryngoscopy should be supplemented by contrast larygography in patients with T1 or small T2 tumors. The radiological examination may add information concerning the anterior commissure, the subglottis, or the laryngeal ventricle that may change the classification of the tumor.

In patients with large T2 or T3 or T4 tumors, contrast laryngography often offers no advantage over plain film examination, tomography, or xeroradiography. Sometimes, cartilage invasion may be diagnosed on plain films or by xeroradiography. In these patients, details of the mucosal extent are less important than the mapping of deep infiltration. Computed tomography is an excellent tool for this purpose and should be used whenever there seems to be a risk of deep spread and cartilage invasion, such as in the types of tumors mentioned above and in tumors crossing the anterior commissure.

In some patients, the clinical examination and ordinary radiography may reveal such a large tumor that the outcome of a CT will not influence treatment.

In patients with tumors that are possibly amenable to partial laryngectomy, both contrast laryngography and CT should be performed. Both methods may give additional information concerning the anterior commissure. Contrast laryngography may add information on the laryngeal ventricles. Computed tomography adds information regarding the preepiglottic space in supraglottic tumors and concerning the posterior commissure, spread lateral to the arytenoid cartilages, and to the laryngeal cartilages in glottic tumors.

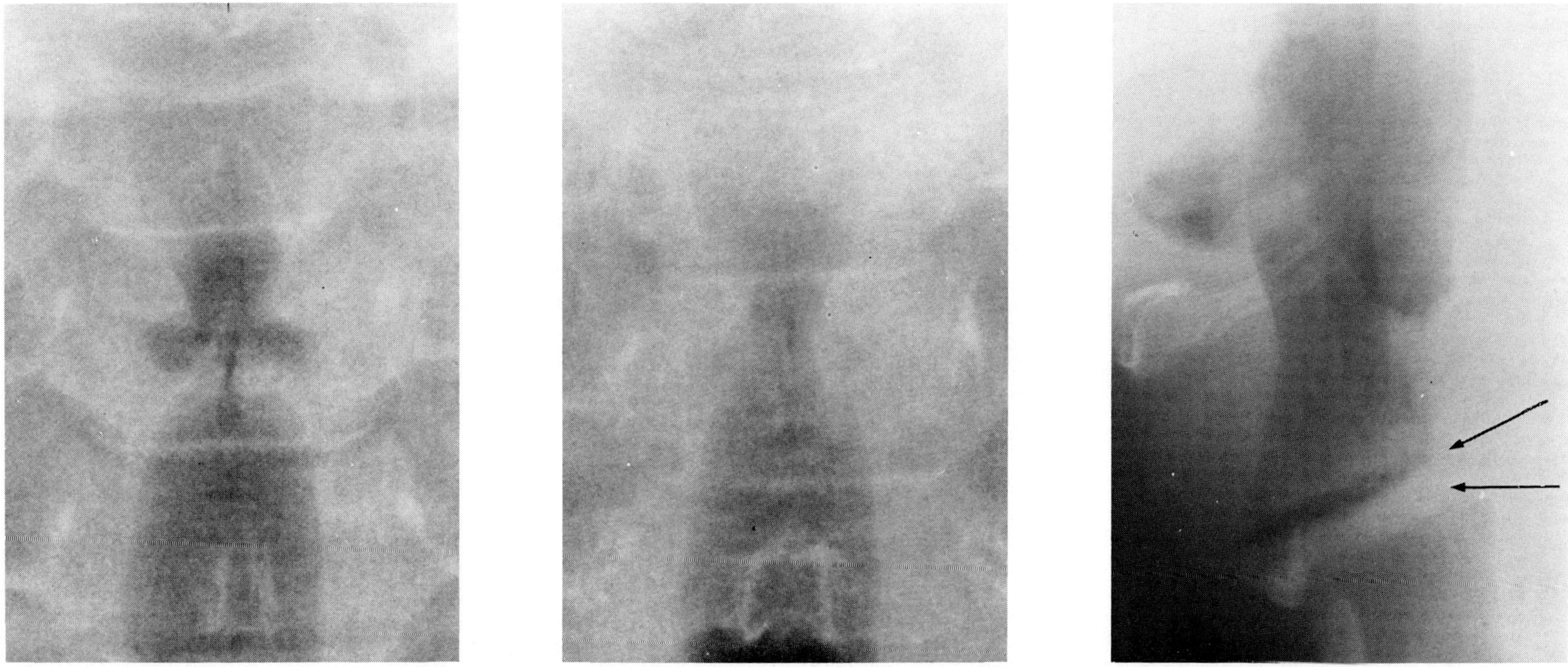

A B C

FIGURE 1. Normal plain films in a 53-year-old man. (A and B) A.p. views; (C) lateral view. Expiratory phonation. Note the difference in the appearance of the cords in (A) and (B), both taken during phonation. The difference is entirely due to the different directions of the incident beams indicated by arrows in (C). The upper arrow indicates the direction of the beam in (B), parallel to the cords, the lower the direction in (A).

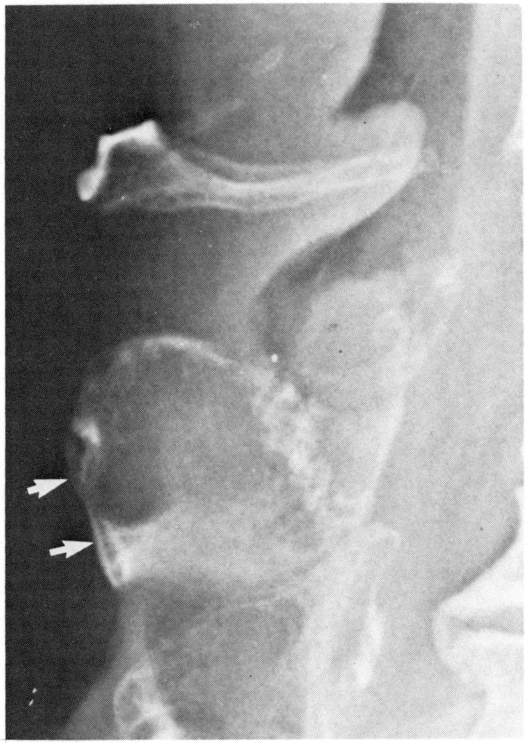

FIGURE 2. Normal larynx in a 57-year-old man. Lateral view. Low-voltage film (55 kV) to show the ossification of the laryngeal cartilages. The ossification is unusually complete in this case. The anterior part of the thyroid cartilage (arrows) is usually ossified in men older than 50 years and forms a figure eight.

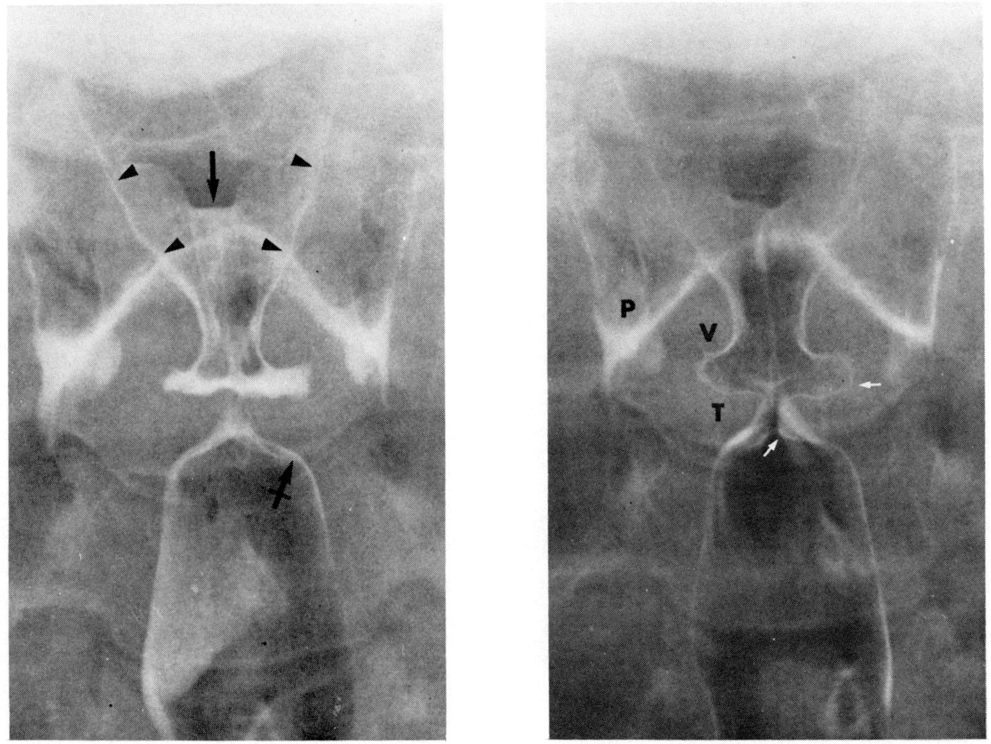

A B

FIGURE 3. Normal contrast laryngography in a 60-year-old man. (A) A. p. view. Expiratory phonation. Arrow indicates interarytenoid notch. Hatched arrow indicates subglottic angle. The arrowheads indicate the lateral wall of the laryngeal vestibule. Note the pooling of contrast in the laryngeal ventricle; (B) a.p. view. Inspiratory phonation. Arrows indicate the upper and lower borders of the glottic region. P = piriform sinus, T = true vocal cord, V = false vocal cord. Note the widening of the laryngeal ventricle and the thin contrast coating of the upper surface of the cords.

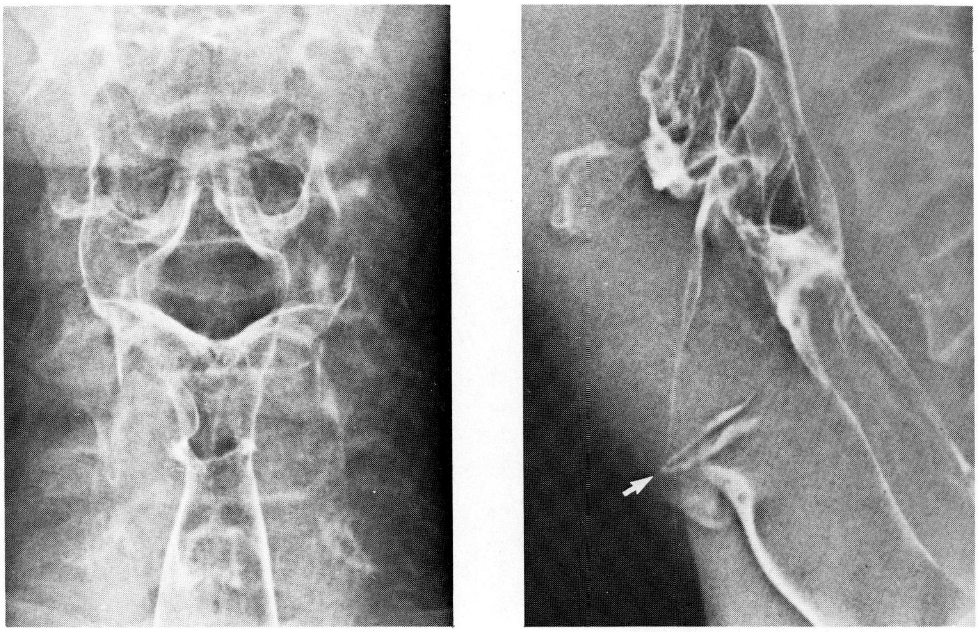

A B

FIGURE 4. Normal contrast laryngography. Quiet inspiration. (A) A.p. view;(B) lateral view. The vocal cords are abducted. The slight bulge of the right true and false vocal cords is probably due to a slightly rotated larynx (A). Arrow indicates the anterior commissure (B). Below the commissure, there is a smooth posterior bulge. The distance between the posterior part of the thyroid cartilage and the laryngeal lumen should not exceed 6 mm.

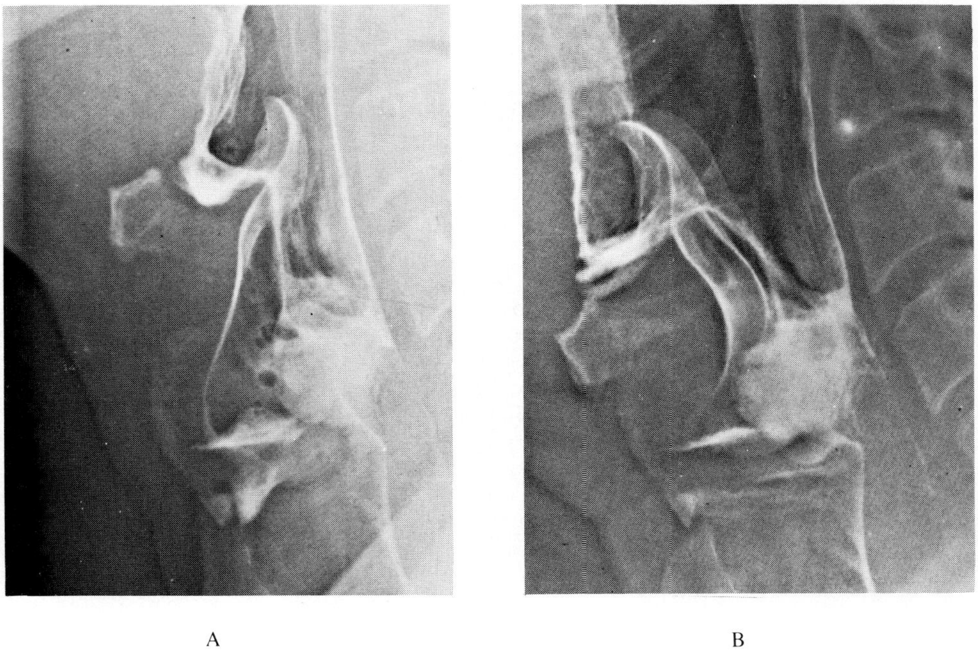

A B

FIGURE 5. Normal contrast laryngography in a 62-year-old man. Lateral views. (A) Quiet inspiration;(B) expiratory phonation. Note the variations in the configuration of the epiglottis. As the vocal cords are not fully abducted in (A), the anterior commissure cannot be evaluated (cf. Figure 1B.) At phonation the hyoid bone approaches the thyroid cartilage.

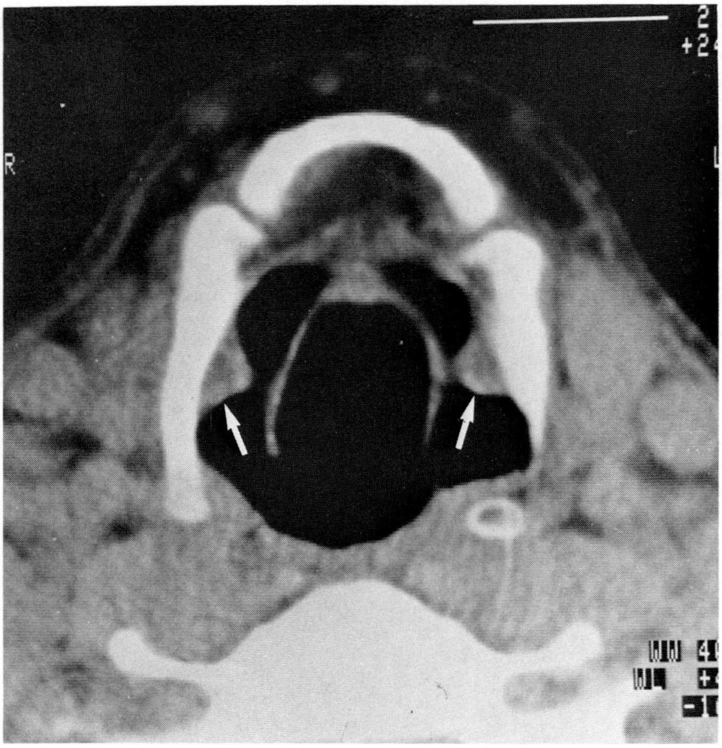

A

FIGURE 6. Computed tomography of normal larynx. Quiet respiration. (A to D) 43 year-old-man; (E) 37 year-old-man. Slice thickens 3 mm, exposure time 4.8 sec. R= right, L = left. (A) Section through the hyoid bone. The posterior part of the left cornu is not completely included in the section. Lateral to the epiglottis, the two lateral glossoepiglottic folds (arrows) separate the piriform sinuses from the valleculae, which are separated from each other by the median glossoepiglottic fold. Part of the tongue base is included anterior to the valleculae; (B) section through the laryngeal vestibule, 20 mm below (A). The thyroid wings are poorly and irregularly ossified. They are separated anteriorly, showing that the section is above the thyroid notch. The aryepiglottic folds (arrows) separate the piriform sinuses from the laryngeal vestibule. There is fat in the preepiglottic space. The tissue of higher attenuation (arrowheads) may represent the body of the epiglottis or be due to artifacts created by the air-tissue interface. Note the marked difference in attenuation of the fat and the extralaryngeal muscles; (C) section through the vocal cords, 15 mm below (B). The slice is not parallel to the true cords. The upper posterior parts of the true cords and the lower anterior parts of the false cords are depicted in this scan. The notch at the free edge marks the transition between the glottic and the supraglottic regions. The soft tissues in the midline anteriorly are thus situated above the anterior commissure. Only the anterior and posterior edges of the thyroid cartilages are ossified. Arrows indicate the arytenoid cartilages; (D) section through the cricoid ring, 22 mm below (E). The cartilage is poorly ossified. Note that the soft tissues inside the cartilage are hardly visible. T = thyroid gland; (E) section through the true cords. At this level the thyroid cartilage is more arched anteriorly. In this man it is completely ossified. Posteriorly it contains fatty bone marrow, which the arytenoid cartilages (A) do too. The left arytenoid is best seen, with the vocal process anteriorly. Arrows indicate the cricoarytenoid joints. The tip of the cricoid signet (C) is irregularly ossified. Note the absence of soft tissues in the anterior and posterior commissures and medial to the arytenoids. The distances between the arytenoids and thyroid cartilages are usually symmetric but may differ by 2 to 3 mm.

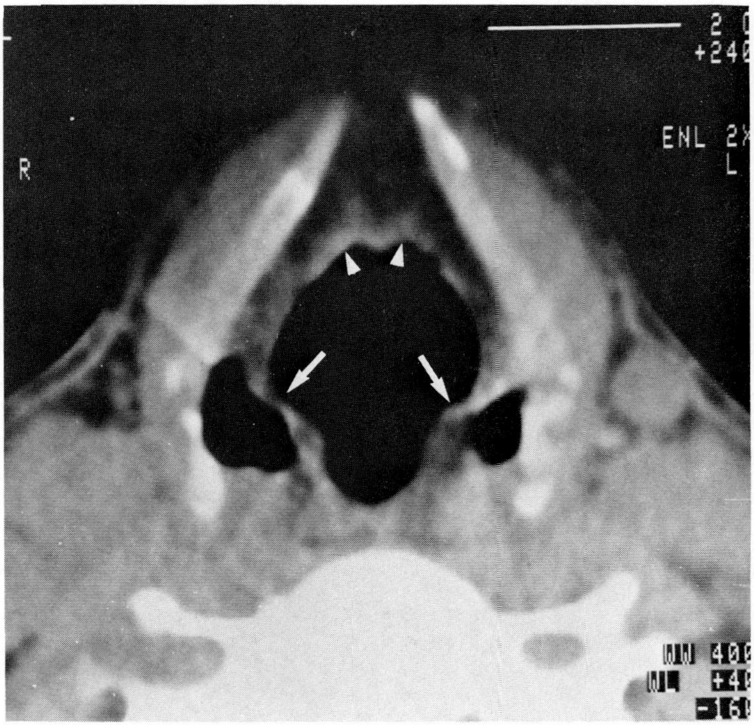

FIGURE 6B

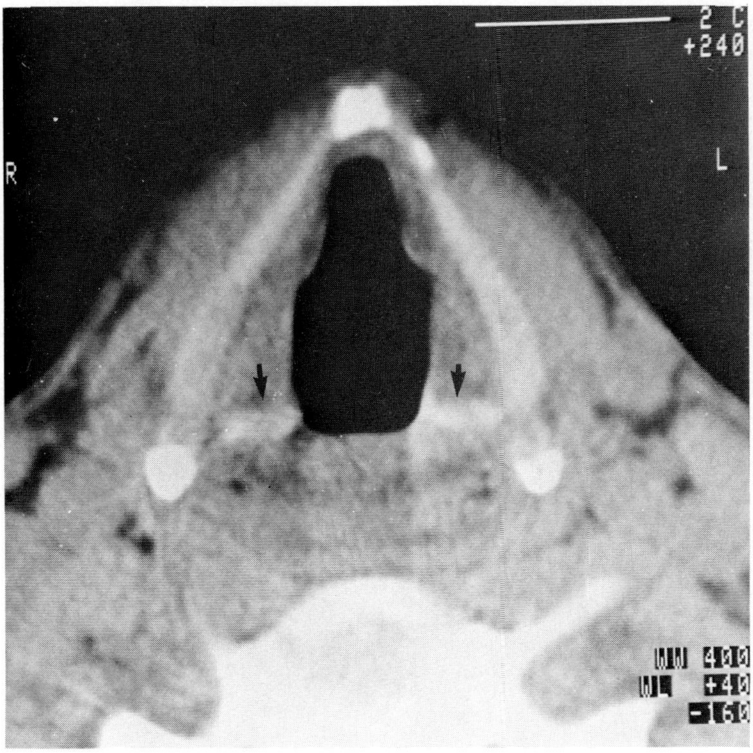

FIGURE 6C

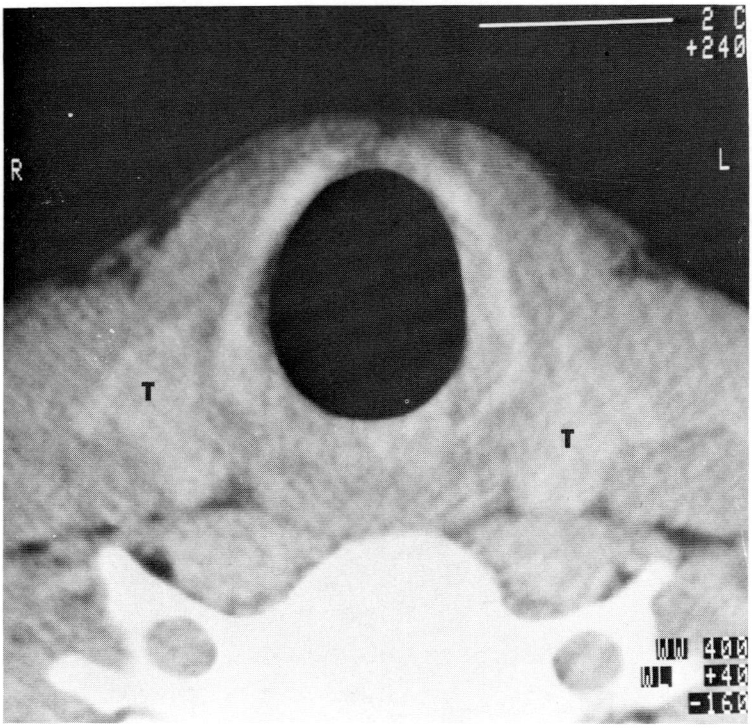

FIGURE 6D

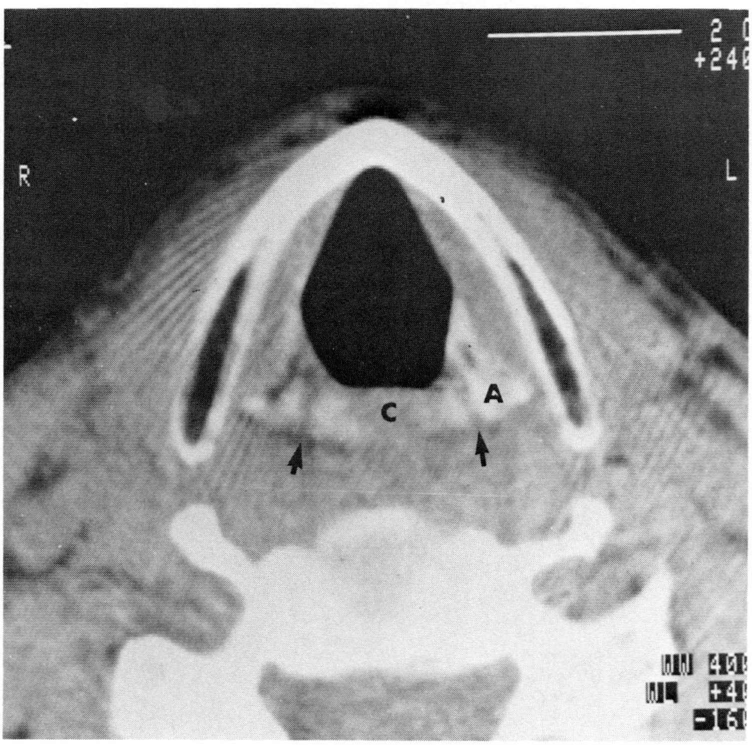

FIGURE 6E

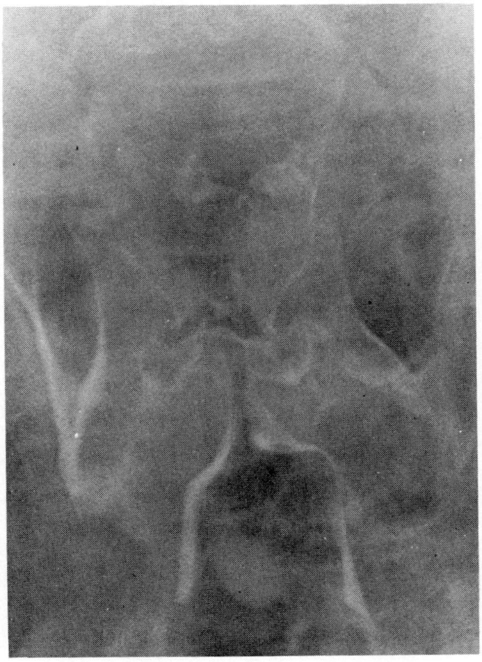

A

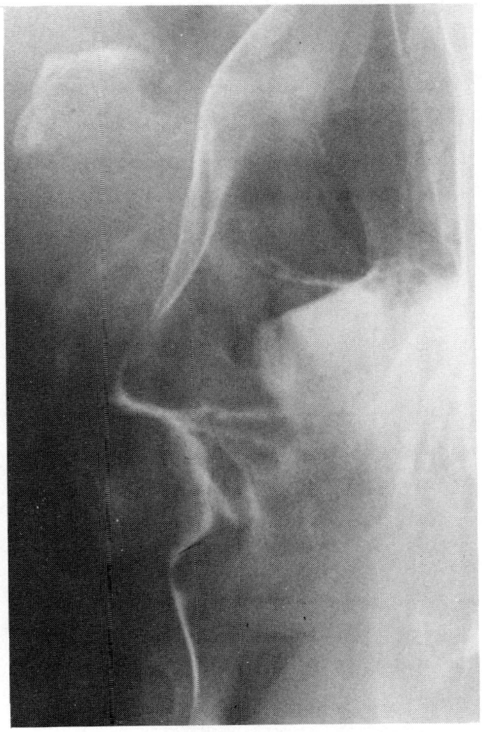

B

FIGURE 7. An 82-year-old man with a right glottic-subglottic carcinoma with spread to the anterior commissure. (A) Laryngography, a.p. view. Expiratory phonation. There is a subglottic tumor extension with flattening of the subglottic angle; (B) laryngography, lateral view. Quiet inspiration. There is tumor in and below the anterior commissure; (C to E) computed tomography. Sections through the vocal cords (C and D) and 3 mm further caudal (E); 3-mm sections, 4.2 sec scanning time. The tumor is seen in (C) and (D) only by the deformation of the free edge of the cord and the increased soft tissues in the anterior commissure. It is not possible to diagnose the tumor by its attenuation, which is entirely different in (C) and (D), probably due to movement artifacts. In (E) there is a slightly increased thickness of the soft tissues anteriorly and below the free margin of the right vocal cord. No evidence of cartilage invasion. Comment: Contrast laryngography gives a good overview of the craniocaudal extent. CT should always be performed in anterior commissure carcinoma to evaluate the laryngeal framework.

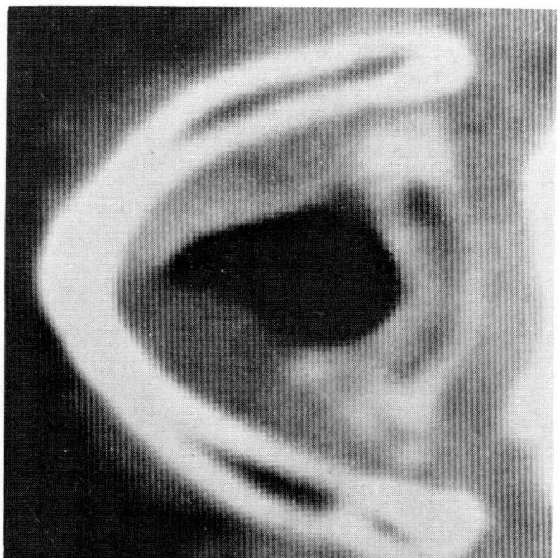

FIGURE 7C

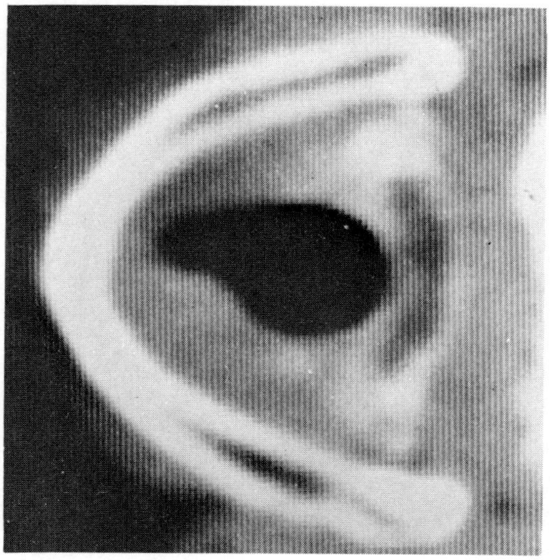

FIGURE 7D

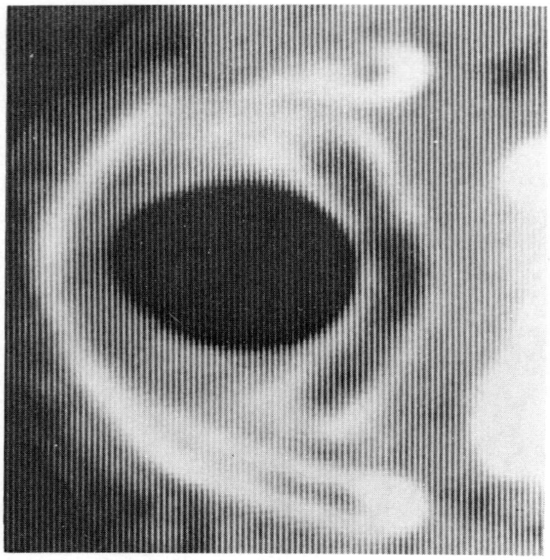

FIGURE 7E

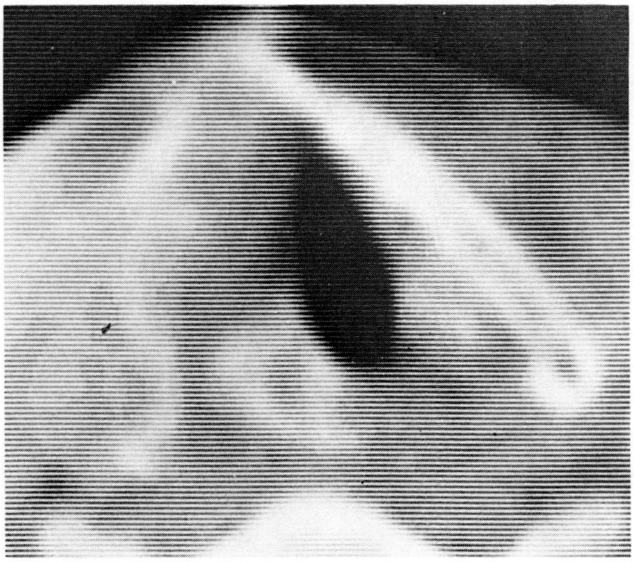

A

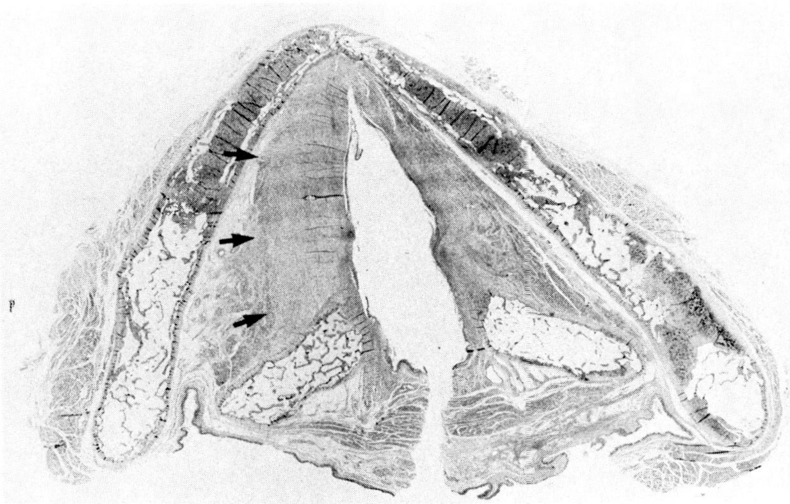

B

FIGURE 8. A 70-year-old man with a glottic-subglottic tumor on the right side with spread to the anterior commissure and with fixation of the vocal cord. (A) Computed tomography; 6-mm section through the vocal cords. The larynx is rotated. There is swelling of the right vocal cord and the anterior commissure. The appearance of the right thyroid wing suggests cartilage invasion; (B) whole organ section at the level of (A). Arrows indicate tumor which invades the thyroarytenoid muscle but not the thyroid cartilage, which is symmetrically ossified. Comment: The asymmetry of the laryngeal framework in (A) was due to tilting of the larynx.

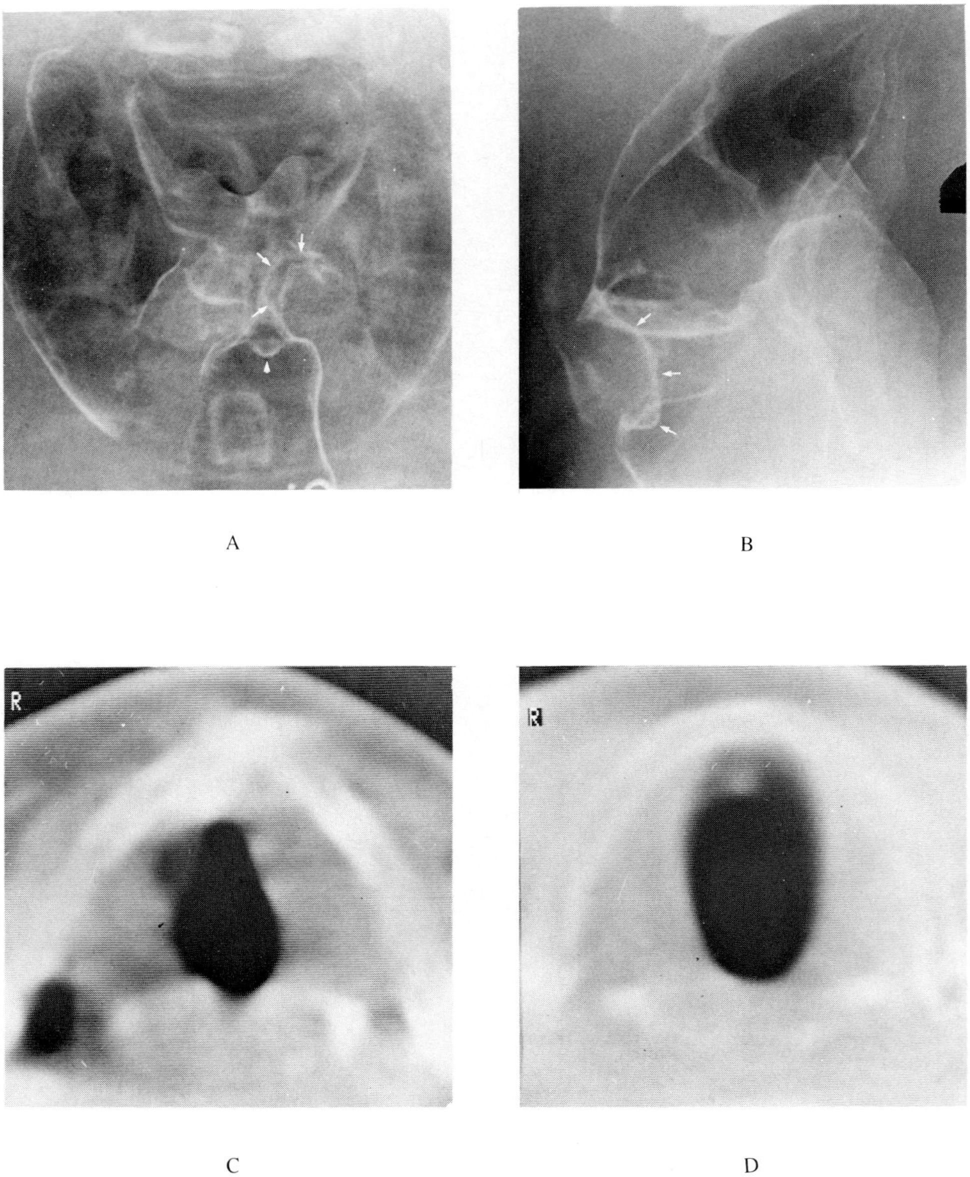

FIGURE 9. Tumor of the left vocal cord and the anterior commissure with extension below the anterior commissure in a 71-year-old man. (A) Laryngography, a.p. view. Arrows indicate the tumor of the left vocal cord. Arrowhead indicates tumor below the anterior commissure. (B) laryngography. Lateral view. Arrows indicate the tumor in and below the anterior commissure. (C) computed tomography; 6-mm section through the vocal cords. There is increased thickness of the left vocal cord and of the soft tissues in the anterior commissure. (D) computed tomography; 6-mm section immediately below (C). Tumor is seen below the anterior commissure. No evidence of cartilage invasion. *Comment:* In this T2 tumor, contrast laryngography gives a good survey of the tumor. CT was performed because of the extensive tumor growth anteriorly. The patient received radiotherapy (64 Gy). He was free from tumor 3 years later, which suggests that there was no cartilage invasion at the time of the CT.

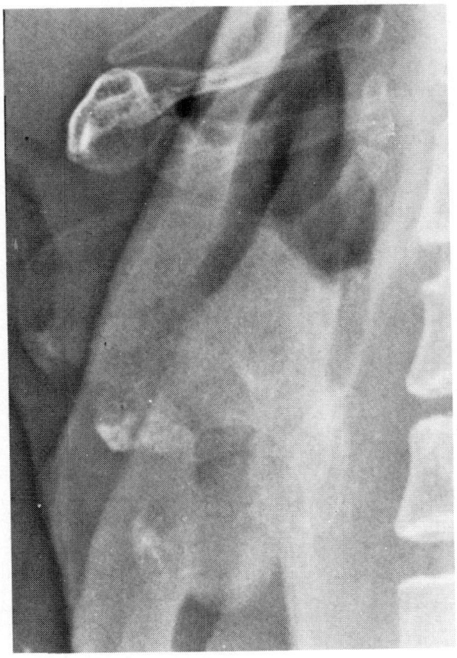

A

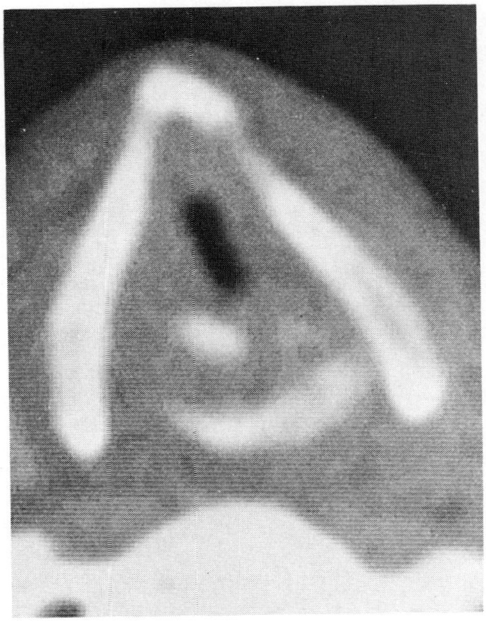

B

FIGURE 10. Glottic tumor with sub- and supraglottic extension on the right side in a 57-year-old man. (A) Plain film, lateral view. Disruption of the normal "figure eight" configuration indicates invasion by the tumor; (B and C) computed tomography; 6-mm sections through the vocal cords (B) and the cricoid ring (C). There is medial and anterior displacement of the right arytenoid and probable destruction of the signet of the cricoid cartilage (B). Subglottic extension of the tumor posteriorly and to the right, with destruction of the cricoid ring and spread outside the larynx (C); (D to F) transverse sections through the lower part of the arytenoid cartilage (A) (D), the vocal cords (E), and the cricoid ring (F). Ulcerated tumor (arrows) of the right hemilarynx, with spread to the anterior part of the thyroid cartilage (T), the thyroarytenoid muscle (E), the interarytenoid muscle (D), the arytenoid cartilage, the cricoid signet to the right, and the cricoarytenoid joint (E). Subglottic extension with destruction of the cricoid ring to the right and spread outside the larynx (F). C = cricoid cartilage. THY = thyroid gland. *Comment:* The invasion of the anterior part of the thyroid cartilage is not well seen in (B) because the section is thick enough to include the lower part of the thyroid cartilage, which is still ossified as can be seen in (A). (From Sökjer, H. and Olofsson, J., *Clin. Otolaryngol.*, 6, 335, 1981. With permission.)

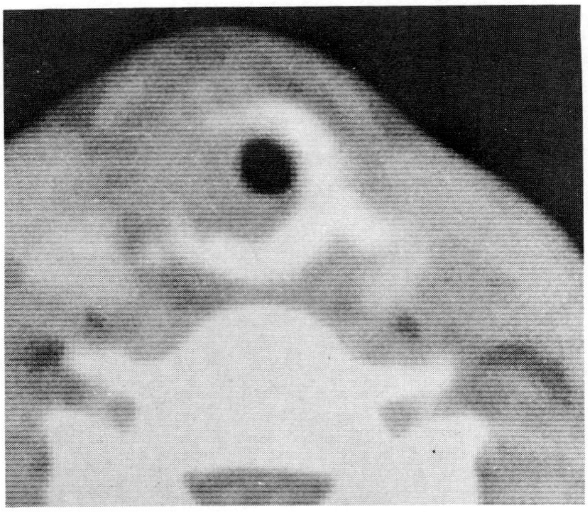

FIGURE 10C

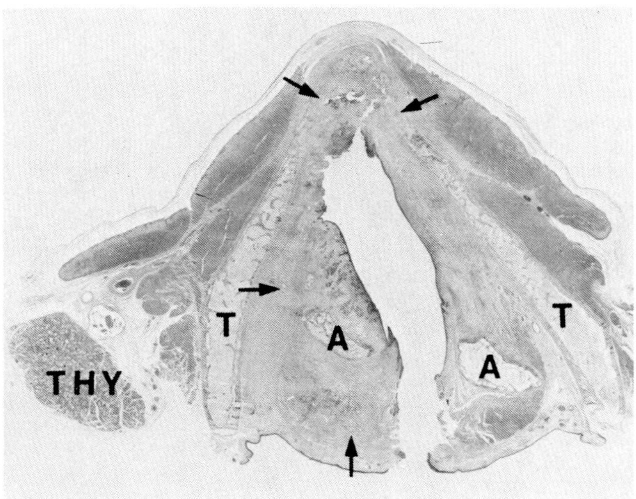

FIGURE 10D

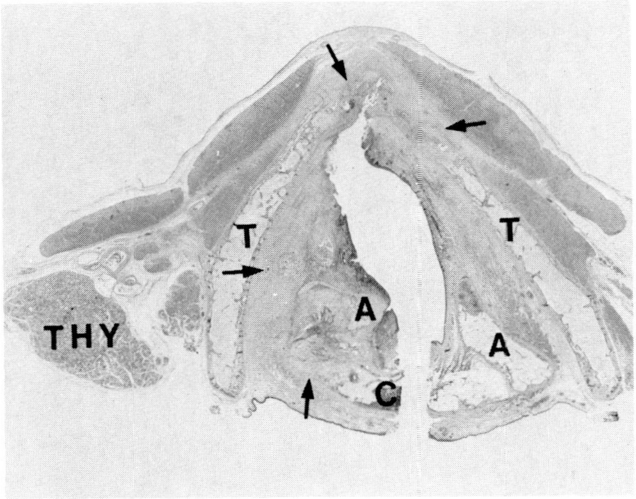

FIGURE 10E

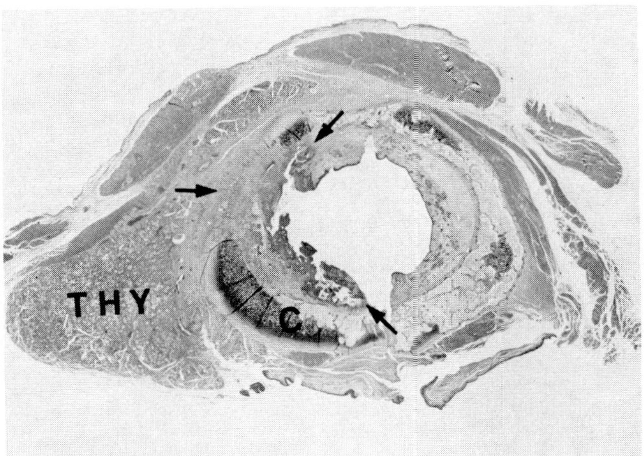

FIGURE 10F

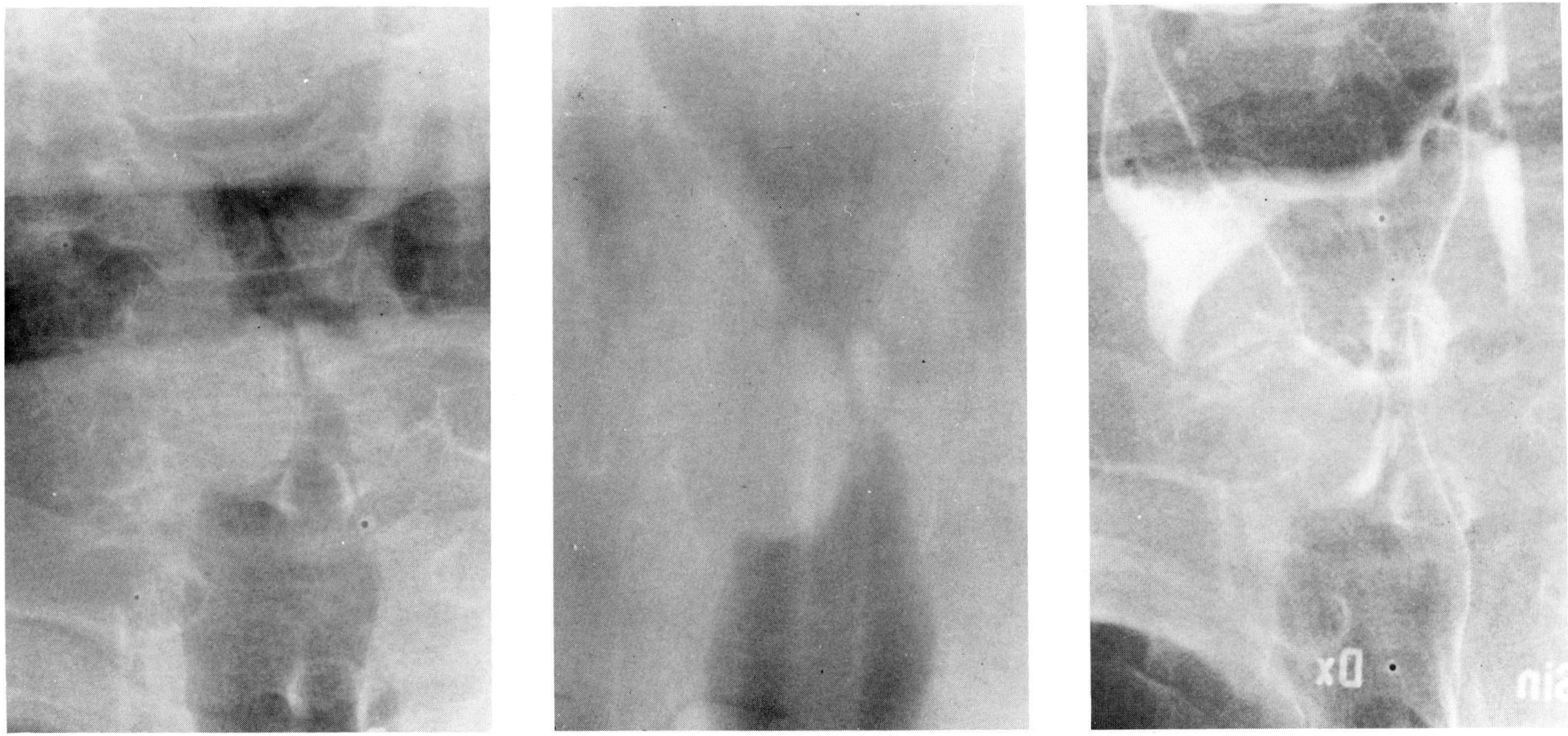

A B C

FIGURE 11. A 55-year-old man with a right glottic tumor with sub- and supraglottic extension and fixation of the cord. CT was not performed. (A) Plain film, a.p. view. Phonation; (B) tomography, a.p. view. Phonation; (C) contrast laryngography. Quiet inspiration. The sub- and supraglottic extension was diagnosed at all three examinations. A laryngectomy was done following preoperative radiotherapy. Whole organ sectioning confirmed the radiological findings. There was also invasion of the cricoid and arytenoid cartilages not diagnosed preoperatively.

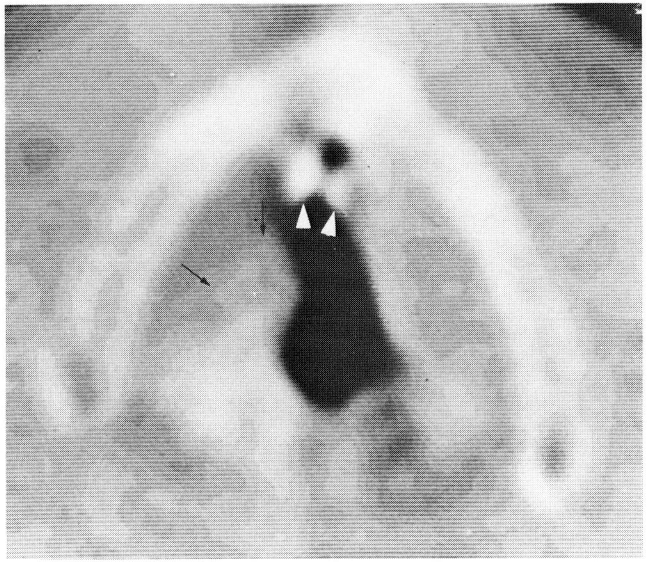

A

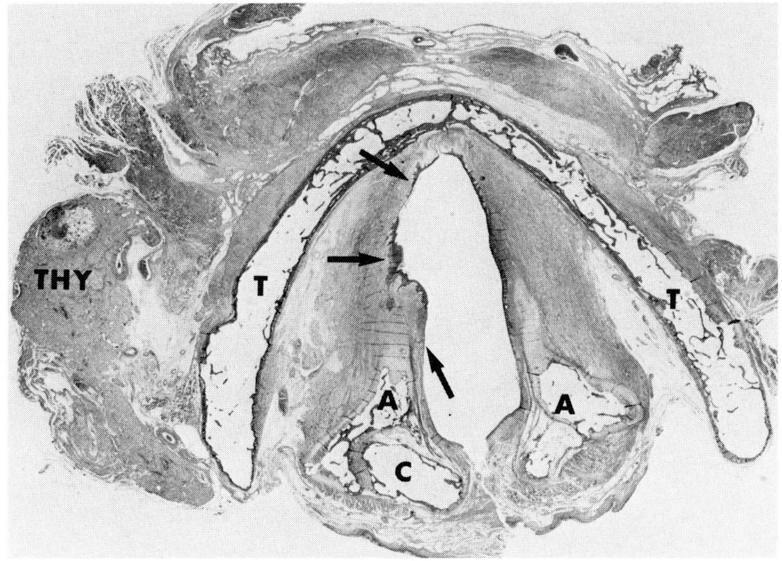

B

FIGURE 12. A 70-year-old man with recurrent tumor following radiotherapy, 1 year earlier for a bilateral glottic tumor (T1B). (A) Computed tomography; 3-mm section through the vocal cords. Tissue with increased attenuation (arrows) is seen anterior to the sclerotic right arytenoid cartilage. This was interpreted as deep tumor spread. Arrowheads indicate residual contrast on the vocal cords following contrast laryngography 1 day before the CT; (B) whole organ section at the level of (A). Arrows indicate tumor which is only superficial. There is fibrotic tissue anterior to the arytenoid cartilage (A). C = cricoid cartilage, T = thyroid cartilage, THY = thyroid gland.

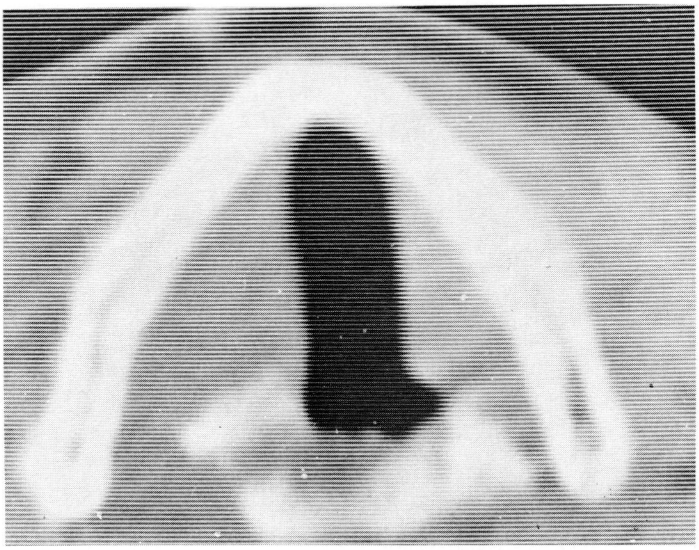

A

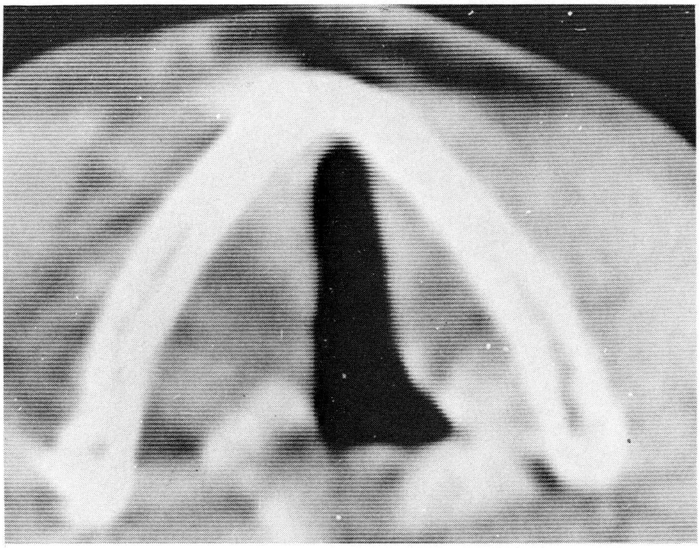

B

FIGURE 13. A 62-year-old man, irradiated 3 years earlier for a left glottic carcinoma (T1). He had a possible chondritis 2 years earlier and was now examined because of a fixed vocal cord on the right side. (A and B) computed tomography. Sections through the vocal cords. Slice thickness: (A) 6 mm, (B) 3 mm. Scanning time: (A) 4.8 sec, (B) 9.6 sec. The vocal cords have homogenous attenuation in (A), but irregular in (B) due to movement artifacts. The asymmetry of the cords is due to fixation of the right cord. Note the straight edge of the cord. The cause for the increased distance between the arytenoid and thyroid cartilages on the right side may be tumor, fibrosis, or vocal cord paresis. Multiple biopsies did not reveal any recurrent tumor.

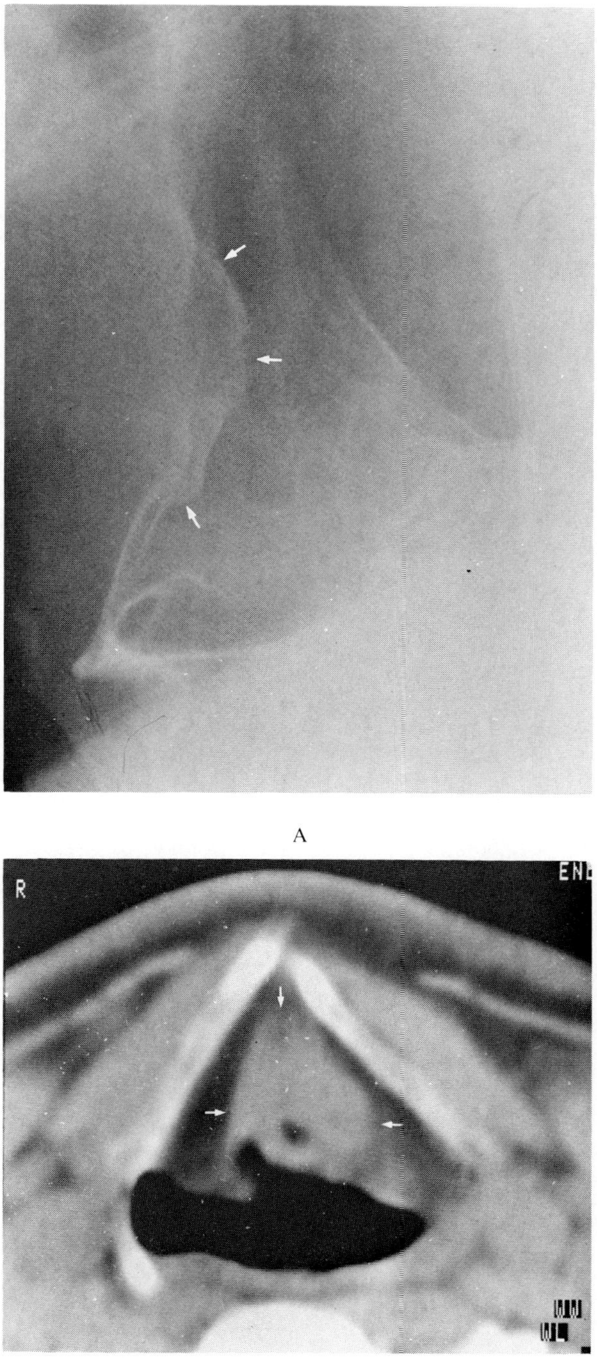

FIGURE 14. A 61-year-old man with a tumor of the epiglottis amenable to horizontal supraglottic laryngectomy. Arrows indicate tumor. (A) contrast laryngography. Lateral view. The tumor does not reach the anterior commissure; (B) computed tomography; 6-mm section through the tumor that invades the preepiglottic space but does not reach the laryngeal framework. *Comment:* Contrast laryngography shows the craniocaudal extent of the tumor. CT outlines the tumor growth in the preepiglottic space and is necessary to exclude tumor spread to the laryngeal framework. Note the normal asymmetry of the thyroid wings.

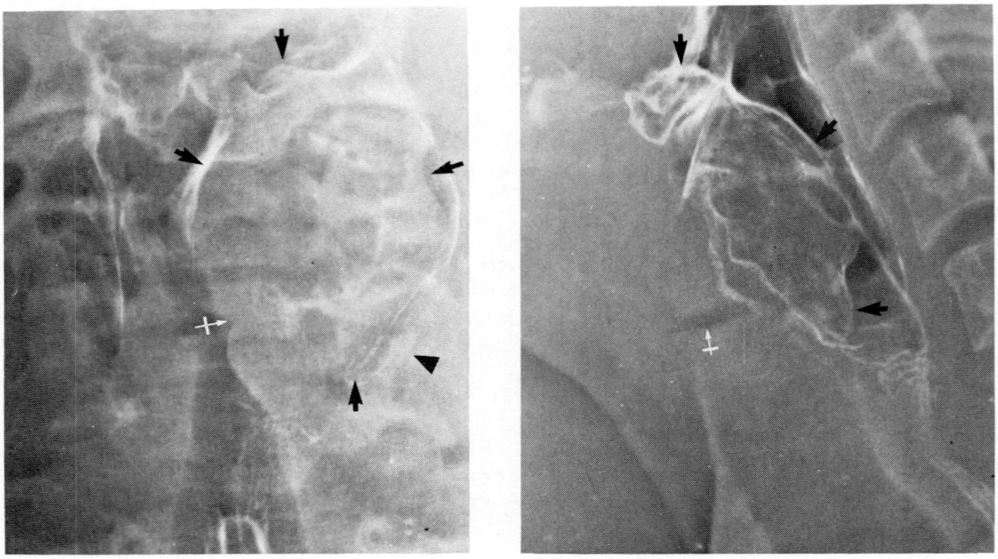

A B

FIGURE 15. A 40-year-old woman with a left supraglottic tumor. (A and B) Barium swallow, a.p. view (A) and lateral view (B). Arrows indicate the tumor that bulges into the left vallecula (upper arrow), invades the anteromedial wall, displaces the lateral wall of the left piriform sinus and the thyroid wing (arrowhead), and reaches below the laryngeal ventricle (cross-hatched arrows); (C to E) computed tomography, 6-mm sections, 4.8 sec scanning time; (C) section through the hyoid bone, showing spread to the left vallecula and suggesting spread lateral to the hyoid bone (arrow); (D) section through the thyroid cartilage above the false cords. There is displacement of the left thyroid wing suggesting invasion, but there is no definitive evidence of spread outside the larynx. Posteriorly the tumor cannot be separated from the posterior wall of the hypopharynx; (E) sections through the true vocal cords. The tumor invades the left cord and has spread posteriorly between the arytenoid (arrow) and the thyroid cartilages. The asymmetry of the ossification of the thyroid cartilage strongly suggests invasion. Note the normal appearance of the anterior commissure. Histology showed this to be an anaplastic carcinoma or, possibly, a lymphoma. There were several nodes in the neck. The patient was treated with a full course of radiotherapy. There is no follow-up.

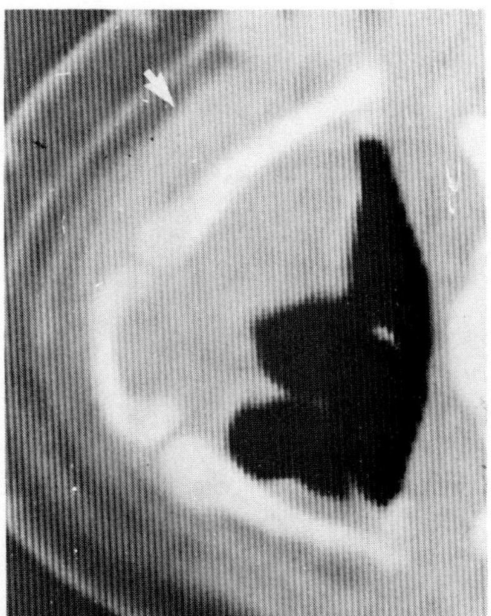

FIGURE 15C

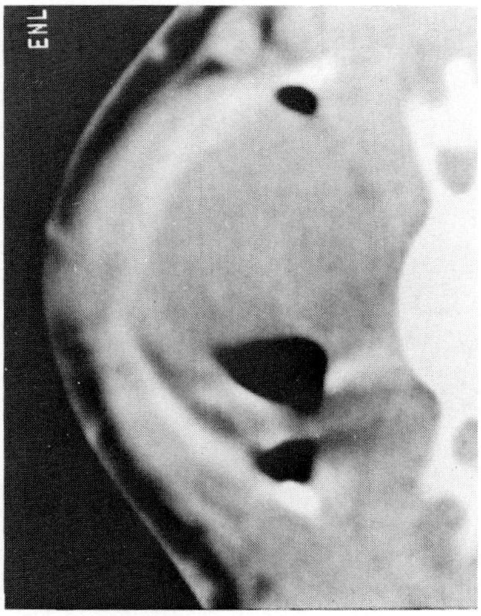

FIGURE 15D

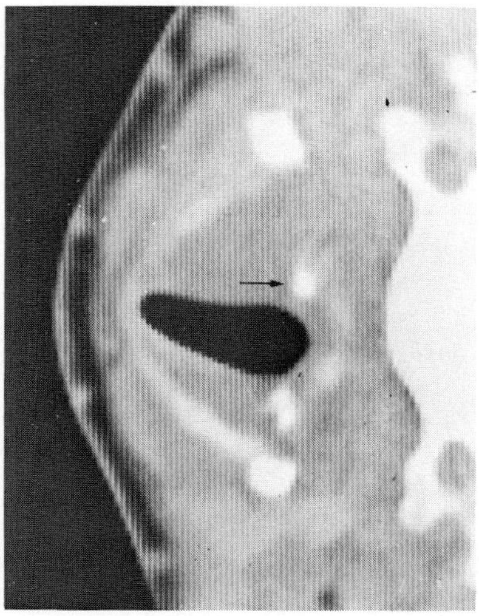

FIGURE 15E

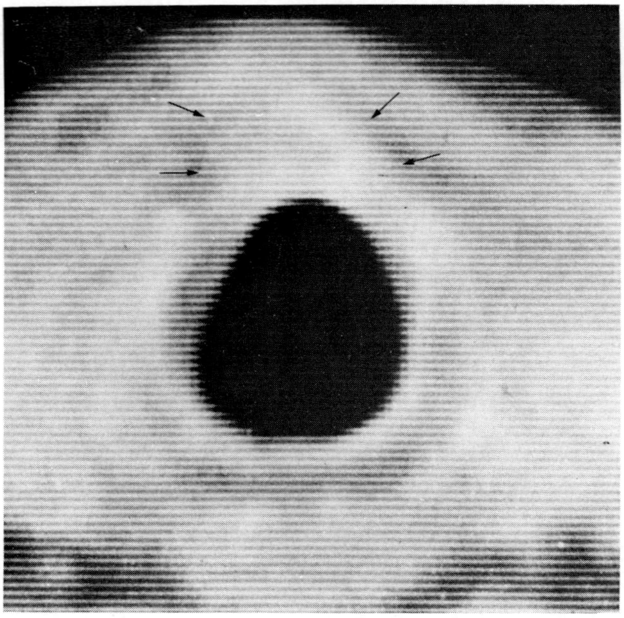

A

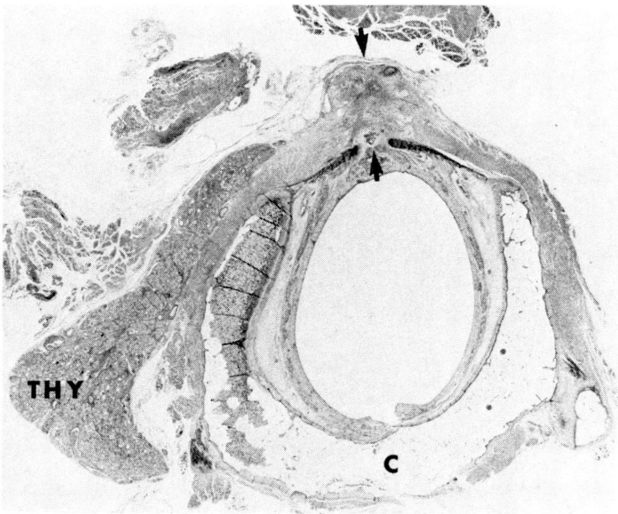

B

FIGURE 16. A 52-year-old man with recurrent tumor following radiotherapy (64 Gy) 8 months earlier for a right glottic-subglottic carcinoma invading the anterior commissure. (A) Computed tomography; 6-mm section through the cricoid cartilage and cricothyroid membrane (CTM). Arrows outline abnormal soft tissue anterior to the CTM, suggesting tumor spread outside the larynx; (B) whole organ section at the level of A. Arrows indicate tumor anterior to the CTM. C = cricoid cartilage, THY = thyroid gland.

REFERENCES

1. **Jörgensen, J., Jorgensen, K., Myhre Jensen, O., Jensen, J. T., Elbrönd, O., and Anderson, A. P.,** Radiography of laryngeal carcinoma. Assessment of value, *Acta Radiol. Diag.*, 16, 367, 1975.
2. U.I.C.C. (Union Internationale Contre le Cancer), TNM classification of malignant tumours, (Larynx. Classified 1972. Confirmed 1978.) Geneva, 1978.
3. **Scheier, M.,** Weitere Mitteilungen über die Anwendung der Röntgenstrahlen in der Rhino- und Laryngologie, *Fortschr. Röntgenstr.*, 1, 59, 1899.
4. **Scheier, M.,** Über die Ossification des Kehlkopks, *Arch. Mikr. Anat.*, 59, 220, 1901.
5. **Thost, A.,** Der normale und kranke Kehlkopf des Lebenden im Röntgenbild, (Archiv und Atlas der normalen und pathologischen Anatomie in typischen Röntgenbildern), *Fortschr. Röntgenstr., Ergänzungsband*, 31, 1913.
6. **Coutard, H.,** Note préliminaire sur la radiographie du larynx normal et du larynx cancéreux, *J. Belge. Radiol.*, 13, 287, 1924.
7. **Baclesse, F.,** Tumeurs malignes du pharynx et du larynx (étude anatomo-topographique et radiographique), 2nd ed., Masson Cie, Paris, 1960, 190, 664.
8. **Baclesse, F.,** Carcinoma of the larynx. Radiotherapy of laryngeal cancer. Clinical, radiological and therapeutic study. Follow-up of 341 cases treated at the Fondation Curie, from 1919 to 1940, *Br. J. Radiol.*, Suppl. 3, 1949.
9. **Lindgren, E.,** Über die Röntgenuntersuchung des Larynx, *Fortschr. Röntgenstr.*, 59, 273, 1939.
10. **Maguire, G. H.,** The larynx: simplified radiological examination using heavy filtration and high voltage, *Radiology*, 87, 102, 1966.
11. **Hemmingsson, A.,** Roentgenologic methods in examination of the larynx. Comparative phantom investigations in the frontal projections, *Acta Radiol. Diagn.*, 12 673, 1972.
12. **Gunsett, A.,** Über die Anwendungsmöglichkeit der Planigraphie bei Erkrankungen des Kehlkopfinneren, inbesondere beim Karzinom des Endolorynx, *Fortschr. Röntgenstr.*, 56, 705, 1937.
13. **Leborgne, F.,** Tomographic study of cancer of the larynx, *Am. J. Roentgenol.*, 43, 493, 1940.
14. **Samuel, E.,** Xerography or conventional radiography for laryngeal examination?, *Can. J. Otolaryngol.*, 4, 59, 1975.
15. **Hemmingsson, A.,** Roentgenologic examination of the larynx. A clinical comparison, *Acta Radiol. Diagn.*, 12, 433, 1972.
16. **Ardran, G. M. and Emrys-Roberts, E.,** Tomography of the larynx, *Clin. Radiol.*, 16, 369, 1965.
17. **Iglauer, S.,** Use of injected iodized oil in roentgen-ray diagnosis of laryngeal, tracheal and bronchopulmonary conditions, *JAMA*, 86, 1879, 1926.
18. **Jackson, C. L.,** The value of roentgenography of the neck, *Trans. Am. Laryng. Assoc.*, 58, 112, 1936.
19. **Powers, W. E., McGee, H. H., and Seaman, W. B.,** Contrast examination of the larynx and pharynx, *Radiology*, 68, 169, 1957.
20. **Powers, W. E., Holtz, S., Ogura, J., Ellis, B. L., and McGavran, M. H.,** Contrast examination of larynx and pharynx. Accuracy and value in diagnosis, *Am. J. Roentgenol.*, 86, 651, 1961.
21. **Powers, W. E., Holtz, S., and Ogura, J.,** Contrast examination of the larynx and pharynx. Inspiratory phonation, *Am. J. Roentgenol.*, 92, 40, 1964.
22. **Landman, G. H. M.,** *Laryngography and Cinélaryngography*, Excerpta Medica, Amsterdam, 1970.
23. **Holinger, P. H., Lutterbeck, E. F., and Bulger, R.,** Xeroradiography of the larynx, *Ann. Otol.*, 81, 806, 1972.
24. **Di Guglielmo, L. and Cherubino, M., Laringe,** in *La Xeroradiografia in Otorinolaringoiatria*, 32 Raduno gruppo alta Italia (Pavia, 29 novembre 1975), Di Guglielmo, L. and Cherubino, M., Eds., Societá italiana di otorinolaringologia e patologia cervico - faciale, Pavia, 23, 1975.
25. **Hemmingsson, A., and Löfroth, P. O.,** Xeroradiography and conventional radiography in examination of the larynx, *Acta Radiol. Diagn.*, 17, 723, 1976.
26. **Nathan, M. D., Sagel, S. S., Gall, A. M., Griffith, R. C., and Ogura, J. H.,** Diagnostic accuracy of xeroradiographic assessment of extent of carcinoma of the larynx, *Trans. Am. Acad. Ophtalmol. Otolaryngol.*, 84, 609, 1977.
27. **Mancuso, A. A., Hanafee, W. N., Juillard, J. F., Winter, J., and Calcaterra, T. C.** The role of computed tomography in the management of cancer of the larynx, *Radiology*, 124, 243, 1977.
28. **Mancuso, A. A. and Hanafee, W. N.,** A comparative evaluation of computed tomography and laryngography, *Radiology*, 133, 131, 1979.
29. **Parsons, C. A., Chapman, P., Counter, R. T., and Grundy, A.,** The role of computed tomography in tumours of the larynx, *Clin. Radiol.*, 31, 529, 1980.
30. **Archer, C. R., Sagel, S. S., Yeager, V. L., Martin, S., and Friedman, W. H.,** Staging of carcinoma of the larynx: comparative accuracy of CT and laryngography, *Am. J. Radiol.*, 136, 571, 1981.
31. **Ward, P. H., Hanafee, W. N., Mancuso, A. A., Shallit, J., and Berci, G.,** Evaluation of computerized tomography, cinelaryngoscopy, and laryngography in determining the extent of laryngeal disease, *Ann. Otol.*, 88, 454, 1979.

32. **Gamsu, G., Webb, W. R., Shallit, J. B., and Moss, A. A.,** CT in carcinoma of the larynx and pyriform sinus: value of phonation scans, *Am. J. Radiol.*, 136, 577, 1981.
33. **Gregor, R. T., Lloyd, G. A. S., and Michaels, L.,** Computed tomography of the larynx: a clinical and pathologic study, *Head Neck Surg.*, 3, 284, 1981.
34. **Sökjer, H. and Olofsson, J.,** Computed tomography in carcinoma of the larynx and piriform sinus, *Clin. Otolaryngol.*, 6, 335, 1981.
35. **Sökjer, H. and Olofsson, J.,** Angiography in laryngeal carcinoma, *Acta Radiol. Diagn.*, 21, 379, 1980.
36. **Hemmingsson, A. and Lundqvist, H.,** Optimum photon energy in ordinary radiography of the larynx, *Acta Radiol. Diagn.*, 12, 305, 1972.
37. **Palva, T., Jokinen, K., Saloheimo, M., and Karvonen, P.,** Ultrasonic nebulizer in local anesthesia for bronchoscopy, *ORL*, 37, 306, 1975.
38. **Mafee, J. F., Schild, J. A., Valvassor, G. E., and Capek, V.,** Computed tomography of the larynx: correlation with anatomic and pathologic studies in cases of laryngeal carcinoma, *Radiology*, 147, 123, 1983.
39. **Mancuso, A. A., Calcaterra, T. C., and Hanafee, W. N.,** Computed tomography of the larynx, *Radiol. Clin. N. Am.*, 16, 195, 1978.
40. **Gamsu, G., Mark, A. S., and Webb, W. R.,** Computed tomography of the normal larynx during quiet breathing and phonation, *J. Comp. Assist. Tomogr.*, 5, 353, 1981.
41. **Hagemann, J., Heller, M., and Lemke, Th.,** Die Computertomographie des normalen Larynx, *Fortschr. Röntgenstr.*, 134, 512, 1981.
42. **Friedman, W. H., Archer, C. R., Yeager, V. L., and Donovan, T. J.,** Computed tomography of the normal larynx, *Head Neck Surg.*, 1, 435, 1979.
43. **Jing, B. -S.,** Roentgen examination of laryngeal cancer: a critical evaluation, *Can. J. Otolaryngol.*, 4, 64, 1975.
44. **Fletcher, G. H., Old, J. W., and Loquvam, G. S.,** A topographic approach to the roentgenologic and pathologic examination of the laryngopharyngeal tumours, *Radiology*, 63, 361, 1954.
45. **Thornbury, J. R. and Latourette, H. B.,** A comparison study of laryngography techniques. 150 KVP plain roentgenography vs. positive contrast roentgenography, *Am. J. Roentgenol.*, 99, 555, 1967.
46. **Ogura, J. H., Powers, W. E., Holtz, S., McGavran, M. H., Ellis, B., and Voorhees, R.,** Laryngograms. Their value in the diagnosis and treatment of laryngeal lesions. A study based on clinical, radiographic and pathologic findings on 99 patients with cancer of the larynx, *Laryngoscope*, 70, 780, 1960.
47. **Olofsson, J. and Sökjer, H.,** Radiology and laryngoscopy for the diagnosis of laryngeal carcinoma, *Acta Radiol. Diagn.*, 18, 449, 1977.
48. **Olofsson, J. and Sökjer, H.,** Radiologic assessment of laryngeal carcinoma. A clinico-pathologic comparison based on whole-organ serial sections, *Acta Radiol. Diagn.*, 20, 789, 1979.
49. **Sökjer, H.,** Radiologic Evaluation of Laryngeal Carcinoma, Linköping University Medical Dissertations, No. 69, Linköping, Sweden, 1979.
50. **Olofsson, J., Williams, G. T., Rider, W. D., and Bryce, D. P.,** Anterior commissure carcinoma. Primary treatment with radiotherapy in 57 patients, *Arch. Otolaryngol.*, 95, 230, 1972.
51. **Hanafee, W. N.,** Radiography of the pharynx and larynx, in *Radiology of the Ear, Nose and Throat*, Valvassori, G. E., Potter, G. D., Hanafee, W. N., Carter, B. L., and Buckingham, R. A., Eds., Springer-Verlag, Stuttgart, 1982, 267.
52. **Sagel, S. S., AufderHeide, J. F., Aronberg, D. J., Stanley, R. J., and Archer, C. R.,** High resolution computed tomography in the staging of carcinoma of the larynx, *Laryngoscope*, 91, 292, 1981.
53. **Olofsson, J., Lord, I. J., and Van Nostrand, A. W. P.,** Vocal cord fixation in laryngeal carcinoma, *Acta Otolaryngol.*, 75, 496, 1973.
54. **Archer, C. R. and Yeager V. L.,** Evaluation of laryngeal cartilages by computed tomography, *J. Comp. Assist. Tomogr.*, 3, 604, 1979.
55. **Archer, C. R., Friedman, W. H., Yeager, V. L., and Katsantonis, G. P.,** Evaluation of laryngeal cancer by computed tomography, *J. Comp. Assist. Tomogr.*, 2, 618, 1978.
56. **Kirchner, J. A.,** One hundred laryngeal cancers studied by serial section, *Ann. Otol.*, 78, 689, 1969.
57. **Olofsson, J. and Van Nostrand, A. W. P.,** Growth and spread of laryngeal and hypopharyngeal carcinoma with reflections on the effect of preoperative irradiation. 139 cases studied by whole organ serial sectioning, *Acta Otolaryngol.*, Suppl. 308, 1973.
58. **Kirchner, J. A. and Som, M. L.,** Clinical and histological observations on supraglottic cancer, *Ann. Otol.*, 80, 638, 1971.
59. **Nathan, M. D., El Gammal, T., and Hudson, J. H.,** Computerized axial tomography in the assessment of thyroid cartilage invasion by laryngeal carcinoma: a prospective study, *Head Neck Surg.*, 88, 726, 1980.
60. **Lloyd, G. A. S., Michaels, L., and Phelps, P. D.,** The demonstration of cartilaginous involvement in laryngeal carcinoma by computerized tomography, *Clin. Otolaryngol.*, 6, 171, 1981.
61. **Sagerman, R. H. and Chung, C. T.,** Computed tomography in the management of head and neck cancer, *J. Comp. Tomogr.*, 5, 229, 1981.

INDEX

D

E

F

G

H

I

J

K

L

M

N

O

P

R

S